Health Program Planning and Evaluation: A Practical, Systematic Approach for Community Health

L. Michele Issel, PhD, RN
Clinical Assistant Professor
School of Public Health
University of Illinois at Chicago

JONES AND BARTLETT PUBLISHERS
Sudbury, Massachusetts
BOSTON   TORONTO   LONDON   SINGAPORE

World Headquarters
Jones and Bartlett Publishers
40 Tall Pine Drive
Sudbury, MA 01776
978-443-5000
info@jbpub.com
www.jbpub.com

Jones and Bartlett Publishers Canada
2406 Nikanna Road
Mississauga, ON L5C 2W6
CANADA

Jones and Bartlett Publishers International
Barb House, Barb Mews
London W6 7PA
UK

Library of Congress Cataloging-in-Publication Data

Issel, L. Michele.
  Health program planning and evaluation : a practical, systematic
approach for community health / L. Michele Issel.
       p. ; cm.
Includes bibliographical references and index.
  ISBN 0-7637-4800-5
  1. Community health services. 2. Health planning.
  [DNLM: 1. Community Health Services—organization &
administration—United States. 2. Health Planning—methods—United
States. 3. Program Development—methods—United States. 4. Program
Evaluation—methods—United States. WA 546 AA1 I86h 2004] I. Title.
  RA427.I75 2004
  3.12
                                                    2003017116

Publisher: Michael Brown
Production Manager: Amy Rose
Associate Editor: Chambers Moore
Marketing Manager: Joy Stark-Vancs
Production Coordination: Jenny Bagdigian
Manufacturing Buyer: Therese Bräuer
Cover Design: Brianna Donahue
Text Design, Art, and Composition: Dartmouth Publishing, Inc.
Printing and Binding: Malloy, Inc.
Cover Printing: Malloy, Inc.

Printed in the United States of America
08 07 06 05   10 9 8 7 6 5 4 3

Table of Contents

Preface

Today's world of health care is influenced by many factors, including the *Healthy People 2010* goals, an emphasis on the outcomes of health care, an emphasis on the evidence-based approach to practice, the use of various total quality management and improvement tools, and the federal legislation regarding performances known as the General Performance and Results Act (GPRA). Under these conditions, health professionals must develop health programs to address a wide variety of health and well-being problems, and deliver an assortment of programmatic health interventions to individuals, families, aggregates, communities, or entire populations. The influencing forces make it insufficient for health professionals to do the "same old" program. It also no longer is acceptable to merely count participants in a program and give minimal anecdotal evidence of program effectiveness. Health programs need to be systematically developed, thoughtfully implemented, and rigorously evaluated in order to compete for funding and support from a broad base of stakeholders. Yet most health professionals receive minimal, if any, training in the areas of program planning, implementation, and evaluation.

This graduate-level text addresses the needs of professionals from a variety of health disciplines who find themselves responsible for developing, implementing, or evaluating health programs. The aim of the text is to assist health professionals not only to become competent health program planners and evaluators, but also to become savvy consumers of evaluation reports and prudent users of evaluation consultants. To that end, throughout the text practical tools and concepts necessary to develop and evaluate health programs are discussed in language understandable to both the practicing and the novice health program planner and evaluator. Health programs are conceptualized as encompassing a broad range of programmatic interventions that range from individual-level health education to population-level health policy programs. Examples of programs used throughout the text are specific yet broadly related to improving health, and fall within the rubric of public health. This focus on public health provides an opportunity to demonstrate how health programs can target different levels within a population, different determinants of the health problem, and different strategies and interventions to address particular health problems. In addition, examples of health programs and references are selected to pique the interests of the diverse students and practicing professionals that comprise the multidisciplinary program teams. Thus, the content and examples are relevant to health administrators, medical social workers, nurses, nutritionists, pharmacists, public health professionals, physical and occupational therapists, and physicians.

The desire and idea for this textbook grew from my teaching experience. In teaching program planning and evaluation to both nurses and public health students, I came to appreciate the extent to which they need and want to directly apply the course content to their work. In large part, the available textbooks were from social services, with little direct relevance to the health programs with which they were more familiar. Existing texts also had very limited applicability to community-based health care settings, to public health issues, or to health problems at a population level. The lack of attention to the distinction between individual patient health and behavior and the interventions needed to address population health hampered students from clinical backgrounds in their efforts to think in terms of aggregates and populations.

In most graduate programs in the health professions, students are required to take a research methods course and a statistics course. Therefore, this evaluation text does not attempt to duplicate content related to research methods and statistics. Instead, it addresses and extends that content into the development, implementation, and evaluation of health programs. In addition, because the use of total quality management and related methodologies has become standard practice in health care, areas of overlap between quality improvement methodologies and traditional program evaluation approaches are acknowledged. This includes ways in which quality improvement methodologies can complement program evaluations. There are times when evaluations are not appropriate. Enthusiasm for providing health programs and conducting evaluations is tempered with thoughtful notes of caution, in the hope that students will avoid potentially serious and costly program and evaluation mistakes.

UNIQUE FEATURES OF THIS TEXT

Three features distinguish this text from other program planning and evaluation textbooks: use of the public health pyramid, consistent use of a program logic model throughout this text, and modeling of evidence-based practice.

The public health pyramid illustrates how health programs can be developed for individuals, aggregates, populations, and service delivery systems. Use of the pyramid is also intended as a practical application of the ecological perspective that acknowledges a multilevel approach to addressing health problems. The public health pyramid contains four levels: direct service to individuals, enabling services to aggregates, population-level services provided to entire populations, and, at the base, the infrastructure level. The pyramid is used as a structure for summarizing the content of each chapter, with specific attention to how key concepts in this chapter might vary across the pyramid levels. It also reinforces the fact that enhancing health and well-being requires integrated efforts across the levels of the pyramid. Health program development and evaluation are relevant for programs targeted to individuals, aggregates, populations, and service delivery systems, and the pyramid is a particularly germane means of tailoring program plans and evaluation designs that are congruent with the level at which the program is conceptualized. In addition, the public health framework helps transcend disciplinary boundaries.

The second unique feature of this text is that one logic model of program planning and evaluation is used throughout the text, with the content of each chapter situated in relationship to the program theory. The logic model becomes a string connecting the content across the chapters and, more importantly, the activities across the planning and evaluation cycle. To this string is added one additional gem that also is used consistently throughout the text: a more detailed model of the effect theory that is used for generating hypotheses related to program effects. Use of the effect theory model draws on the notions of action and intervention hypotheses posed by Rossi and Freeman (1986) but dropped from later editions of their text (Rossi, Freeman, & Lipsey, 1999). These notions have been adapted and extended in this text because I believe they were onto something with their effort to distinguish among the pathways leading from a problem to an impact and outcome.

The current norm of using logic models, program theories, and flow diagrams makes a return to Rossi and Freeman's ideas very fruitful. Their earlier notions of hypotheses have been integrated into public health techniques and language, resulting in a model for describing relationships among health antecedents, health determinants, program interventions, and health impacts. The hypotheses that constitute the effect theory need to be understood and explicated to plan a successful health program and to evaluate the "right" elements of the program. This text highlights the usefulness of the effect theory model throughout the planning and evaluation cycle. For example, the model is used as a means of linking program theory to impact evaluation designs and data collection. The logic model becomes an educational tool by serving as an example of how the program theory manifests through the stages of planning and evaluation, and by reinforcing the value of carefully articulating the causes of health problems and the consequences of programmatic interventions. Experience with students has shown that while they have an intuitive sense of the connection, they are not skilled at articulating those connections and relationships in ways that program stakeholders can readily grasp.

The third unique feature of the text is the intentional modeling of evidence-based practice. The use of published, empirical evidence as the basis for practice, whether it be clinical practice or program planning practice, has become the professional standard. Thus, the substantive examples that are liberally used in each chapter come from the published scientific health and health-related literature. Relying on the literature for examples of programs, evaluations, and issues raised is consistent with the espoused preference for using scientific evidence as the basis for making programmatic decisions. Each chapter has multiple examples from the health science literature that substantiate the information presented in the chapter and, as much as possible, show a practical relevance of the chapter content to planning, providing, and evaluating health programs.

ORGANIZATION OF THE BOOK

The book is organized into five sections, each covering a major phase in the planning and evaluation cycle. Section 1 provides a context in which health programs and evaluations occur. Chapter 1 begins with an overview of definitions of health, followed by a historical context. The public health pyramid is introduced and presented as an ecological framework for thinking of health programs. An overview of community is provided and discussed as both the target and the context of health programs. The role of community members in health programs and evaluations is introduced. Emphasis is given to community as context and to strategies for community participation throughout the program development and evaluation process. Chapter 2 provides a discussion of the role that diversity has in the planning and evaluation cycle—in other words, how diversity affects the delivery and evaluation of health programs. Although material on diversity could have been added to each chapter, the sensitive nature of the topic and its importance to a successful health program warranted it being covered early in the text and as a separate chapter. Cultural competence is discussed, particularly with regard to the organization providing the health program and the program staff. Chapter 3 focuses on the activities, perspectives, and history of health program planning. Based on the belief that effective health program developers are self-aware, six perspectives drawn from public administration and philosophy are reviewed. The perspectives provide a reference point for understanding diverse preferences regarding how to prioritize health needs and expenditures, thus enabling health program planners to reflect on the process of planning as it unfolds. Based on that reflection, they can tailor planning actions to best fit the situation.

The chapters in Section 2 deal with planning and developing a health program. Chapter 4 begins with an overview of four perspectives that can be used to conduct a community health assessment. Building on this overview, distinct types of assessments are discussed—namely organizational assessments, marketing, needs, and community. These assessments are foundational to decision-making about the future health program. Essential steps involved in conducting a community health and needs assessment are outlined, with particular attention to the use of appropriate statistical methods. The generic model of relationships among health antecedents, health determinants, and health impacts is introduced. The chapter concludes with a discussion of how the "problem" can be stated. Chapter 5 explains what theory is and how it provides a cornerstone to programs and to evaluations, as well as the distinction between process and outcome. This chapter introduces the concept of the program theory and explains its component elements of process theory and effect theory. The program theory becomes the basis for the logic model that is used to organize ideas presented in subsequent chapters, in particular the development of interventions and strategies and the evaluation of processes and program effects. Chapter 6 goes into detail on developing goals and objectives for the program, with particular attention given to articulating the interventions provided by the program. A step-by-step procedure is presented for deriving numeric targets for the objectives from existing data, which makes the numeric targets more defendable and programmatically realistic.

The two chapters in Section 3 focus on launching the program and monitoring its implementation. Chapter 7 provides an in-depth review of key elements that comprise the process theory. The process theory contains not only the organizational plan and service utilization plan (Rossi et al., 1999), but also, more specifically both inputs and outputs to each of those plans. Enumerating the inputs and outputs of the process theory is a prerequisite to the development of a process evaluation plan. Chapter 8 details how to evaluate the outputs of the organizational plan and the service utilization plan. The practical application of measures of coverage is provided, along with an emphasis on connecting the results of the process evaluation to programmatic changes.

The chapters in Section 4 are specific to conducting the effect evaluations. Rather than having a focus on research methods, these chapters focus on the realities of the program effect evaluation. Here, students' prior knowledge of research methods and epidemiology is brought together in the context of health program and service evaluation. Chapter 9 highlights the importance of refining the evaluation questions and provides information on how to clarify the questions with stakeholders. Earlier discussions about program theory are brought to bear on the development of the evaluation questions. Issues such as data integrity and survey construction are addressed with regard to the practicality of program evaluation. Chapter 10 takes a fresh approach to evaluation design by organizing the traditional experimental and quasi-experimental designs and epidemiological designs into three levels of program evaluation design based on the design complexity and purpose of the evaluation. The discussion of sampling retains the emphasis on being practical for program evaluation, rather than taking a more pure research approach. However, sample size and power are discussed, as these have a profound relevance to program evaluations. Chapter 11 reviews data management, analysis of data with attention to application to programs with small numbers, and issues in interpreting the statistical findings. The data analysis is linked to interpretation and potential flaws in how numbers are understood. Chapter 12 provides a review of six qualitative designs and methods, with a discussion of their use in health program development and evaluation.

The final section, Section 5, includes two chapters. Chapter 13 addresses the topic of cost analyses, providing basic comparative descriptions of cost-effectiveness, cost-benefit, cost-utility, and sensitivity analyses with sufficient detail so that thoughtful and realistic program and evaluation decisions can be made. There is no attempt to make the reader an expert; rather, the intent is to help the reader be savvy and skeptical about cost studies that might be influencing program decision making. Again, the program theory is used to organize thinking about cost evaluations. Chapter 14 discusses the use of evaluations for making decisions regarding existing and future health programs. Practical and conceptual factors related to the ethical issues that program evaluators face are addressed. The chapter also includes a review of how to assess the quality of evaluations and summarizes the relevance of quality improvement methodologies to program monitoring and evaluation.

Each chapter concludes with discussion questions that are intended to be provocative and to generate critical thinking. At a graduate level, students need to be encouraged to engage in independent thinking and to foster their ability to provide rationales for decisions. The discussion questions are developed from this point of view. Given the critical role that funding sources play in the formulation of health programs, issues related to funding are addressed as they relate to the content of each chapter.

References

Rossi, P. H., & Freeman, H.E. (1993). *Evaluation: A Systematic Approach* (5th ed.) Newbury Park, CA: Sage Publications.

Rossi, P. H., Freeman, H.E., & Lipsey, M. W. (1999). *Evaluation: A Systematic Approach* (6th ed.) Thousand Oaks, CA: Sage Publications.

Acknowledgments

Like all authors, I am indebted to many who supported and aided me in this endeavor. First and foremost, I owe a great debt to the numerous students over the years who asked questions that challenged me to find new explanations. It was through their quest to learn that I learned there is no one way to explain the complex. I was also motivated by the way the topic of planning and evaluating health programs captured their imaginations and gave them a forum for making a difference. I am especially grateful to one student in particular, Nicole Miller, who did a yeoman's job of keeping the references straight, editing, and providing insights into the understandability of the text from a novice's perspective. Other students helped along the way, especially Kusuma Madama, who helped in the final days of sending the manuscript to the publisher.

Like the master's students I now teach, as a student I was intrigued by the mystery of how to do the seemingly impossible: evaluate prevention of illnesses. One of my teachers, Frannie (Frances Marcus Lewis at the University of Washington School of Nursing), suggested that I pursue a doctorate as the route to doing evaluation. I followed her suggestion. I now consult with agencies and conduct health program evaluations. She also was a wonderful role model for how to always have one foot in evaluation while being an academic. Recent inspiration came from Bernard Turnock at the University of Illinois at Chicago School of Public Health, who encouraged me to contact the publisher. I have him to thank for getting me started down this path of authorship.

Several colleagues helped to fine-tune this text. On a day-to-day basis, several colleagues provided intellectual support and encouragement, one being Lou Rowitz for his understanding of the work of being a book author. Both Arden Handler and Noel Chavez deserve acknowledgment for being the best office neighbors one could hope to have. I am especially indebted to Arden for taking time to contribute to the development of one chapter. Her devotion to quality and clarity added richness to otherwise dry material. I am also deeply indebted to Deborah Rosenburg, also of the University of Illinois at Chicago School of Public Health, for innovative and quintessentially useful work on developing targets for program impact and outcome objectives. Many thanks are also due to Amy Rose for her careful work, and an anonymous reviewer whose thoughtful suggestions led to substantive improvements in the text.

Many friends and family members also are due a huge thanks for putting up with my anxiety and helping me to keep a larger perspective on my work. I particularly thank my sister, Debbie Mier, and my mother, Helen Issel, both for having faith in me and for being unabashedly proud. I thank Ruth Anderson for actively demonstrating her love of research and inspiring me to bring that love of data and intellectual challenge to this text. And finally, thanks to my friend Gil for listening more than anyone.

Section 1

The Context of Health Program Development and Evaluation

CHAPTER 1

Health Program
Development and Evaluation

Health is not a state of being that can easily be achieved through isolated, uninformed, individualistic actions. Health of individuals, of families, and of populations is a state in which physical, mental, and social well-being are integrated so that optimal functioning is possible. From this perspective, achieving and maintaining health across a lifespan is a complex, complicated, intricate affair. For some, health is present irrespective of any special efforts or intention. For most of us, health requires, at a minimum, some level of attention and specific information. It is through health programs that both attention and information are provided or made available. That, however, does not guarantee that the attention and information are translated into actions or behaviors needed to achieve health. Thus, those providing health programs, however large or small, need to understand not only the processes whereby those in need of attention and information can receive what is needed, but also the processes of learning from their experiences of providing the health program.

The processes of health program planning and evaluation are the subject of this textbook. The discussion begins with a brief overview of the historical context. This sets the stage for appreciating the growing numbers of publications on the topic of health program planning and evaluation in recent years, and the professionalization of evaluators. The use of the term "processes" to describe the actions involved in health program planning and evaluation is intended to denote action, cycles, and open-endedness. This chapter introduces the planning and evaluation cycle, and the interactions and iterative nature of this cycle are stressed throughout the text. Because health is both an individual and an aggregate phenomenon, health programs need to be conceptualized for both individuals and aggregates. The public health pyramid, introduced in this chapter, is used throughout the text as a tool for conceptualizing and actualizing health programs for individuals, aggregates and populations.

HISTORY AND CONTEXT

Reflection on and understanding of what is "health" is an appropriate starting point for this textbook, as is having a basic appreciation for the genesis of the fields of health program planning and evaluation. These are elements of becoming an evaluation professional.

Concept of Health

It is crucial to begin a textbook on planning and evaluating health programs by first reflecting on the meaning of health. Both explicit and implicit meanings of health can dramatically influence what is considered the health problem and the subsequent direction of a program. The most widely accepted definition of health is that of the World Health Organization (WHO) (WHO, 1947), in which health, for the first time, was defined as more than the absence of illness, but also the presence of well-being. Since the publication of the WHO definition, health has, indeed, come to be viewed across the health professions as a holistic concept that encompasses the presence of physical, mental, developmental, social, and financial capabilities, assets, and balance. This does not preclude each health profession from having a particular aspect of health to which it primarily contributes. For example, a dentist contributes primarily to a patient's oral health, knowing that the state of that patient's teeth and gums has a direct relationship to that patient's physical and social health. Thus, the dentist might say the health problem is caries. Throughout this text, the term "health problem" is used, rather than "illness," "diagnosis," or "pathology," in keeping with the holistic view that there can be problems, deficits, and pathologies in one component of health while the other components remain "healthy." Using the term "health problem" also makes it easier to think about and plan health programs for aggregates of individuals. A community, a family, and a school can each have a health problem that is the focus of a health program intervention. The extent to which the health program planners have a shared definition of health and have defined the scope of that definition will influence the nature of the health program.

Health is a matter of concern for more than just health professionals. For many Americans, the concept of health falls within the category of a right, along with civil rights and liberties. The right to health is often translated by the public and politicians into the perceived right to have or to access health care. This political aspect of health is the genesis of health policy at the local, federal, and international levels. The extent to which the political nature of health underlies the health problem of concern and is programmatically addressed will also have an influence on the final nature of the health program.

History of Health Program Planning

The history of planning health programs has a different historical lineage than that of program evaluation. It is only relatively recently, in historical terms, that these lineages have begun to overlap, with resulting synergies. Planning for health programs has the older history, if public health is considered. Rosen (1993) argued that public health planning began approximately four thousand years ago with planned cities in the Indus Valley that had covered sewers. Particularly since the Industrial Revolution, planning for the health of populations has progressed, and it is now considered a key characteristic of the discipline of public health. Blum (1981) related planning to efforts undertaken on behalf of the public well-being to achieve deliberate or intended social change, as well as providing a sense of direction and alternative modes of proceeding to influence social attitudes and actions. Others (Dever, 1980; Rohrer, 1996; Turnock, 2001) have similarly defined planning as an intentional effort to create something that has not occurred previously for the betterment of others and for the purpose of meeting desired goals. The purpose of planning is to assure that a program has the best possible likelihood of being successful in terms of being effective with the least possible resources. Planning encompasses a variety of activities undertaken to meet this purpose.

The quintessential example of planning is the development and use of the Healthy People goals. In 1979, *Healthy People* (US Department of Health, Education, and Welfare [DHEW], 1979) was published as an outgrowth of the need to establish an illness prevention agenda for the nation. The companion publication, *Promoting Health/Preventing Disease* (US Department of Health and Human Services [DHHS], 1980), was the first time that goals and objectives regarding specific areas of the nation's health were made explicit, with the expectation that these goals would be met by the year 1990. *Healthy People 1990* became the framework for the development of state and local health promotion and disease prevention agendas. Since its publication, the goals for the nation have been revised and published as *Healthy People 2000* (DHHS, 1991), *Healthy Communities 2000* (American Public Health Association [APHA], 1991), and *Healthy People 2010* (DHHS, 2000).

The evolution of the Healthy People goals also reflects the accelerating rate of emphasis on nationwide coordination of health promotion and disease prevention efforts and a reliance on systematic planning to achieve this coordination.

The development of the Healthy People publications also reflects the underlying assumption of most planners that planning is a rational activity that can lead to results. However, with regard to many health problems, the nation has not yet achieved the objectives set for 1990; this fact reflects the colossal potential for planning to fail. Given this potential, this text provides techniques to help future planners of health programs be more realistic in the goals set and less dependent upon a linear, rational approach to planning. The *Healthy People 1990* objectives were developed by academics and clinician experts in illness prevention and health promotion. In contrast, the goals and health problems listed in *Healthy People 2010* were based on and incorporated ideas generated at public forums and through Internet commentary, and were finally revised by expert panels. The shift to a greater participation of the public in the planning stage of health programs is a major change that is now considered the norm. In keeping with the emphasis on participation, the role and involvement of stakeholders are stressed at each stage of the planning and evaluation cycle.

History of Health Program Evaluation

The history of evaluation, from which the evaluation of health programs grew, is far shorter than the history of planning, beginning roughly in the early 1900s, but it is equally rich in important lessons for future health program evaluators. The first evaluations were done in the field of education, particularly as student assessment and evaluation of teaching strategies gained interest (Patton, 1997). Assessment of student scholastic achievement is a comparatively circumscribed outcome of an educational intervention. For this reason, early program evaluators were from education, and it was from the fields of education and educational psychology that many methodological advances were made and statistics developed.

Guba and Lincoln (1987) summarized the history of evaluations by proposing generational milestones or characteristics that form distinct generations, and Swenson (1991) built on their concept of generations by acknowledging that subsequent generations will occur. Each generation incorporates the knowledge of early evaluations and extends that knowledge based on current broad cultural and political trends. Guba and Lincoln called the first generation of evaluations in the early 1900s the technical generation. During this time, scientific management, statistics, and research methodologies were nascent and were being used to test interventions. Currently, evaluations continue to incorporate the rationality of this generation by using activities that are systematic, science based, logical, and sequential. Rational approaches to evaluations focus on identifying the best-known intervention or strategy given the current knowledge, measuring quantifiable outcomes experienced by program participants, and deducing the degree of effect from the program.

The second generation, which lasted until the 1960s, focused on using goals and objectives as the basis for evaluation, in keeping with the managerial trend of management by objectives. Second-generation evaluations were predominantly descriptive. With the introduction in the 1960s of broad innovation and initiation of federal social service programs, including Medicare, Medicaid, and Head Start, the focus of evaluations shifted to establishing the merit and value of the programs. Because of the political issues surrounding these and similar federal programs, there was a growing awareness of the need to determine whether the social policies were having any effect on people. Programs needed to be judged on their merits and effectiveness. The US General Accounting Office (GAO) had been established in 1921 for the purpose of studying the utilization of public finances, assisting Congress in decision making with regard to policy and funding, and evaluating government programs. The second-generation evaluation emphasis on quantifying effects was spurred, in part, by reports from the GAO that were based on the evaluations of federal programs.

Typically, the results of evaluations were not used in the "early" days of evaluating education and social programs. That is, federal health policy was not driven by whether the programs were found successful. Evaluations grew in scientific rigor, but not in usefulness. Beginning in the 1980s, the third generation of evaluations began—namely, the negotiation or responsiveness generation. Evaluators began to acknowledge that they were not autonomous and that their work needed to be responsive to the needs of those being evaluated. As a result of this awareness, several lineages have begun. One is utilization-focused evaluation (Patton, 1997), in which the evaluator's primary concern is with developing an evaluation that will be used by the stakeholders. Utilization-focused evaluations are built on the following premises (Patton, 1987): concern for use of the evaluation pervades the evaluation from beginning to end, evaluations are aimed at the interests and needs of the users, users of the evaluation must be invested in the decisions regarding the evaluation, and a variety of community, organizational, political, resource, and scientific factors affect the utilization of evaluations. Utilization-focused evaluation differs from evaluations that are focused on outcomes (Exhibit 1.1). Another lineage is participatory evaluation (Whitmore, 1998), in which the evaluation is merely guided by the expert and is actually generated by and conducted by those invested in the health problem. A participatory or empowerment approach invites a wide range of stakeholders into the activity of planning and evaluation, providing those participants with the skills and knowledge to contribute substantively to the activities and fostering their sense of ownership of

Exhibit 1.1   Comparison of Outcome-Focused and Utilization-Focused Evaluations

	Outcome-Focused	Utilization-Focused
Purpose	Show program effect	Get stakeholders to use evaluation findings for decisions regarding program improvements and future program development
Audience	Funders, researchers, other external audience	Program people (internal audience), funders
Method	Research methods, external evaluators (usually)	Research methods, participatory

the product. These lineages within the responsiveness generation account for the current diversity in types, emphases, and philosophies regarding program evaluation.

The next generation of evaluation, emerging in the mid 1990s, seems to be meta-evaluation, which is the evaluation of evaluations done across similar programs. This trend in program evaluation is consistent with the trend in social science toward the use of meta-analysis of existing studies to better understand theorized relationships. It is also consistent with the trend across the health professions toward the use of meta-analysis of existing research for the development of evidence-based practice.

This new generation is possible because there now exists a culture of evaluation that pervades the health sciences, and thus huge data sets now exist for use in the meta-evaluations. One indicator of the evaluation culture is the mandate from United Way, a major funder of community-based health programs, for grantees to conduct outcome evaluations. To help grantees meet this mandate, United Way has published a user-friendly manual (United Way of America, 1996) that could be used by nonprofessionals to develop basic program evaluations. The culture of evaluation is most evident in the explicit requirement of federal agencies that fund community-based health programs that such programs include evaluations conducted by local evaluators.

Despite the complexities involved in this latest stage of evolution, most people have an intuitive sense of what evaluation is. The purpose of evaluation can be to measure the effects of a program against the goals set for it, in order to contribute to subsequent decision making about the program (Weiss, 1972). Alternatively, evaluation can be "the systematic application of social research procedures for assessing the conceptualization, design, implementation, and utility of intervention programs" (Rossi & Freeman, 1993). Others (Herman, Morris, & Fitz-Gibbon, 1987) have defined evaluation as judging how well policies and procedures are working, or as assessing the quality of a program. Inherent in these understandings of evaluation is an element of being judged against some criteria. This implicit understanding of evaluation leads those involved with the health program to feel as though they will be judged or found not to meet those criteria and will subsequently experience some form of repercussions. They may fear that they as individuals or as a program will be labeled a failure, unsuccessful, or inadequate. Such feelings must be acknowledged and addressed early in the planning cycle. Throughout the planning and evaluation cycle there are opportunities for the program planners to engage and involve program staff and stakeholders in the evaluation process. Taking advantage of these opportunities goes a long way in abetting the concerns of program staff and stakeholders about the judgmental quality of the program evaluation.

EVALUATION AS A PROFESSION

A major development in the field of evaluation has been the professionalization of evaluators. Founded in 1986, the American Evaluation Association (AEA) serves evaluators primarily in the United States. Several counterparts to the AEA exist, such as the Society for Evaluation in England and the Australian Evaluation Society. The existence of these professional organizations whose members are evaluators, and the presence of health-related sections within these organizations, demonstrate a field of expertise and of specialized knowledge regarding the evaluation of health-related programs.

As the field of evaluation has evolved, so have the numerous approaches that can guide the development of evaluations. Currently, 22 different approaches to evaluation have been identified, falling into 3 major groups (Stufflebeam, 2001). One group of evaluations is oriented toward questions and methods, such as objectives-based studies and experimental evaluations. The second large group of evaluations is oriented toward improvements and accountability and includes consumer-oriented and accreditation approaches. The third group of evaluations consists of those that have a social agenda or advocacy approach, such as responsive evaluation, democratic evaluation, and utilization-focused evaluation. Several concepts are common across the types of evaluations: pluralism of values, stakeholder constructions, fairness and equity regarding stakeholders, the merit and worth of the evaluation, a negotiated process and outcomes, and full collaboration. These concepts have been formalized into the standards for evaluations that were established by the Joint Committee on Standards for Educational Evaluation in 1975. Currently, this Joint Committee includes many organizations in its membership, such as the AEA and the American Educational Research Association.

The four standards of evaluation are utility, feasibility, propriety, and accuracy (Exhibit 1.2) (AEA, 2002). The utility standard specifies that an evaluation must be useful to those who requested the evaluation. Usually an evaluation is useful when it shows ways to make improvements to the intervention, increase the efficiency of the program, or enhance the possibility of garnering financial support for the program. The feasibility standard denotes that the ideal may not be practical. Evaluations that are highly complex or costly will not be done by small programs with limited capabilities and resources. Propriety is the ethical and politically correct component of the standards. Evaluations can invade privacy or be harmful to either program participants or program staff, and they must uphold the standards. Finally, accuracy is essential and is achieved through the elements that constitute scientific rigor. The established and accepted standards for

---

Exhibit 1.2   Table of Evaluation Standards Established by the Joint Commission on Standards for Educational Evaluation

Standard	Description
Utility	To ensure that the evaluation will meet the content needs of those involved
Feasibility	To ensure that the evaluation will be realistic, prudent, diplomatic, and frugal
Propriety	To ensure that the evaluation will be conducted in a legal and unbiased way, with special attention paid to the integrity of everyone involved in the evaluation process and the implementation of its results
Accuracy	To ensure that the evaluation will communicate appropriate and accurate information concerning the standards that determine the usefulness of the program under consideration

Adapted from American Evaluation Association (2002).

evaluations reflect current norms and values held by professional evaluators and deserve attention in health program evaluations. The existence and acceptance of standards is truly an indication of the professionalism of evaluators.

Achieving these standards requires that those involved in the program planning and evaluation have experience in at least one aspect of planning or evaluation: whether that be experience with the health problem; experience with epidemiological, social, or behavioral science research methods; or skill in facilitating processes that involve diverse constituents, capabilities, and interests. Program planning and evaluation can be done in innumerable ways; there is no one right way. This degree of freedom and flexibility can be uncomfortable. As with any skill or activity, until experience is acquired, program planners and evaluators feel intimidated by the size of the task or by the experience of others involved. To become a professional evaluator thus requires a degree of willingness to learn, to grow, and to be flexible.

PLANNING AND EVALUATION CYCLE

Although planning and evaluation are commonly described in a linear, sequential manner, they constitute a cyclical process. In this section, the cycle is described along with an emphasis on factors that enhance and detract from that process being effective.

Interdependent and Cyclic

A major premise running through this text is that activities comprising program planning and program evaluation are cyclical and interdependent (Exhibit 1.3), and that the activities occur more or less in stages or sets of activities. The stages are cyclical to the extent that the end of one program or stage flows almost seamlessly into the next program or planning activity. The activities are interdependent to the extent that the learning, insights, and ideas that result at one stage are likely to influence the available information and thus the decision making and actions of another stage. Interdependence of activities and stages is ideally a result of information and data feedback loops that connect the stages. Naturally, not all of the possible interactions among program planning, implementation, and evaluation are shown in Exhibit 1.3. In reality, the cyclical or interactive nature of health program planning and evaluation exists in varying degrees. Ideally, interactions, feedback loops, and reiterations of process would be reflected throughout this textbook. For the sake of clarity, the cycle is presented in a linear fashion in the text, with

Exhibit 1.3 The Planning and Evaluation Cycle

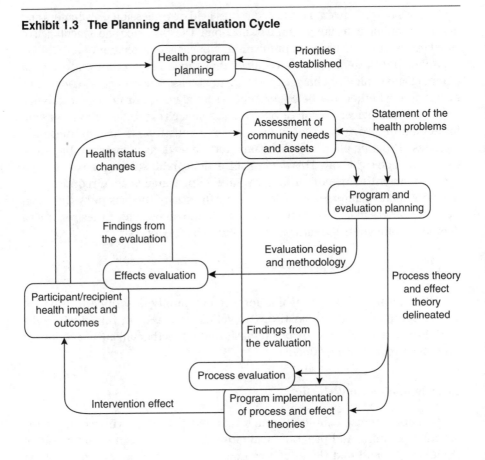

steps and sequences covered in an orderly fashion across the progression of chapters. This pedagogical approach belies the true messiness of health program planning and program evaluation. Because the planning and evaluation cycle is susceptible to and affected by external influences, to be successful as a program planner or evaluator requires a substantial degree of flexibility and creativity in recovering from these influences.

The cycle begins with a trigger event, such as awareness of a health problem, a periodic strategic planning effort, or newly available funds for a health program. This trigger event or situation leads to the collection of data about the health problem, the characteristics of the people affected, and their perceptions of the health problem. These data, along with additional data on available resources, constitute a community needs and assets assessment. Based on the data from the needs assessment, program development begins. Problems and solutions are prioritized. The planning phase includes developing the program theory, which explicates the connection between what is done and the intended effects of the program. Assessing organizational and infrastructure resources for implementing the program, such as garnering resources to implement and sustain the program, is a component of the planning. Another major component of program planning is setting goals and objectives that are derived from the program theory.

After the resources necessary to implement the program have been secured and the activities that comprise the program intervention have been explicated, the program can be implemented. The logistics of implementation include marketing the program to the target audience, training and managing program personnel, and delivering or providing the intervention as planned. During implementation of the program, it is critical to conduct an evaluation of the extent to which the program is provided as planned; this is the process evaluation. The data and findings from the process evaluation are key feedback items in the planning and evaluation cycle, and they can and ought to lead to revisions in the program delivery.

Ultimately, the health program ought to have an effect on the health of the individual program participants or on the recipients of the program intervention if provided to the community or a population. The evaluation of this effect can be an impact evaluation of immediate and closely causally linked programmatic effects or an outcome evaluation of more temporally and causally distal programmatic effects. Both types of evaluations provide information to the health program planners for use in subsequent program planning. The evaluation of the effect of the program provides data and information that can be used to alter the program intervention. These findings can also be used in subsequent assessments of the need for future or other health programs.

When Not to Evaluate

Situations and circumstances do exist that are not amenable to conducting an evaluation, despite a request or the requirement for having an evaluation. Specifically, there are four circumstances when it is not advisable to evaluate: when there are no questions about the program, when the program has no clear direction, when stakeholders cannot agree on the program objectives, and when there is not enough money to conduct a sound evaluation (Patton, 1997). In addition to these, Weiss (1972) recognized that sometimes evaluations are requested and conducted for less than legitimate purposes; namely postponing program or policy decisions, avoiding the responsibility of making the program or policy decision, making a program look good as a public relations effort, or fulfilling program grant requirements. As these lists suggest, those engaged in program planning and evaluation need to be purposeful in what is done and should be aware that external forces can influence the planning and evaluation processes.

Since Weiss made this observation in 1972, funders have begun to require program process and effect evaluations and conducting these evaluations to meet that requirement is considered quite legitimate. This change has occurred as techniques for designing and conducting both program process and effect evaluations have improved, and the expectation is that even mandated evaluations will be useful in some way. Nonetheless, it remains critical to consider how to conduct evaluations legitimately, rigorously, inexpensively, and fairly. In addition, if the AEA standards of utility, feasibility, propriety, and accuracy cannot be met, it is not wise to conduct an evaluation (Patton, 1997).

Interests and the degree of influence held by stakeholders can change. Such changes affect not only the way in which the evaluation is conceptualized, but also whether evaluation findings are used. In addition, the priorities and responsibilities of the organizations and agencies providing the program can change during the course of delivering the program, which can then lead to changes in the program implementation that have not been taken into account by the evaluation. For example, if withdrawal of resources leads to a shortened or streamlined evaluation, subsequent findings may indicate a failure of the program intervention. However, it will remain unclear whether the ineffective intervention was due to the design of the program or of the evaluation. In addition, unanticipated problems in delivering the program interventions and the evaluation will always exist. Even rigorously designed evaluations face challenges in the real world of staff turnover, participant nonparticipation, bad weather, or any of a host of other factors that might hamper achieving the original evaluation design. Stakeholders will need to understand that the evaluator attempted to address challenges as they arose if they are to have confidence in the evaluation findings.

Use as the Cyclical Link

Before embarking on either a process or an effect evaluation, it is important to consider who will use the results, because, in being used, evaluation results are perpetuating the program planning and evaluation cycle. The usefulness of evaluations depends on the extent to which questions that need to be answered are in fact answered. However, different stakeholder groups that are likely to use evaluation funding will be concerned with different questions.

One stakeholder group is the funding organizations, whether federal agencies or private foundations. Funders may use process evaluations for program accountability and effect evaluations for determining the success of broad initiatives and individual program effectiveness. Another stakeholder group is the project directors and managers, who will use both process and effect evaluation findings as a basis for seeking further funding, as well as for making improvements to the health program. The program staff is another stakeholder group that is likely to use both the process and the effect evaluation as a validation of their efforts and as a justification for their feeling about their success with program participants or recipients. Scholars and health professionals constitute another stakeholder group that accesses the findings of effect evaluations through the professional literature. They are likely to use effect evaluations as the basis for generating new theories about what is effective in addressing a particular health problem, and why it is effective.

Policy makers are yet another stakeholder group that uses both published literature and final program reports regarding process and effect evaluation findings when formulating health policy and making decisions about program resource allocation. Finally, community action groups, community members, and the program participants and recipients form another group of stakeholders. This stakeholder group is most likely to advocate for a community health assessment and to use process evaluation results to advocate for additional resources or to hold the program accountable.

Thus far, this discussion has taken the positive perspective that the evaluations will be used. It is just as possible, however, that evaluations, no matter how sound, will not be used. The stakeholder groups may suppress, ignore, or discredit evaluations that are not favorable. This reality gains the most visibility in the health policy arena. An example will illustrate this point. Mathematica, a private research firm, was hired by the Federal Maternal and Child Health Bureau (MCHB) of the Health Resources Services Administration to evaluate the effect of the Healthy Start Initiative programs funded by the MCHB (Howell, 1997). The Healthy Start Initiative funded local programs designed to reduce infant mortality and the rate of low birth weight births; each local Healthy Start had a local evaluation. Mathematica evaluated a range of programmatic interventions in more than 20 locations, using much of the data from the local evaluations in addition to other data sources. The Mathematica meta-evaluation revealed a lack of evidence that the Healthy Start programs had an effect on the rates of infant mortality or low birth weight. These findings were not used by the MCHB in subsequent requests to Congress for funds for the Healthy Start Initiative. This story illustrates the tension that exists between health policy, which may be driven by beliefs about what will work, and the "cold, hard facts" of an evaluation. The political considerations involved in situations like these can be problematic. Regardless of the source of the political issues, planners and evaluators will encounter the occasional unexpected "land mine."

PROGRAM LIFE CYCLE

Feedback loops contribute to the overall development and evolution of a health program, giving it a life cycle. In the early stages of an idea for a health program, the program may begin as a pilot. That is, the program does not rely upon any existing format or theory, and so simple trial and error is used. These pilot programs are likely to be small and somewhat experimental because a similar type of program has not been developed or attempted. If the program is successful and doable, as documented by both the process and effect evaluations, it may evolve into a model program. A model program has interventions that are formalized, or explicit, with protocols that standardize the intervention, and the program is delivered under conditions that are controlled by the program staff and developers. The model program, because it is provided under ideal rather than realistic conditions, is difficult to sustain over time. Evaluating the effects of this type of program is easier than in a pilot program, however, because there are more stringent procedures for enrollment and follow-up of program participants. If the model program shows promise for addressing the health problem, it can be copied and implemented as a prototype program. A prototype program is implemented under realistic conditions and thus is easily replicated and tailored to the organization and the specifics of the local target audience.

If the prototype health program is successful and stable, it may become institutionalized within the organization as an ongoing part of the services provided. It is possible for successful programs that are institutionalized across a number of organizations in a community to gain wide acceptance as standard practice, with the establishment of an expectation that a "good" agency will provide the program. At this last stage, the health program has become institutionalized within health services.

Regardless of the stage in a program's life cycle, the major planning and evaluation stages of community assessment and evaluation are carried out. The precise nature and purpose of each activity varies slightly as the program matures (Exhibit 1.4). Being aware of the stage of the program being implemented can help tailor the community assessment and evaluation.

This life cycle of a health program is reflected in the evolution of hospice care. Hospice, care for the dying in a home and family setting, began in London

Exhibit 1.4   Assessment, Implementation, and Evaluation Across the Program Life Cycle

Stage of Program	Community Assessment	Program Implementation	Program Evaluation
Pilot	Generic, global information about the health problem and the target audience	Small number of participants; strict guidelines and protocols for intervention	Rigorous impact evaluation; rigorous process monitoring
Model	Greater information about the target audience	Realistic number of participants; use previously set procedures	Impact and outcome assessment; rigorous process monitoring
Prototype	Very specific information about the local target audience and local variations of the health problem	Some flexibility and adaptation to local needs; realistic enrollment	Impact and outcome assessment; routine process monitoring
Organizationally institutionalized	More attention on assessment of organizational resources for program sustainability	Use standard operating procedure; organization specific	Impact and outcome assessment based on objectives; routine process monitoring
Professionally institutionalized	Rarely any detail; more assessment of competitors and professional norms	Standard for professional practice; certification may be involved	Use professionally set standards as benchmarks of impact and outcome assessment

in 1967 as a grassroots service that entailed trial and error (pilot) for how to manage the dying patient (Kaur, 2000). As its advocates saw the need for reimbursement for the service, they began to systematically control what was done and who was "admitted" to hospice. Once evaluations of these hospice programs began to yield findings that demonstrated their positive benefits, they became the model for more widespread programs that were implemented in local agencies or by new hospice organizations (prototypes). As the prototype hospice programs became accepted as a standard of care for the dying, the hospice programs became standard, institutionalized services for organizations. Now the availability and use of hospice services for terminally ill patients is accepted as standard practice, and most larger health care organizations or systems have a hospice program. The evolution of hospice is but one example of how an idea for a "better" or "needed" program can gradually become widely available as routine care.

TYPES OF EVALUATION

There are six major types of activities that can be and sometimes are classified as evaluations. Each type of activity requires a specific focus, purpose, and set of skills. The six are introduced here as an overview of the field of planning and evaluation, although each receives far greater discussion in subsequent chapters.

Community needs assessment or community health assessment is one type of evaluation. The community needs assessment is done to collect data about the health problems of a particular group, and those data are used to tailor the health program to the needs and distinctive characteristics of that group. A community needs assessment is a major component of program planning, done at an early stage in the program planning and evaluation cycle. However, community assessments may be required to be completed on a regular basis. For example, many states do five-year planning of programs based on state needs assessments.

Another type of evaluation starts at the beginning of the program; it is a process evaluation. Process evaluations focus on the degree to which the program has been implemented as planned and on the quality of the program implementation. Process evaluations are also known as monitoring evaluations. The underlying framework for designing a process evaluation comes from the process theory component of the overall program theory developed during the planning stage. The process theory delineates the logistical activities, resources, and interventions needed to achieve the health change in program participants or recipients. Information from the process evaluation is used to further plan, revise, or improve the program.

The third type of evaluation seeks to determine the effect of the program—in other words, to demonstrate or identify the program's effect on those who participated in or received the program. Effect evaluations answer the key question of whether the program has made a difference. The effect theory component of the program theory is used as the basis for designing this evaluation. For the most part, evaluators seek to use the most rigorous and robust designs, methods, and statistics possible and feasible when conducting an effect evaluation. Thus, several chapters of this text are devoted to various aspects of conducting these evaluations, with particular attention to the methods needed to achieve scientific rigor, as well as practical suggestions for conducting effect evaluations. Findings from effect evaluations are used to revise the program and may be used in subsequent initial program planning activities.

Effect evaluations are more commonly known as impact or outcome evaluations. Impact evaluations are those that focus on the more immediate effects of the program, whereas outcome evaluations may have a more long-term focus. However, this language is not used consistently in the evaluation literature, and the terms "impact evaluation" and "outcome evaluation" seem to be used interchangeably. Summative evaluations, in the strictest sense, are done at the conclusion of a program to provide a conclusive statement regarding program effects. Unfortunately, the term "summative evaluation" is sometimes used to refer to either an impact or outcome evaluation, thus adding confusion to the evaluation terminology and vernacular language. Program planners and evaluators must be vigilant with regard to how they and others are using terms, and should not hesitate to clarify meanings and address any underlying misconceptions or misunderstandings.

A fourth type of evaluation focuses on efficiency and the costs associated with the program. Cost evaluations encompass a variety of more specific cost-related evaluations, namely cost-effectiveness evaluations, cost-benefit evaluations, and cost-utility evaluations. For the most part, cost evaluations are done by researchers because cost-benefit and cost-utility evaluations, in particular, require expertise in economics. Nonetheless, small-scale and simplified cost-effectiveness evaluations can be done if good cost accounting has been maintained by the program and a more sophisticated impact evaluation has been done. The similarities and differences among these three types of cost studies are reviewed in greater detail in the text so that program planners can be, at minimum, savvy consumers of published reports of cost evaluations. Because cost evaluations are done late in the planning and evaluation cycle, results are not likely to be available in time to make program improvements or revisions. Instead, cost evaluations are generally used during the planning stages to gather information for prioritizing program options.

Comprehensive evaluations, the fifth type of evaluation, involve analyzing needs assessment data, process evaluation data, effect evaluation data, and cost evaluation data as a set of data. It is not uncommon for program staff to have each of these types of data; it is relatively uncommon, however, for the program to use all of these data to draw more sweeping conclusions about the effectiveness and efficiency of the program. In addition, for larger, more complex health programs, a comprehensive evaluation can be quite costly and challenging, and is therefore less likely to be planned as an evaluation activity. It is possible to create a comprehensive evaluation from existing process and effect evaluations done over time, if the data can be collated and interpreted as a complete set of information. Comprehensive evaluations are more likely to be done for model or prototype programs, as a point of reference and to document the value of the program.

A sixth type of evaluation is a meta-evaluation. A meta-evaluation is done by combining the findings from previous outcome evaluations of various programs for the same health problem. The purpose of a meta-evaluation is to gain insights into which of the various programmatic approaches has had the most effect and to determine the maximum effect that a particular programmatic approach has had on the health problem. This type of evaluation relies upon the availability of existing information about evaluations and on the use of a specific set of methodological and statistical procedures. For these reasons, meta-evaluations are less likely to be done by program personnel and instead are generally done by evaluation researchers. Meta-evaluations that are published are extremely useful in program planning because they indicate which programmatic interventions are more likely to succeed in having an effect on the participants. Published meta-evaluations can also be valuable in influencing health policy and health funding decisions.

THE PUBLIC HEALTH PYRAMID

As part of the Government Performance and Results Act (GPRA) of 1993, federal agencies were directed to evaluate their services and effectiveness. The MCHB administers several entitlement programs, including Title V, which provides funds to states for maternal and child health improvement programs. One step toward complying with the GPRA was the development of standard performance measures for the Title V programs. In order to address the range of health issues covered under Title V, a model was developed under the leadership of the director, Pete Van Dyke, in which the range of services could be categorized. The model became known as "the pyramid" among the state and local maternal and child health programs that received Title V funds. Although the pyramid was developed for use with state maternal and child health programs, it has applicability and usefulness as an overarching framework for health program planning and evaluation.

The pyramid is divided into four sections (Exhibit 1.5). The top section of the pyramid contains direct health care services, such as medical care, psychological counseling, hospital care, and pharmacy services. At this level of the pyramid, programs are delivered to individuals, whether patients, clients, or even students. Generally, programs at the direct services level have a direct, and often fairly immediate, effect on individual participants in the health program. Direct services are at the tip of the pyramid to reflect that, overall, the smallest proportion of a population receives them.

At the second level of the pyramid are enabling services, which are those health and social services that support or supplement the health of aggregates. Aggregates are used to distinguish between individuals and populations; they are groups of individuals who share a defining characteristic, such as mental illness or a terminal disease. Thus, examples of enabling services are mental health drop-in centers, hospice programs, financial assistance programs that provide transportation to medical care, community-based case management for AIDS patients, nutrition education programs provided by schools, and workplace child care centers. As this list of programs demonstrates, the

Exhibit 1.5 The Public Health Pyramid

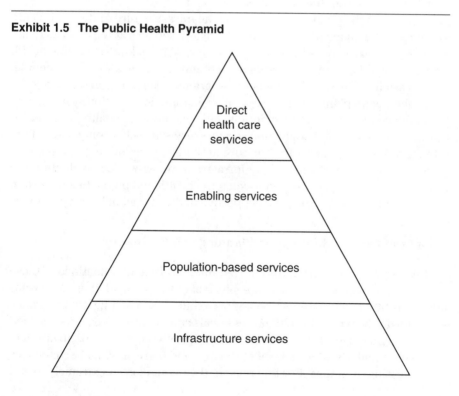

services at this level may directly or indirectly contribute to the health of individuals, families, and communities and are provided to aggregates.

The next, more encompassing level of the pyramid is population-based services. At the population level of the pyramid, services are delivered to an entire population, such as all persons residing in a city, state, or nation. Examples of population services include immunization programs for all children in a county, newborn screening for all infants born in a state, food safety inspections carried out under the auspices of federal regulations, workplace safety programs, nutrition labeling on food, and the Medicaid program for pregnant women who are below poverty guidelines. As this list reflects, the distinction between an aggregate and a population can be blurry. Programs at this level typically are intended to reach an entire population, sometimes without the conscious involvement of individuals. In this sense, individuals receive a population-based health program, such as water fluoridation, rather than participating in the program, as they would in a smoking cessation class. The terms "participant" and "recipient" are used throughout the text to denote the level of the pyramid at which the program was designed and delivered. The population-level programs contribute to the health of individuals and, cumulatively, to the health status of the population.

Supporting the pyramid at its base is the infrastructure of the health care system and the public health system. The health services at the other pyramid levels would not be possible unless there were skilled, knowledgeable health professionals, laws and regulations pertinent to the health of the people, quality assurance and improvement programs, leadership and managerial oversight, health planning and program evaluation, information systems, and technological resources. The planning and evaluation of health programs at the direct, enabling, and population services levels is itself a component of the infrastructure; these are infrastructure activities. In addition, planning programs to address problems of the infrastructure, as well as evaluating the infrastructure itself, are needed to keep the health and public health system infrastructure strong, stable, and supportive of the myriad of health programs.

Use of the Pyramid in Program Planning and Evaluation

Health programs exist across the pyramid levels, and evaluations of these programs are needed. However, at each level of the pyramid, there are issues unique to that level that must be addressed in developing health programs. Accordingly, the types of health professionals and the type of expertise needed varies by pyramid level, reinforcing a need to match program, participants, and providers. Similarly, at each level of the pyramid there are unique challenges for evaluating programs. For this reason, the pyramid is an extremely useful framework to help illuminate those differences, issues, and challenges, as well as to reinforce that health programs are needed across the pyramid levels if the *Healthy People 2010* goals and objectives are to be achieved. Thus, at the end of each chapter in this text, the pyramid is used as a framework to identify and discuss potential or real issues related to the topic of the chapter.

In a more general sense, the pyramid provides a reminder that various aggregates of potential audiences exist for any health problem and program, and that health programs are needed across the pyramid. Depending on the health discipline and the environment in which the planning is being done, direct service programs may be the natural or only option. The pyramid provides a rationale for thinking about only those programs needed to improve the health of the people that are appropriately at the direct services level. It is hard and expensive to reach the same number of persons with a direct services program as with a population-based program.

The pyramid also serves as a reminder that there will be stakeholder alignments and allegiances that may be specific to a level of the pyramid. For example, a school health program, an enabling-level program, will have a different set of constituents and concerned stakeholders than a highway safety program, a population-level program. In other words, the savvy program planner considers not only the potential program participants at each level of the pyramid, but also the stakeholders that are likely to make themselves known during the planning process.

The pyramid has particular relevance for public health agencies concerned with addressing the core public health functions (Institute of Medicine, 1988): assessment, assurance, and policy. These core functions are evident, in varying forms, at each level of the pyramid. Similarly, the pyramid can be applied to the strategic plans of organizations in the private health care sector. For optimal health program planning, each health program being developed or implemented ought to be considered in terms of its relationship to services, programs, and health needs at other levels of the pyramid. For all of these reasons, the public health pyramid is used throughout this textbook as a framework for summarizing specific issues and applications of chapter content to each level of the pyramid.

The Pyramid as an Ecological Model

Individual behavior and health are now understood to be influenced by the social and physical environment of individuals. This recognition is reflected in the growing use of the ecological approach to health services and public health programs. The ecological approach, which stemmed from systems theory applied to individuals and families (Bronfenbrenner, 1970), postulates that individuals can be influenced by factors in their immediate social and physical environment. The individual is viewed as a member of an intimate social network, usually a family, which is a member of a larger social network, such as a neighborhood or community. The way in which individuals are nested within these social networks has consequences for the health of the individual.

The pyramid, by distinguishing and recognizing the importance of enabling and population services, can be integrated with an ecological view of health and health problems. If one were to look down on the pyramid from above, the levels would appear as concentric squares (Exhibit 1.6)—direct services for individuals nested within enabling services for families, aggregates, and neighborhoods, which are nested within population services for all residents of cities, states, or nations. This is similar to individuals being nested within the

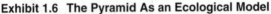

Exhibit 1.6 The Pyramid As an Ecological Model

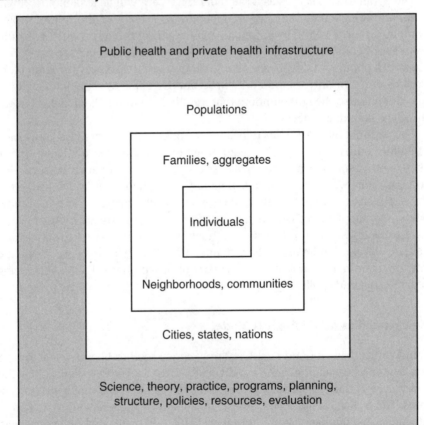

enabling environment of their family, workplace setting, or neighborhood, all of which is nested within the population environment of factors such as social norms and economic and political environments. The infrastructure of the health care system and public health system is the foundation and supporting environment for promoting health and preventing illness and disease.

At the end of each chapter, a summary of the chapter contents is presented in the form of challenges or issues related to applying the chapter content to each level of the pyramid. This is done to reinforce that each level of the pyramid has value and importance to health program planning and evaluation. In addition, there are unique challenges that are specific to each level of the pyramid. The chapter summary by levels is an opportunity to acknowledge and address the issues related to the levels.

COMMUNITY

The use of the ecological model and the pyramid lead naturally to considering community and its role in health program planning and evaluation. Community is a concept that has been the subject of debate and deliberation by sociologists, beginning with Tonnies in 1897 (Bell & Newby, 1971). The term "community" is increasingly used to refer to almost any group of people, which results in a lack of conceptual clarity. This, in turn, can lead to conflicts and confusion during program planning. Thus, it is worth considering what is and is not a community, as a prelude to articulate thinking and as a foundation for better planning of health programs.

Delineating Community

Community encompasses people, some form of proximity or place that enables interaction, and interaction that leads to shared values or culture (Bell & Newby, 1971) (Exhibit 1.7). A defining characteristic of a community is people with the potential for interaction. Without the potential for interaction, the sharing of values and norms is not possible. In today's world of electronic communication, interactions can be virtual as well as in person. To the extent that interacting individuals share values and culture, a community exists. Virtual communities that exist via electronic media contrast with the traditional, anthropological notions of community that grew from the study of tribes and villages. Another defining characteristic of community is that the members have shared values and norms of behavior. The prerequisite that a community have commonly held values precludes, in many instances, a census tract, a zip code, a telephone area code, a consortium of health agencies, or a catchment

Exhibit 1.7   Three Elements of Community, with Examples

People	Place	Interaction
Values, beliefs, behaviors, size, membership, demographic characteristics, social and economic status, sense of power or influence, sense of belonging	Geography, boundaries, housing, industry, air, water, land, virtual presence	Communication, familial, education, religious based, political, recreational, virtual

area for a health service from being a community in the more pure sense. In contrast, active members of a church or residents of a small and homogeneous neighborhood might be a community.

This distinction between a convenient geographic designation and an actual community is important for planning how to have participation by community members in the planning process. However, some convenient locations can be mobilized into a community. In one study (Hedly, Keller, Vanderkooy, & Kirkpatrick, 2002), seniors at a recreation center were mobilized to become active in planning a nutrition program. Their involvement in the program planning led to increased rates of program participation and to their taking increasing responsibility for planning and providing the program.

Shared values are the basis for the cultural unity of a community, which is the basis for the perception of being connected and belonging to a community. From that sense of belonging stems the subsequent behaviors that might be attributed to members of a particular community. What constitutes a "sense of community" can include membership based on membership boundaries, influence over what occurs within the community, shared values and needs fulfillment, and a shared emotional connection (Chavis, Hogge, McMillan, & Wandersman, 1986). As this list of the elements fostering a sense of community connotes, community and its associated emotional and cultural components creates complexities for health program planning and evaluation. When one is planning health programs for small populations, the sense of community can be a key factor in gaining support for the program and for maximizing the health effects of some programs.

Community in Planning and Evaluation

Distinguishing one community from another, while perhaps necessary from the perspective of a health planner, may lead to artificial delineations. Program planners must clarify the purpose for which "the community" is being delineated. A community, as a unit of individuals with some degree of cultural cohesion, can be both the target of a health program as well as the context in which a health program is provided and evaluated.

When a community is the target of a health program, some or all of the community members are the intended recipients of the health program. Thus, to establish the size of the health problem, it is necessary to delineate the community boundaries. In this sense, a community becomes akin to a population. Community assessments or community needs assessments are processes by which the health problem is more fully understood and described. The word "community" is used irrespective of whether a community or a population is being assessed. However, if an actual community, in contrast to a population or an aggregate, is the focus, it is necessary to clarify the boundaries of the community membership to understand the specific health and social conditions within that community.

There are two ways to view the community as the context of the program. Every community has myriad sociopolitical and economic factors that can influence the program plan and implementation. Because there may not be program resources to address these influences directly, it may be possible only to acknowledge, articulate, and take into account these influences as contextual to the program. Another way to address these community influences is to devote some program planning resources to identifying influential individuals from the community to invite to participate in program development and in the program evaluation. From this perspective, community members involved in the planning process become an immediate, intimate context of the program intervention.

Community as target and as context are not mutually exclusive. An example helps demonstrate their interactive nature. At a university health promotion program, students, faculty, and university staff were involved in planning the program, and they also received the wellness program (Reger, Williams, Kolar, Smith, & Douglas, 2002). They were community as target to the extent that all those working and going to school on campus were the intended recipients of the wellness program and were assessed as a unit to identify health problems. They were community as context to the extent that the values, norms, social structure, and university bureaucracy were influences on the program, the university community. To address the contextual influences, the program initiators included and promoted participation by members of the university community in planning the wellness program. In so doing, they overcame institutional barriers and mobilized resources for the program. The synergies achieved by involving community members were possible because the university community was understood not as a single thing nor as a simple geographic location, but as a group of individuals. In other words, to involve "the community" in program planning actually requires having influential, energetic, devoted individuals as representatives of or from that group actively participate in discrete activities.

Collaboration between health program planners and formal or informal leaders from a community, and their participation in the development and evaluation of a health program, are increasingly valued. In fact, such collaboration is increasingly mandated or required by funding agencies as a prerequisite to being considered for funding. Collaboration creates interaction, which can intensify the sense of community, as well as the synergy among the community representatives, the agency sponsoring the health program, and the program staff (Exhibit 1.8). The interactions and influences occur in two directions, with ideas and energy flowing toward the health program and results and respect flowing from the health program.

Exhibit 1.8   Connections Among Program, Agency, and Community

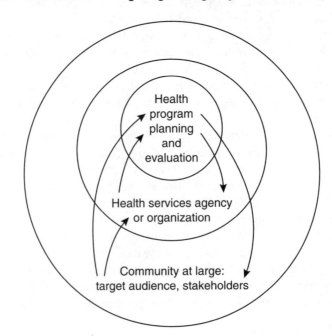

Health program planning and evaluation

Health services agency or organization

Community at large: target audience, stakeholders

Defining "Based," "Focused," and "Driven"

There are three additional terms that deserve defining. "Community-based" is an adjective describing where a program or service is provided. A health program is community-based if it is delivered at locations considered within the boundaries of the community, rather than at a centralized location outside the community boundaries. Generally this translates into a program being delivered in local churches, schools, recreation centers, clinics, or libraries. "Community-focused" refers to the way in which the program is designed. Health programs that seek to affect the community as a whole, as a unit, are best described as community-focused. A community-focused program may seek to change the norms or behaviors of the members of a community that contribute to the health problem, or it may seek to reach all members of the community. In contrast, if a health program is the result of the involvement of community members and is driven by their expressed preferences, it ought to be referred to as "community-driven." A community-driven program has its genesis, its design and implementation, in the involvement, persistence, and passion of key representatives or members from the community.

It is worth noting that the designations of "based," "focused," and "driven" can also apply to families, populations, or other aggregates. Thus, family-based programs could be provided to individuals but within the theoretical or physical presence of families, family-focused programs would be designed to enhance the family as a unit, and family-driven programs would be the result of a group of families advocating for or demanding the programs. These distinctions can be important in terms both of describing health programs and of conceptualizing the nature of a program. Whether a health program is based or focused on a unit ought to flow from an understanding of the health problem and the best strategy for addressing it.

WHO DOES PLANNING AND EVALUATIONS?

A variety of different types of health professionals and social scientists can be involved in health program planning and evaluation. At the outset of program planning and evaluation, one trepidation revolves around who ought to be the planners and evaluators. In a sense, virtually anyone with an interest and a willingness to be an active participant in the planning or evaluation process could be involved, including health professionals, business persons, paraprofessionals, and advocates or activists.

Planners and evaluators may be employees of the organization about to undertake the activity, or they may be external consultants hired to assist in all phases or just a specific phase of the planning and evaluation cycle. Internal and external planners and evaluators each have their advantages and disadvantages. Regardless of whether an internal or external evaluator is used, professional stakes and allegiances ought to be acknowledged and understood as factors that can affect the decision making.

Planners and evaluators from within the organization are susceptible to biases, consciously or not, in favor of the program or some aspect of the program, particularly if their involvement can positively affect their work. On the positive side, internal planners and evaluators are more likely to have insider knowledge of organizational factors that can be utilized or may have a positive effect on the delivery and success of the health program. Internal evaluators may experience divided loyalties, such as between the program and their job, between the program staff and other staff, or between the proposed program or evaluation and their view of what would be better.

A source of internal evaluators can be members of quality improvement teams, particularly if they have received any training in program development or evaluation as they relate to quality improvement. The use of total quality management (TQM), continuous quality improvement (CQI), and other quality improvement methodologies by health care organizations and public health agencies is supportive of health program evaluation. The quality improvement impetus of health care has been fueled by the use of standard measures of performance, such as the National Council on Quality Assurance's Health Employer Data Information System (HEDIS). The wide use of HEDIS is not only a source of data for health program planners and evaluators, but demonstrates the social value that is currently placed on data and on the evaluation of services, albeit for competitive purposes.

External evaluators can bring a fresh perspective and a way of thinking that generates alternatives not currently in the agencies' repertoire of approaches to the health problem and program evaluation. Compared to internal evaluators, external evaluators are less likely to be biased in favor of one approach, unless, of course, they were chosen for their expertise in a particular area, which would naturally bias their perspective to some extent. External program planners and evaluators can, however, be expensive consultants.

The question of who does evaluations can also be answered by looking at who funds health program evaluations. The answer thus is not about individual planners and evaluators but about organizations that do evaluations as a component of their business. Although most funding agencies prefer to fund health programs rather than stand-alone program evaluations, there are some exceptions. For example, the Agency for Healthcare Research and Quality (AHRQ) funds health services research about the quality of medical care, which is essentially effect evaluation studies. Other federal agencies, such as the National Institutes of Health and the bureaus within the Department of Health and Human Services, fund evaluation research of pilot health programs. However, the funding priorities of these federal agencies change with changes in federal health policy. Thus, organizations funding and conducting health program evaluations evolve over time. There is another type of organization that does health program evaluations—namely for-profit research firms, such as Mathematica and the Alpha Center. These organizations receive contracts to evaluate health program initiatives and conduct national evaluations, which require sophisticated methodology and considerable resources.

ROLES OF EVALUATORS

Evaluators may be required to take on various roles, given that they are professionals involved in a process that very likely involves others. For example, as the evaluation takes on a sociopolitical process, the evaluators become mediators and change agents. If the evaluation is a learning–teaching process, evaluators become both teacher and student of the stakeholders. To the extent that the evaluation is a process that creates a new reality for stakeholders, program staff, and program participants, evaluators are reality shapers. There will be times when the evaluation has an unpredictable outcome, and at such times, evaluators are human instruments that gauge what is occurring and analyze events. Ideally, evaluations are a collaborative process, and evaluators are collaborators with the stakeholders, program staff, and program participants. If the evaluation takes the form of a case study, the evaluators may become illustrators, historians, and storytellers. These are but a few examples of how the roles of the professional program evaluator evolve and emerge from the situation at hand. One's role in the planning and evaluation activities may not be clear at the time that the project is started. Roles will develop and evolve as the planning and evaluation activities progress.

ACROSS THE PYRAMID

At the direct services level, health program planning and evaluation focuses on individual clients or patients, on developing programs that are provided to those individuals, and on assessing the extent to which those programs make a difference in the health of the individuals who receive the health program. Health is defined in individual terms, and program effects are measured as individual changes. From this level of the pyramid, community is most likely viewed as the context affecting individual health.

At the enabling services level, health program planning and evaluation focuses on the needs of aggregates of individuals and on the services that the aggregate needs to maintain health or make health improvements. Enabling services are often social, educational, or human services that have an indirect effect on health, thus warranting their inclusion in planning health programs. Health continues to be defined and measured as an individual characteristic to the extent that enabling services are provided to individual members of the aggregate. However, program planning and evaluation focuses not on individuals but on the aggregate as a unit. At this level of the pyramid, community can be either the aggregate that is targeted for a health program or the context in which the aggregate functions and lives. How community is viewed will depend upon the health problem being addressed.

At the population-based services level, health program planning and evaluation focuses on the needs of all members of a population. At this level of the pyramid, health programs are at a minimum population-driven, meaning that data on the health of the population drives the decisions about the health program. This will result in having programs that are population-focused and ideally, but not necessarily, population-based. It is worth noting that population-focused programs tend to have a health promotion or health maintenance focus, rather than a focus on treatment of illnesses. At a population level, health is defined in terms of population statistics, such as mortality and morbidity rates. In this regard, the *Healthy People 2010* objectives (Exhibit 1.9) are predominantly at the population level of the pyramid. Community is more likely to be a population targeted by the health program.

At the infrastructure level, health program planning and evaluation is an infrastructure activity of both the public health system and the health care system. Infrastructure includes organizational management, acquisition of resources, and development of health policy. A significant document reflecting health policy is *Healthy People 2010*, the goals and objectives for the health of the people of the United States. These national objectives are used in setting priorities and are used by many federal and nongovernmental funding agencies in requiring that a health program identify which *Healthy People 2010* objectives are being addressed. To the extent that health planners and evaluators are familiar with these objectives, they are better able to design appropriate programs and then to argue the relevance of that program. At the infrastructure level, health can be defined in terms of the individual workers in the health care sector (an aggregate). But more to the point, because program planning and evaluation are infrastructure activities, it is actually at the infrastructure level that the decisions are made on the definition of health to be used in the program. Similarly, the way that community is viewed is determined at the infrastructure level.

Exhibit 1.9   A Summary of the *Healthy People 2010* Priority Areas

Healthy People 2010: 28 Focus Areas	
1. Access to quality health services	15. Injury and violence prevention
2. Arthritis, osteoporosis, and chronic back conditions	16. Maternal, infant, and child health
3. Cancer	17. Medical product safety
4. Chronic kidney disease	18. Mental health and mental disorders
5. Diabetes	19. Nutrition and overweight
6. Disability and secondary conditions	20. Occupational safety and health
7. Educational and community-based programs	21. Oral health
8. Environmental health	22. Physical activity and fitness
9. Family planning	23. Public health infrastructure
10 Food safety	24. Respiratory diseases
11. Health communication	25. Sexually transmitted diseases
12. Heart disease and stroke	26. Substance abuse
13. HIV	27. Tobacco use
14. Immunization and infectious diseases	28. Vision and hearing

Source: DHHS website: www.healthypeople.gov/about/hpfact.htm (accessed 8/12/03).

DISCUSSION QUESTIONS

1. When and under what conditions might it be advisable not to conduct an evaluation?

2. Oral health is a major health problem, especially for children in poverty. Describe how an oral health program developed at each level of the public health pyramid would differ and how the considerations would differ.

3. Conduct a literature search using words such as "planning," "evaluation," "program," and a health condition of interest to you. Which journals publish articles about health program planning and health program evaluations? What are the current trends in the field as reflected in the published literature that you reviewed?

4. Access and review the material in the following document and compare it with the perspective given in this chapter:

   Centers for Disease Control and Prevention (1999). *Framework for program evaluation in public health.* MMWR, 48 (RR-11): i–41. www.cdc.gov/mmwr/indrr_99.html

REFERENCES

American Evaluation Association (2002). *The program evaluation standards: Summary of the standards.* www.eval.org/EvaluationDocuments/progeval.html (accessed 8/12/03).

American Public Health Association (1991). *Healthy communities 2000: Model standards.* Washington, DC: American Public Health Association.

Bell, C., & Newby, H. (1971). *Community studies: An introduction to the sociology of the local community.* London: George Allen & Unwin.

Blum, H. L. (1981). *Planning for health: Generics for the eighties* (2nd ed.). New York: Human Sciences Press.

Bronfenbrenner, U. (1970). *Two worlds of childhood.* New York: Russell Stage Foundation.

Chavis, D. M., Hogge, J. H., McMillan, D. W., & Wandersman, A. (1986). Sense of community through Brunswick's Lens: A first look. *Journal of Community Psychology, 14,* 24–40.

Dever, G. E. (1980). *Community health analysis: A holistic approach.* Germantown, MD: Aspen Publishers.

Guba, E. G., & Lincoln, Y. S. (1987). Fourth generation evaluation. In D. J. Palumbo (Ed.), *The politics of program evaluation.* (pp. 202–204). Newbury Park, CA: Sage Publications.

Hedley, M. R., Keller, H. H., Vanderkooy, P. D., & Kirkpatrick, S. I. (2002). Evergreen Action nutrition: Lessons learned planning and implementing nutrition education for seniors using a community organization approach. *Journal of Nutrition for the Elderly, 21*, 61–73.

Herman, J. L., Morris, L. L., & Fitz-Gibbon, C. T. (1987). *Evaluators' handbook.* Newbury Park, CA: Sage Publications.

Howell, E., Devaney, B., Foot, B., Harrington, M., Schettini, M., McCormick, M. C., Hill, I., Schwalberg, R., & Zimmerman, B. (1997). *The implementation of Healthy Start: Lessons for the future.* Mathematica Policy Research, Inc. Unpublished Report.

Institute of Medicine, National Academy of Sciences. (1988). *The future of public health.* Washington, DC: National Academy Press.

Kaur, J. (2000). Palliative care and hospice programs. *Mayo Clinic Proceedings, 75*, 181–184.

Patton, M. Q. (1987). *How to use qualitative methods in evaluation.* Newbury Park, CA: Sage Publications.

Patton, M. Q. (1997). *Utilization-focused evaluation: The new century text* (3rd ed.). Thousand Oaks, CA: Sage Publications.

Reger, B., Williams, K., Kolar, M., Smith, H., & Douglas, J. W. (2002). Implementing university-based wellness: A participatory planning approach. *Health Promotion Practice, 3*, 507–514.

Rohrer, J. (1996). *Planning for community-oriented health systems.* Washington, DC: American Public Health Association.

Rosen, G. (1993). *A history of public health* (Expanded ed.). Baltimore: Johns Hopkins University Press.

Rossi, P. H., & Freeman, H. E. (1993). *Evaluation: A systematic approach.* Newbury Park, CA: Sage Publications.

Stufflebeam, D. L. (2001). Evaluation models. *New Directions for Evaluation, 89*, 8–98.

Swenson, M. M. (1991). Using fourth generation evaluation. *Evaluation and Health Professions, 14*(1), 79–87.

Turnock, B. (2001). *Public health: What it is and how it works.* Gaithersburg, MD: Aspen Publishers.

United Way of America. (1996). *Measuring program outcomes: A practical approach.* Alexandria, VA: United Way of America.

US Department of Health and Human Services. (1980). *Promoting health/preventing disease: Objectives for the nation.* Washington, DC: DHHS-PHS.

US Department of Health and Human Services. (1991). *Healthy people 2000: National health promotion and disease prevention objectives.* Washington, DC: DHHS-PHS. Publication No. PHS 91–50212.

US Department of Health and Human Services. (2000). *Healthy people 2010.* Washington, DC: DHHS-PHS. www.healthypeople.gov/publications (accessed 8/12/03).

US Department of Health, Education, and Welfare. (1979). *Healthy people: The surgeon general's report on health promotion and disease prevention.* DHEW, PHS Publication No. 79–55071.

Weiss, C. (1972). *Evaluation.* Englewood Cliffs, NJ: Prentice Hall.

Whitmore, E. (Ed.). (1998). *Understanding and practicing participatory evaluation: New directions for evaluation.* San Francisco: Jossey-Bass.

World Health Organization. (1947). Constitution of World Health Organization. *Chronicle of World Health Organization, 1*, 29–43.

CHAPTER 2

Relevance of Diversity and Disparities to Health Programs

The health status of individuals and populations is influenced not only by the biological process, but also by lifestyle behaviors and circumstances. The intersection of biology, lifestyle, and circumstances leads to disparities in health status, with some groups having lower morbidity and mortality rates than others. At the root of the heath disparities is diversity in biological characteristics and diversity in social, cultural, ethnic, linguistic, and economic characteristics of individuals and populations. In the late 1990s, President Clinton put race, racism, and ethnic diversity on the public agenda. As a consequence, federal agencies, including the National Institutes of Health and the Department of Health and Human Services, began to explicitly fund research into understanding and eliminating racial and ethnic disparities in health status. Private foundations and other agencies funding health programs followed suit by requiring grantees to explicitly state how the program contributes to reducing racial and ethnic health disparities. The high level of attention given to health disparities means that program planners and evaluators must appreciate the sources of disparity, notably diversity, understand key aspects of diversity and how those aspects are relevant to health programs, and know what strategies can be used to address diversity so that the health program will be successful. This chapter begins to address these issues.

A current urban legend exemplifies the influence of culture on health care decisions and the importance of having culturally competent staff. A woman from Africa was in labor with her first child in an American hospital. Her labor was not progressing, and the physician wanted to deliver the baby by cesarean section in an effort to minimize the potential brain damage that was likely to result from a vaginal delivery. The woman and her husband refused the surgery, opting for a difficult vaginal delivery. The couple explained that they needed to make their decision based on what their life would be like when they returned to Africa. In their home village, a woman who has a history of a cesarean section would be in grave danger if she were to have another baby because of the lack of surgical services for delivery in her home village. The life and health of the woman were paramount. The child would be loved and cared for by the entire village, even if it were mentally retarded from the difficult delivery. Whether the story is true has been lost in the telling, but it brings into contrast cultures and how cultural values and norms of behavior are critical to health discussions.

The topic of diversity is addressed early in this text because of its relevance throughout the planning and evaluation cycle (Exhibit 2.1) and for its pervasive effects on programs (Lientz & Rea, 2002). Diversity is relevant with regard to assessment of the health disparities to be addressed. It also affects the intervention choice and delivery, a component of which is the issue of

Exhibit 2.1 Effects of Diversity Throughout the Planning and Evaluation Cycle

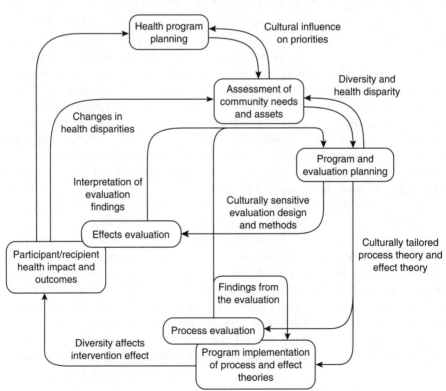

diversity of health providers. Exhibit 2.2 provides examples of considerations that need to be weighed throughout the health program planning and evaluation cycle. The culture of the health care organization and the cultural competence of the program staff are directly related to the ability to culturally tailor programs, as is the formation of coalitions.

HEALTH DISPARITIES

"Health disparities" is a term for the important differences in health status among racial and ethnic groups. This definition of disparities was used in the

Exhibit 2.2   Examples of Cultural Tailoring Throughout the Program Planning and Evaluation Cycle

Stage in the Planning and Evaluation Cycle	Examples of Tailoring for Cultural and Ethnic Diversity
Community needs assessment	Definitions of health and illness; willingness to reveal needs or wants; self-definition in terms of culture, race, or ethnicity; health disparities; experience of disparities in access to or quality of health care
Program theory and development	Identification of contributing and determinant factors of the health disparities; role of discrimination and culturally bound health behaviors in the disparities; culturally acceptable and appropriate interventions
Process or program implementation	Culturally and ethnically adjusted program object targets; cultural, racial, and ethnic representations and appropriateness of materials developed or chosen, such as visual representations, colors used, language or languages, location, media used, modality of distribution, enticement used; culturally appropriate enticements to participate
Program intervention delivery	Type of intervention; length of time participants receive intervention (i.e., session length); amount of intervention (i.e., number of sessions)
Program effect evaluation	Language or languages of survey questionnaires; access to culturally and ethnically equivalent "control" groups

Institute of Medicine report on disparities in health care (Smedley, Stith, & Nelson, 2002). Smedley et al. (2002) defined disparities in health care as differences by race or ethnicity in the quality of health care that are not due to the health or clinical needs or preferences of the person. Well-documented health disparities exist. Blacks have higher rates of low birth weight infants (Martin, Hamilton, Ventura, Menacker, & Park, 2002) and infant mortality (MacDorman, Minion, Strobino, & Guyer, 2002) than whites. Black, poor children have higher rates of morbidity due to asthma than nonpoor black, white poor, or white nonpoor children (Akinbami, LaFleur, & Schoendorf, 2002). White adolescents have higher rates of deaths caused by unintentional injury than blacks (National Vital Statistics Report, 2002). Disparities also exist for chronic illnesses; native Hawaiians are 2.4 times more likely to have diabetes mellitus than non-Hispanic whites of a similar age (National Diabetes Statistics, 2003). Black women have higher mortality rates from breast cancer than Hispanics or whites (National Cancer Institute, 2003). These are a few examples of health disparities that could be addressed by individual practitioners but perhaps more appropriately by health programs across the public health pyramid.

The causes of health disparities are under research, but current theories regarding health disparities posit that they have multiple, interactive, not mutually exclusive causes that are biological, socioeconomic, and cultural. The interactive causes of health disparities either can be primary targets for health programs or can constitute a contextual environment for the health program. In either case, at the heart of addressing health disparities in a practical manner and for developing successful health programs is the need to understand the relationship of diversity to health disparities.

Diversity and Health Disparities

Diversity, in the context of health, refers to the numerous ways in which individuals and groups differ in their beliefs, behaviors, values, backgrounds, preferences, and biology. Diversity is most often described in terms of language, culture, ethnicity, and race. Each of these aspects, along with biological diversity within the human population, have health implications.

Culture is a learned set of beliefs, values, and norms that are shared by a group of people; it is a design for how to live (Spector, 1991). As a set of behavioral norms or expectations, cultural beliefs influence a wide range of behaviors, including dietary choices, hygiene practices, sexual practices, and illness behaviors. Through such behaviors, culture has an effect on health and thus is relevant to health programs. Cultures can be difficult to define and distinguish, particularly when subcultures rather than the dominant culture are the target. Assigning a label to a culture is less important than seeking information about unique or distinct culturally bound patterns of behavior that have health implications. For example, it is not as important to be able to identify a person as being from a Hopi versus Navajo culture as it is to ask about daily consumption of meats and fresh vegetables and how they are prepared. Culture, as the sharing of similar beliefs, values, and norms, contributes to a sense of unity among the members of the culture. The cultural cohesion and sense of belonging to a cultural group is a powerful force in creating conflicts as well as in creating opportunities. Both the Hopi and the Navajo have strong cultural identities that present an opportunity for health program planners to build that cultural identity into the program. The strong cultural identity, however, also can create conflicts between program planners and the Hopi or Navajo if the program is perceived as threatening their culture or being inconsistent with their cultural beliefs.

The relationship between culture and illness is recognized as having distinct manifestations, especially in mental health. The DSM-IV, the diagnostic manual of mental health problems, includes a category for "culture-bound syndromes" (Guranaccia & Rogler, 1999), which are patterns of behaviors and symptoms that are unique to specific and well-defined cultural groups. The existence of culture-bound syndromes lends credence to the theory that illness is, at least in part, socially and culturally constructed. The interaction of culture and illness extends into physical illnesses: it is generally accepted that pain tolerance or intolerance is also influenced by cultural norms (cf. Carragee, Vittum, Truong, & Burton, 1999; Rotheram-Borus, 2000; Sabbioni & Eugster, 2001). The message is that diversity in culture is related to diversity in illness manifestations and responses to illnesses, but these differences are likely to be identified only through cross-cultural comparisons and astute observations. If program planners lack direct personal knowledge of the culture, they will need to rely on published reports of cultural influences on illness manifestations that are specific to the target audience.

Diversity also exists with regard to the economic well-being of individuals, as measured through socioeconomic status (SES). The relationship between SES and a wide variety of health status indicators is well documented (Kosa & Zola, 1975; Polednak, 1997) but not completely understood (Ford & Cooper, 1995; Nickens, 1995; Schulman, Rubenstein, Chesley, & Eisenberg, 1995). The correlation between SES and health status applies both across racial groups and within racial groups. For example, Shakoor-Abdullah, Kotchen, Walker, Chelius, and Hoffman (1997) compared moderate and low-income African-American communities. Compared to the moderate SES African-American community, they found significantly more obesity in the very low SES African-American community and significantly more women with high blood pressure. The fact that individuals in lower SES groups, regardless of other characteristics, have poorer health suggests that health programs may need to target specific SES groups, not just specific cultural, racial, or ethnic groups.

The attention given to cultural and ethnic diversity is driven, in part, by the numbers. In 1998, more than 660,400 individuals immigrated to the United States, with over two-thirds of the immigrants coming from 20 countries (Department of Justice, 1999). By 2050, the population of the United States will be 53% non-Hispanic white, 25% Hispanic, and 14% African-American (Day, 1996). Although these numbers reflect a dramatic shift in the racial composition of the United States population, they do not reflect possible shifts in the distribution of cultures or ethnicities. Changes in the cultural and ethnic composition of the United States cannot be as easily predicted, given that cultures evolve over time and ethnicity can be subsumed into the dominant culture.

DIVERSITY AND HEALTH PROGRAMS

As this very brief introduction to health disparities suggests, the extent of diversity within a target population can have multiple effects on how health programs are developed and provided. The three main areas affected by diversity are measurement done during planning and evaluating the health program, design and implementation of the health program intervention, and the heath care organization and program itself, including cultural competence and coalition formation. Each of these is addressed in some detail in the sections that follow.

Measurement

Measurement occurs throughout the planning and evaluation cycle. Measurement of health status and of factors contributing to the health problem occur during the community needs assessment phase. Program delivery and participation measurement occur during the process evaluation phase. Measurement of program effects occurs during program evaluation. At each of these points in the planning and evaluation cycle, diversity in the target audience and in program participants or recipients has ramifications for what is measured, what data are collected, and how data are collected.

The first consideration is, however, the purpose of measuring an aspect of diversity. The purpose of measuring diversity is paramount in deciding how it is measured. Imagine that in a statewide community needs assessment, an atheist born in San Francisco and a Muslim born in Palo Alto were grouped into one ethnic category. Stated in this way, it seems strange to assign these two individuals the same ethnicity. But grouping these individuals together makes sense if the purpose of the assessment is to have data on Mexican immigrant culture. Given that ethnicity denotes a set of religious, racial, national, linguistic, or cultural characteristics that define a group, the ethnicity measure was based on religion as Catholic or not and on birthplace as California or not. Thus, non-Californian Catholics were assigned a Mexican ethnicity. This example was intentionally contrived to demonstrate the importance of purpose in developing indicators of diversity and the profound effect the variables used have on the indicator and findings.

Culture is often implicit, tacit, and not expressed as a distinct factor, making it difficult to measure. In addition, because a dominant culture exists at a societal level, measures of culture are less useful in health programs than indicators of more discrete, smaller subpopulations, such as those that might be defined by ethnicity or nationality. Thus, ethnicity is used as a proxy for cultural identity. The extent of language diversity and religious diversity makes constructing a comprehensive measure of ethnicity very difficult. For example, religious diversity is reflected in the large number of religions, religious sects, and churches listed in the U.S. military's *Ministry Team Handbook*, each of which has specific dietary practices, clothing, health practices, religious practices, and birth, marriage, and death rituals. Health researchers are attempting to understand the relationship between health status and mainstream religious beliefs and practices (Mathews et al., 1998). Typically, ethnicity is measured with a single item rather than a more valid multifactorial set of items that encompass religion, language, and race. Nonetheless, using a valid and reliable measure of ethnicity is key to having good data for planning and evaluating health programs.

Nationality, the place of birth of the individual or the parents, is a more straightforward measure. Because cultural identity and ethnicity can be difficult to measure, nationality by birth or birthplace of the parents is sometimes used as an indicator of culture and ethnicity. Many countries, however, have multiple ethnic groups, making it problematic to equate nationality with ethnicity or culture. Thus, if nationality is measured, another measure, such as primary language, may be needed to have a more accurate measure of ethnicity and culture.

The following example demonstrates the importance of carefully choosing indicators of diversity, such as measures of ethnicity or culture, for planning health programs. In one neighborhood of Chicago, a large percentage of the residents belong to a specific sect of Judaism. In this neighborhood, the food stores are kosher, the women's clothing is consistent with their religion, and friendships are built around synagogue membership. Less than half a mile away is another neighborhood with a large percentage of residents with ties to the Indian subcontinent. In this neighborhood, the food stores stock food for their cultural cuisine, the women wear their traditional clothing, and the social structure is built around the dominance of the male head of the house-hold. The health statistics for the Jewish neighborhood are relatively good, but the health statistics for the Indian neighborhood reveal women's health problems due to high rates of domestic violence and chronic illness related to alcoholism. Unless the data from the two neighborhoods are separated, the health statistics for the area as a whole mask some of the women's health problems and understate the mens' health problems related to alcoholism. This description of two actual neighboring ethnic groups shows the extent to which program planners need to be familiar not only with the data but, more importantly, with the community characteristics. These characteristics include the cultural beliefs of the residents and the degree to which ethnic and religious diversity coexist, rather than overlap. Having this level of under-standing about the cultural and ethnic diversity of a community facilitates appropriate interpretation of community health status data.

Race has long been considered a physical characteristic. From a biological perspective, race has historically been associated with specific genetic dis-eases, including sickle cell anemia, thalassemia, and some forms of lactose intolerance. Race has also been used as a proxy measure of culture, ethnicity, and SES. To the extent that race has been used as a risk factor for specific genetically transmitted health conditions, it has been of some medical value. However, little agreement exists regarding which categories ought to be used to measure race (Exhibit 2.3). Several authors (Bhopal & Donaldson, 1998; Lin & Kelsey, 2000; McKenny & Bennett, 1994; Williams, 1996) argue that the ways in which race data are collected have limited value from the perspective of health, particularly given that many indicators used to identify race are also indicators of culture or ethnicity. As progress on the human genome project continues and the field of genomics matures (Khoury, 2003), specific genetic markers that are more specific than race may be identified for genetic dis-eases. As tests for these more specific markers become available and afford-able, race, as currently measured, may have less medical value. It is not hard to imagine a day when the current measures of race will no longer be medical-ly relevant. Until the future arrives, however, race will continue to be used as a measure in planning health promotion and disease prevention programs.

The cultural and ethnic background of program participants affects the development or choice of questionnaires, as well as the interpretation of

Exhibit 2.3   Indicators Used to Measure Race in Different Surveys, As Indicated by the Shaded Areas

Category Used	Census 2000[1]	Birth Certificate[2]	National Health Interview Survey[3]	National Hospital Discharge Survey[4]
Question(s) are phrased to ask about:	Race	Hispanic origin; race	National origin or ancestry; race	Race
White	▓	▓	▓	▓
Black		▓	▓	▓
Black, African-American, Negro	▓		▓	
Hispanic	▓		▓	
Mexican, Mexican-American, Chicano	▓		▓	
Mexican-American			▓	
Chicano			▓	
Mexican		▓	▓	
Puerto Rican	▓	▓	▓	
Cuban	▓	▓	▓	
Cuban-American			▓	
Central and South American			▓	
Other Spanish, Hispanic, Latino	▓		▓	
Other Latin American			▓	
Other Spanish or Hispanic		▓	▓	
Native American				▓
American Indian		▓	▓	
Eskimo		▓	▓	
Aleut		▓	▓	
American Indian or Alaska Native	▓		▓	
Asian Indian	▓	*	▓	
Asian or Pacific Islander (API)		▓	▓	▓
Chinese	▓	▓	▓	
Filipino	▓	▓	▓	
Japanese	▓	▓	▓	
Korean	▓	*	▓	
Vietnamese	▓	*	▓	
Hawaiian		▓	▓	
Native Hawaiian	▓		▓	
Guamanian or Chamorro	▓	*	▓	

Exhibit 2.3   Indicators Used to Measure Race in Different Surveys *(continued)*

Samoan		*		
Other Pacific Islander		*		
Other				
Refused				
Don't know				

* Nine states (California, Hawaii, Illinois, Minnesota, New Jersey, New York, Texas, Virginia, and Washington) report data on these API categories.

Sources: [1] US Census, Form D-GIA. *http://www.census.gov* (accessed 8/28/03).
   [2] US Standard Certificate of Live Birth. *http://www.cdc.gov/nchs/data/dvs/birth1-acc.pdf* (accessed 8/28/03).
   [3] *National Health Interview Survey (NHIS) CAPI Specifications: 2001 Instrument.* *ftp://ftp.cdc/gov/pub/Health_Statistics/NCHS/Survey_Questionaires/NHIS/2001/ qhoushld.pdf* (accessed 8/28/03).
   [4] Medical Abstract–National Hospital Discharge Survey. (2000). *http://www.cdc.gov/NCHS/data/Series/SR_01/Sr0R01_039.pdf* (accessed 8/28/03).

results. In the development of scientifically sound and rigorous data collection tools, the language and culture of the intended respondents must be considered. To assure that a questionnaire is culturally and linguistically appropriate and understood requires that the questionnaire be translated from the primary language into the second language and then translated back into the primary language. The back-translated version is then compared with the original version of the questionnaire to determine the accuracy of the translation. Translation of words is not sufficient; both the ideas embodied in the questionnaire and the wording of each item need to be translated (Ferketich, Phillips, & Verran, 1993). The questionnaire needs to be culturally equivalent, so that the ideas and the expressions are the same, not just the words.

The following is an example of the measurement challenges program planners and evaluators could face. A questionnaire developed in the United States for the mainstream culture regarding group functioning in a work unit was chosen for use with Taiwanese employees. The questionnaire was translated into Chinese by three Taiwanese researchers and then translated back by three other Taiwanese researchers. The back-translated version was considerably different from the original English version. In trying to understand what had happened, the researchers found that two factors had come into play. The lack of a future tense in some Chinese languages made it impossible to directly translate the English items that asked about the future actions of the respondent. The other factor was that the questionnaire had been designed to measure the degree of individual and group functioning, based on the American value of individualism. Thus, the questionnaire was difficult to translate both linguistically because of the future tenses and conceptually because of the individualist versus collectivist values of the two cultures. This example hints at the potential complexity of using a survey questionnaire designed for one culture with a second culture. It also highlights the potential ethnocentrism involved in thinking that what is valued in the American culture—in this example, individualism—would be relevant in other cultures. This translation story helps explain why such extensive publications exist for the SF-12, a 12-item measure of overall health, one of the most widely translated health questionnaires. These publications document its psychometric properties when translated and used in different countries, demonstrating that even a widely used and researched questionnaire requires a considerable amount of work to assure that a measure is culturally and linguistically appropriate with each culture.

Cultural diversity also affects the interpretation of findings based on the data collected. Stakeholders involved in the health program who come from different backgrounds and cultures hold different values and ideas. Their culturally based interpretations may be quite different from the interpretations of health professionals who have their own professional culture. Culture influences how meaning is attributed to findings and how data are collected for program evaluation. For example, a violence prevention program measured its effectiveness in terms of the lack of gang tags spray-painted on walls in a neighborhood that was next to a city park. When residents of the neighborhood were presented with the findings, they interpreted the findings in a skeptical manner. They explained that for them the lack of gang tags did not mean the lack of gangs, just that they no longer knew the gang boundaries and thus where it was safe to go, including whether it was safe to go the park for exercise. This actual example exemplifies both the powerful influences of culture on interpreting data and the value of involving stakeholders in any data interpretation.

Interventions

Program interventions are the actions done intentionally to have a direct effect on program participants or recipients. The interventions used in health programs must be tailored to the target audience if the program is to be successful in achieving the desired health effects. The choice of interventions and manner of intervention delivery ought to be based on both the sociocultural diversity of the target audience and the biological diversity within the target audience. Three overall approaches dominate the development of program interventions. In addition, the diversity of health professionals and of health sectors plays a role in the effectiveness of program interventions.

Influences of Sociocultural Diversity on Interventions

Understanding how to tailor the program given cultural differences begins with having or collecting information about differences across and within cultural groups. Legge and Sherlock (1991) found differences in substance abuse patterns among three different Asian cultural groups and differences by gender in the three Asian cultures studied. Navarro, Wilson, Berger, and Taylor (1997), in providing Native American students with a program to prevent alcohol and substance abuse, found that tribal differences and conflicting religious themes among tribes were important to those participating in the program. Lew et al. (1999) found the need to use posters that varied in color theme and facial characteristics of those portrayed when targeting Koreans, Taiwanese, and Japanese. They were also able to increase participation by Asian Americans/Pacific Islanders in a walkathon by having community participation, bilingual/bicultural staff, and culturally tailored publicity and programs. Studies such as these highlight the inadequacy of broad cultural classifications when developing a program for specific cultural or ethnic groups. The specificity with which a cultural group was defined made a difference in the delivery strategies and interventions chosen. The health program interventions must be congruent with the values, norms, and expectations of the participants' cultural group.

A trend in health programs is the incorporation of faith into health program planning and to have parish-based health programs (Trofino et al., 2000). This trend has implications for health programs. One implication related to intervention development is that incorporating religious ethnic elements into the program intervention can help address health disparities described in terms of a religion. The other implication is that being able to define a health disparity in terms of religion provides an opportunity to work with members of that religion for delivery of the health program.

Interventions may result in immediate or permanent changes, but most health behavior interventions are intended to change behaviors that must be sustained over time. Culture affects whether behaviors are sustained. Rossiter (1994) evaluated a language- and culture-specific educational program designed to increase breastfeeding among immigrant Vietnamese women. She found that while the program increased breastfeeding, participants did not continue breastfeeding for six months postpartum. These findings hint at two program planning challenges when health programs are tailored to specific cultural groups. Different culturally appropriate interventions may be needed for initiation versus continuation of program effects. Also, program impact objectives need to be culturally appropriate, with correspondingly appropriate target levels.

The sociocultural influences on intervention may occur in unanticipated ways, such as through program participants themselves. For example, program participants bring their culture to the program in ways that can affect the intervention and its effectiveness. Higginson (1998) studied adolescent mothers in a high school program to examine their competitive culture. Higginson concluded that the competitive culture among adolescent mothers in the program was shaped by their social class, age, and race and that their competitive culture also pervaded the beliefs and norms of the health program in which they participated. These adolescents socialized new program participants into the competitive culture, thus creating a "program culture." Kohn and Bryan (1998) argued that one way to understand the culture of a program is to analyze the ceremonies and rituals. They also suggested intentionally building ceremony and rituals into programs for high-risk groups that need a sense of belonging that comes with having a program culture, in order to retain them as active program participants. These are some examples of how diversity can affect program interventions.

Influences of Biological Diversity on Interventions

For some health conditions, physiological responses may vary by race, gender, or age and thus affect decisions about type and intensity of interventions used in the health program. Generational differences in values, norms, beliefs, and health problems all contribute to diversity. From the perspective of health program planning, age distribution is an important factor in reaching the intended audiences of a program. Gender and sexual orientation are other dimensions of physical diversity that have ramifications for program development. Disability, whether physical, mental, or developmental, is another dimension of diversity but is less often mentioned. Nonetheless, it may be extremely relevant for some health programs. The distribution of physical characteristics within a population or community influences decisions during health program planning and later during program evaluation. Take age as an example. Imagine that a county board wants to increase the physical activity of all residents. The age distribution in the community will affect the nature and content of the communitywide media messages. Messages that will be relevant to the physical abilities of the elderly will need to be quite different from messages that address the physical abilities of school-age children. Similar considerations would be needed for the other types of physical diversity.

Approaches to Developing Programs

Various perspectives exist on explaining patterns of health behavioral differences by culture, ethnicity, and race. Kim, McLeod, and Shantzis (1992) suggested that there are three approaches used in health-related programs: cultural content approaches, cultural integration approaches, and cultural conflict approaches. In the cultural content approach, cultural backgrounds and norms are viewed as leading to behaviors and illnesses. Kleinman (1980), a medical anthropologist, explained that illness is cultural in that sickness and symptoms are saturated with specific meaning and are given patterns of human behavior. The notion that illness is cultural, not just biological, affects the degree to which individuals accept professional explanations of health and illness.

Cultural integration approaches to developing health programs focus on acculturation. Acculturation, the adoption and assimilation of another culture, affects behavior in that the less dominant group takes on behaviors of the dominant group. When planning programs, planners need to consider the degree of acculturation because it affects health beliefs and behaviors. Behavior is also affected when individuals identify with more than one culture to varying degrees, such that bicultural individuals have health beliefs and behaviors that are a blend of the dominant and less dominant cultures. When targeting groups or individuals who identify with more than one culture, planners need to understand their health beliefs and behaviors as a "new" culture. This is particularly relevant for health programs targeting former immigrants or first-generation United States citizens.

Cultural conflict approaches underscore conflict as the genesis of behaviors. There are several areas of potential cultural conflict. One area stems from the generation gap, which leads to family conflict and unhealthy behaviors and illnesses. Differences between the role expectations of different cultures are another source of cultural conflict and unhealthy behaviors. Racism, oppression, and lack of political power lead to alienation and identity conflict and subsequent unhealthy behaviors and illnesses. From a psychological perspective, individuals who are experiencing conflicts such as these are more likely to be in some form of crisis and thus have less attention and energy to engage in health-promoting behaviors. Thus, an assessment of the target population ought to assess the degree of cultural conflict. Program planners need to address the immediate causes of the cultural conflict in order to develop appropriate interventions for the health program.

Profession and Provider Diversity

Health program planning and evaluation draws upon the expertise of individuals from a multitude of health disciplines, including medicine, nursing, pharmacy, social work, nutrition, physical therapy, and dentistry, as well as social science disciplines, including health education, health psychology, social demography, and medical sociology. Each discipline has specialized knowledge, different values, and different professional norms. Planning, implementing, and evaluating health programs requires working on teams that bring together the strengths of the different professions and that respect the different educational backgrounds (Exhibit 2.4). Each health discipline has a slightly different professional language, different beliefs about how to identify and address health problems, and different perspectives on what constitutes a health outcome. To tap into the wealth available through professional diversity requires that the team develop a common language and shared goals for the health program.

Health professionals do not reflect the diversity profile of the population of the United States in terms of cultural, racial, and ethnic diversity. For example, the percentage of registered nurses who are black is 4.3%, yet blacks make up 12% of the overall population. Similarly, the percentage of registered nurses who are Hispanic is 1.7%, compared to 10% of the overall population that is Hispanic (Spratley, Johnson, Sochalski, Fritz, & Spence, 2000; Day, 1996). This same pattern of minorities being underrepresented is consistent across the health professions. The lack of racial and ethnic diversity among health professionals creates a cultural gap between professionals and patients, clients, and program participants. The extent of the cultural gap between planners and the program target audience contributes to a reduced understanding of the target audience, a greater need to become informed about the target audience, and, potentially, tensions between the planners and advocates for or from the target audience. The more comprehensive the health program and the greater the cultural diversity of the target population, the greater the need to have parallel diversity among those planning and providing the program.

Health Provider Sectors

From an anthropological perspective, diversity of health providers can be understood in terms of three sectors of the health–illness system from which individuals seek help when experiencing illness (Kleinman, 1980). Each sector has direct implications for planning, implementing, and evaluating health programs. One sector consists of allopathic, naturopathic, and other formally

Exhibit 2.4   Professional Diversity Among Health Professionals

Health Discipline	Average Education	Primary Focus	Licensure/ Certificate	Programmatic Contribution	Estimated Number in U.S.
Dentistry	Dental doctorate (3 to 4 years after baccalaureate)	Diagnosis and treatment of conditions of the teeth and gums	Licensure	Oral health knowledge	168,000 in 2000[1]
Health administration	Master's degree	Leadership and management of health care organizations	Certificate	Management and administration	N.A.[2]
Health education	Baccalaureate	Development and delivery of materials and curriculum designed to impart health knowledge and change behavior	Certificate	Social and behavioral knowledge	N.A.[2]
Medicine	Medial doctorate (4 years after baccalaureate), plus residency of 3 to 4 years	Differential diagnosis and treatment of illnesses	Licensure and certificate	Medical, pathology, and treatment knowledge	782,200 in 2000[1]
Nursing	Baccalaureate (associate degree minimum requirement)	Promotion of health and well-being based on scientific knowledge	Licensure and certificate	Integration of behavioral and medical knowledge	2,201,800 in 2000[1]
Nutrition	Baccalaureate	Dietary and nutritional elements necessary for health	Licensure and certificate	Nutritional knowledge, influence of nutrition on health	90,000 in 2003[3]

| Physical therapy | Baccalaureate | Restoration and mainte-nance of body strength and flexibility for the purpose of maximizing physical capabilities | Licensure | Focus on enhancing capability within limitations | 130,000 in 2000[3] |
| Social work | Master's degree | Address basic needs; help people manage environmental forces that create prob-lems in living | Licensure | Focus on family and psychological factors | 96,268 in 1998[4] |

Source: U.S. Health Workforce Personnel Factbook. (2000). *http://www.bhpr.hrsa.gov/healthwork-force/reports/default.htm* (accessed 8/28/03).
[1] Table 101 in U.S. Health Workforce Personnel Factbook
[2] Data not available on these health disciplines
[3] Table 601 in U.S. Health Workforce Personnel Factbook
[4] Table 701 in U.S. Health Workforce Personnel Factbook

trained health professionals that comprise the medical health care system. Physicians, nurses, pharmacists, naturopathic physicians, chiropractors, and licensed massage therapists function within this sector. Professionals from this sector have legally sanctioned practice parameters. The insurance industry interacts and to some extent intersects with this sector. Although not the most widely used sector, it is the most expensive in societal terms. The field of health program planning falls within this sector, as do the methods and knowledge about health program planning and evaluation. In addition, the preponderance of health programs are designed in accordance with theories and knowledge generated from this sector.

Another sector from which individuals seek help is the folk health care sector, which encompasses nonprofessional, secular, or sacred healers who have not received formal education but who are very likely to have received training through some type of apprenticeship. A wide variety of traditional healers make up this sector: curanderos, espiritualistos, santerias, singers, shamans, and root-workers, among others. Some of these healers and their treatments are now referred to as complementary or alternative medicine. Evidence of the presence of folk healers can be found when visiting neighborhoods that are ethnically isolated or that maintain folkloric traditions. Individuals may consult healers from this sector while receiving more modern or Western health care. The theories of illnesses and diseases that are the basis of folk health practices can conflict with allopathic theories and thus may diminish the effectiveness of interventions based on an allopathic frame of reference. The role of folk healers in community health behaviors and in addressing health problems can be central for some health programs, especially those targeting individuals who have maintained "the old ways."

The third and largest sector of health providers is the popular or lay sector, consisting of family and friends. There is no doubt that most of us talk to a family member or friend about our illness before seeking either professional or folk health care. This almost invisible sector is the most relied upon, from receiving the latest news disseminated through the mass media to getting a mother's recipe for chicken soup. Health information is spread through the lay sector through social networks, making it a powerful sector for influencing health knowledge and behavior. Health programs that seek to change social norms or population-level behaviors are essentially seeking to change the lay health care sector.

Diversity Within Health Care Organizations and Programs

From a systems theory perspective, an organization that is internally diverse will be better able to respond to externally diverse needs and demands. This concept has been formalized into the concept of requisite variety (Weick, 1979). The concept of requisite variety suggests that health care organizations with a culturally diverse and culturally competent workforce are better suited to provide services that meet culturally diverse health needs. The need for requisite variety is a fundamental reason for having a culturally and ethnically diverse health professions sector.

ORGANIZATIONAL CULTURE

Different types of organizations offer health programs, such as state or local health agencies, for-profit acute care networks, not-for-profit community-based agencies, and academic institutions. Each organization has a unique set of values, norms, and beliefs that are collectively held by its members and that are passed on to new employees; this constitutes the organizational culture (Deal & Kennedy, 1982; Schein, 1995). Organizational culture has been studied (Mallak, 2001; Smith, Francovich, & Gieselman, 2000), including in health care (Scott, Mannion, Davies, & Marshall, 2003). Common examples of organizational culture are the norms about starting meetings on time and the willingness to help other employees accomplish tasks. The relevance of organizational culture to health programs is that it is recognized as influencing the performance of an organization, and it reflects the goal of the organization with regard to being culturally competent.

Program managers need to be sensitive to the degree of fit between the organizational culture and the goals of the health program. Not all good ideas for programs are good for the organization. A good match or fit between how the organization views its mission and philosophy—in other words, its beliefs and values—and the purpose of the health program may be important to the success of the health program in terms of financial, personnel, and other organizational support. In a similar vein, the integration and sustainability of a program within an organization are also affected by organizational culture. For example, Gager and Elias (1997) found that to sustain a mental health program in a school, a determinant factor was having the program become part of the school's culture.

Another implication of organizational culture for program managers is that staff with work experience hold some of the values and norms of the prior organizational culture. These values and norms can be shaped; in other words, new employees need to become acculturated into the new organization, a process that begins with orientation. Cox (2001), an expert on multicultural organizations, defined diversity within an organization as the variation in the social and cultural identities of people existing together. For organizations, diversity is value added because it increases respect, improves problem solving, increases creativity and ideas, increases organizational flexibility, improves the quality of employees, and improves marketing strategies. Diversity within organizations not only creates benefits but also poses challenges for managing and enhancing that diversity.

An essential element contributing to a health care organization's cultural competence is the ability for self-assessment of cultural competence. This requires having an understanding of the cultural competency continuum.

Cultural Competency Continuum

Accompanying the emphasis on diversity and health disparities is the emphasis on cultural competency, the extent to which individuals are able to live or work in a culture other than their own. Cultural competence, by its nature, has shades of less and more that extend along a continuum (Cross, Bazron, Dennis, & Isaacs, 1989; Orlandi, 1992) (Exhibit 2.5). It is possible for health professionals and program staff to be at different points along the continuum, depending upon a variety of factors, such as the specific circumstances and their experiences with cultures other than their own. While the prevailing norm and politically correct stance is to be as culturally sensitive and as competent as possible, acceptance of different values and beliefs can be difficult, particularly of cultures that are dramatically different than one's own.

Exhibit 2.5   Cultural Continuum with Examples of the Distinguishing Features of Each Stage

	Cultural Destructiveness	Cultural Incapacity	Cultural Blindness	Cultural Openness	Cultural Competence	Cultural Proficiency
Attitude toward other cultures	Hostility	Dislike, separate but equal	Ambivalence, treat all alike	Curious, cultural awareness	Respect and tolerance, cultural sensitivity	Fully comfortable, cultural attunement
Knowledge of other cultures	Active avoidance of knowledge	None	Little or none	Some	Fair amount	Extensive
Degree of integration across cultures	None	None	None	Contemplation of potential benefits of integration	Some integration, some elements of multicultural integration	Extensive integration, fully multicultural, fusion of cultures
Implications for health program of participants at each stage	Programs address consequences of cultural destructiveness	Need to have programs provided to separate groups	If have multicultural elements, may need to justify and explain	Can provide program to participants from multiple cultures but will need to provide information and role modeling of competence	Can provide program to participants from multiple cultures with minimal adjustments	Can provide multilingual, multicultural interventions in one program

At the least tolerant end of the continuum is cultural destructiveness (Orlandi, 1992), which includes a set of attitudes and practices that explicitly promote one culture over another based on the notion of one being superior to the other. The attitude of superiority of one's culture over the inferior culture stems from the notion of the other being different or distasteful. Often physical characteristics that are visible are used as the basis for cultural destructiveness, especially race, gender, sexual orientation, and age. While it is unlikely that the staff of a health program would be at this end of the continuum, it is possible that health programs are needed by and being planned for individuals who would be at this end of the continuum. In fact, many of the global conflicts that lead to humanitarian crises and refugees have their roots in cultural destructiveness. International health programs are likely to be dealing directly with the consequences of cultural destructiveness. For programs within the United States, program planners will need to have an "insider" understanding of factors that would make the health program acceptable to culturally destructive groups.

Individuals at the next stage, cultural incapacity, also promote one culture over another, although more implicitly than those at the cultural destructiveness stage. Cultural incapacity is manifested in the doctrine of "separate but equal," with the accompanying segregation and discrimination. In the United States, both cultural incapacity and cultural destructiveness have been made illegal through constitutional, federal, and various state statutes.

Cultural blindness, the next stage, is a perspective of being unbiased, such that people are viewed as being alike and thus are treated alike. However, the "alike" is based on the dominant culture, giving cultural blindness ethnocentric overtones. Historically, health programs sought and delivered universal solutions without regard to different communication patterns of different cultures (Airhihenbuwa, 1994). Treating everyone in an unbiased manner would seem to be a reasonable premise for a health program. Cultural blindness, however, does not lead to effective programs. One explanation, from educational psychology, centers on the role of the dominant culture. Boekaerts (1998) suggested that because culture affects self-constructs, it also affects key features of how individuals learn and process information. Thus, what may be an effective learning environment for those from the dominant culture may not be effective for those from the less dominant culture who are being treated like those from the dominant culture. This theory implies that health programs, especially those with education or learning components that are based on a cultural blindness perspective are not likely to be effective for those not from the dominant culture. Another way of thinking about the consequences of cultural blindness is its failure to recognize that ideas and concepts are not the same across cultures, due to the differences in self-constructs and learning. From this perspective, the earlier discussion of the need to translate concepts used in questionnaires is another example of how to overcome cultural blindness and its potential consequences for health program planning and evaluation.

Cultural openness is the attitude of being receptive to different cultures and to active learning about other cultures. Although other cultures are valued and some knowledge of other cultures exists, cultural openness does not include any integration of cultures or cross-pollination of cultural ideas. In this regard, cultural openness is similar to cultural awareness. Each culture is valued and understood as separate and distinct. An example of being culturally open is someone from the dominant white culture going to a local American Indian pow-wow simply to observe what happens. Cultural openness in health programs would be evident in hiring staff to have a balance of cultures, having minority representation on community or advisory boards for the health program, using consultants with expertise in cultural awareness, and providing cultural sensitivity training for staff. Such culturally open practices increase the likelihood that the health program will be culturally appropriate, but they do not assure its appropriateness. To assure that the health program is culturally appropriate requires actively seeking information and integrating that information into the design, delivery, and evaluation of the health program. This process requires cultural competence.

Cultural competence encompasses not only respect for other cultures, but also actively seeking advice and consultation from members of the less dominant cultural group for suggestions on being culturally appropriate from their perspective. Acting in a culturally competent manner requires various skills that one needs to intentionally acquire. These skills are more specific than listening and being respectful. Continuing with the American Indian example, if a tribal shaman is consulted and included as a full member in the planning team for a health program intended for members of his tribe, then the health planning team is exhibiting culturally competent behaviors, especially if the shaman's approach to healing is included in the program. Generally, cultural competence is understood as an individual characteristic of providers. For example, in a study of psychotherapy, Sue (1998) found cultural competence to exist if the psychotherapist was scientifically minded, had dynamic-sizing skills, and had culture-specific expertise.

One challenge to understanding what constitutes cultural competence is that other terms are used, such as cultural sensitivity and cultural attunement. Both sensitivity and attunement can be viewed as elements of cultural competence. Hoskins (1999) proposed five principles of cultural attunement: acknowledging the pain of oppression by the dominant culture, engaging in acts of humility, acting with reverence, engaging in mutuality, and coming from a place of "not knowing." Hoskins' principles are notably developed for members of the dominant culture, with the implicit expectation that members of the dominant culture need to become culturally competent. In other words, it is incumbent upon members of the dominant culture to strive for cultural competence. The principles also reveal that cultural competence, as a set of behaviors, may be difficult to attain or maintain over time.

The Bureau of Primary Health Care, in its document on cultural competence (2003), listed domains of cultural competence for heath care organizations. One domain is the values and attitudes of mutual respect and regard, and acceptance of the role that values and beliefs play in health and illness. Another domain is a communication style of being sensitive and aware of cultural nonverbal language. Community and consumer involvement and participation in decision making is the third domain. The fourth domain is the cultural appropriateness of the physical environment, materials, and resources. Use of posters and brochures with representatives from different races and ethnicities falls into this domain. The fifth domain encompasses policies and procedures of the organization that lead to having staff that reflect the linguistic and cultural diversity of the community. Another domain is the self-awareness the health professional has of his or her own beliefs, values, and knowledge about diversity. The last domain is the training and professional development provided to staff to assure cultural competence across the organization. This list of domains hints at the corresponding amount of work needed to achieve and maintain a culturally competent organization and workforce. These same domains clearly apply to health programs.

At the most culturally capable end of the continuum is cultural proficiency, which involves not only proactively seeking knowledge and information about other cultures but also educating others about other cultures. Cultural proficiency, as with any end point on a continuum, is difficult to achieve and may not be sustained for a long period of time. Those few individuals who can move among cultures, be accepted in those cultures, and be an ambassador of multiple cultures would be considered culturally proficient. Being multicultural, fully accepting and integrating two or more sets of cultural values and beliefs, is a manifestation of cultural proficiency. Multiculturalism in an organization or program (Cox, 1991) is the extent to which different cultures are fully integrated, and would be manifested in programs as integrating folk or professional practitioners and treatment options, having predominantly bicultural staff, celebrating holidays important to cultural groups involved in the program, and synthesizing different cultural beliefs into the program plan and implementation.

Enhancing Cultural Competence

Program managers can enhance cultural sensitivity, cultural awareness, and cultural competencies through several strategies besides hiring consultants or sending staff for cultural competency training. Cox (2001) stressed that to have a diverse, friendly organization, workplace, or program requires making systemwide changes, from hiring policies to the physical structure of the workplace, that are aligned with valuing and respecting the diversity of personnel. For example, before making plans for organizational system changes, an organizational or program self-assessment of cultural competence is warranted. Although various assessment tools have been used in research

(Dana, 1998), the National Center for Cultural Competence (Cohen & Goode, 1999) developed a checklist (Exhibit 2.6) for use by program planners, as well as by other individuals who have roles in shaping policy at the federal, state, or local levels. Use of the checklist can help determine which areas are in need of attention (Goode, Jones, & Mason, 2002) in order to enhance the cultural competence of staff and the program as a whole.

Enhancing the cultural competence of health professionals begins during professional training. For example, Katz, Conant, and Inui (2000), in a program to teach medical residents on a geriatric rotation, described the process used to build a dialogic relationship among participants from different generational

---

Exhibit 2.6   Checklist to Facilitate Development of Culturally and Linguistically Competent Primary Health Care Policies and Structures

Does the health care organization, primary health care system, or program have:

❏ A mission statement that articulates its principles, rationale, and values for culturally and linguistically competent health care service delivery?

❏ Policies and procedures that support a practice model that incorporates culture into the delivery of services to racially, ethnically, culturally, and linguistically diverse groups?

❏ Structures to assure consumer and community participation in the planning, delivery, and evaluation of its services?

❏ Processes to review policy and procedures systematically to assess their relevance for the delivery of culturally competent services?

❏ Policies and procedures for staff recruitment, hiring, and retention that will achieve the goal of a diverse and culturally competent workforce?

❏ Policies and resources to support ongoing professional development and in-service training (at all levels) for culturally competent health care values, principles, and practices?

❏ Policies to assure that new staff are provided with training, technical assistance, and other supports necessary to work within culturally and linguistically diverse communities?

❏ Position descriptions and personnel performance measures that include skill sets related to cultural competence?

❏ Fiscal support and incentives for the improvement of cultural competence at the board, agency, program, and staff levels?

❏ Methods to identify and acquire knowledge about health beliefs and practices of emergent or new populations in service delivery areas?

❏ Policies and allocated resources for the provision of translation and interpretation services?

❏ Requirements for contracting procedures, announcement of funding resources, and/or development of requests for proposals that include culturally and linguistically competent practices?

❏ Policies for and procedures to review periodically the current and emergent demographic trends for the geographic area it serves?

❏ Policies and resources that support community outreach initiatives for limited English proficient and/or nonliterate populations?

Source: Cohen and Goode (1999).

---

cultures, as well as among lay and medical cultures. They learned that a special kind of listening was required that included a high degree of paying attention to the speaker. Their findings suggest that specific efforts and skills are required to overcome the cultural differences between professionals and lay individuals.

One strategy to use with individual program staff is to make it acceptable to ask questions about cultural beliefs and practices and norms so that they can acquire the information necessary to become more culturally competent. Program staff need to be able to express their comfort, as well as discomfort, with other cultures, as a step toward receiving whatever information or counseling is needed to overcome the discomfort. Out of respect, cultural labels ought to be avoided, using instead objective descriptors or names of individuals. Not all staff will be equally accepting and competent with all other cultures, depending upon their cultural background. Some cultures are more accepting and seeking of new experiences than others. Being alert to cultural differences within program staff is an important step toward developing and assuring organizational and program cultural competence. Ignoring the difficulties inherent in having diversity can lead to further problems; therefore, the challenges inherent in moving an organization, a program, or an individual toward cultural competence need to be acknowledged and addressed in a forthright yet sensitive manner.

Another strategy for enhancing the cultural competence of staff is to make diversity visible. This might include displaying posters or cultural artifacts. It may also include having professional journals with a health and culture focus available to staff, such as *American Indian Culture and Research Journal*, *Ethnicity and Disease*, *International Journal of Intercultural Relations*, *Journal of Black Psychology*, *Journal of Cross Cultural Psychology*, *Journal of Health Care for the Poor and Underserved*, and *Journal of Multicultural Counseling and Development*. Making diversity visible in the workplace becomes a symbol that reflects the organizational culture of valuing and respecting cultural diversity.

Fong and Gibbs (1995) acknowledged three factors that influence the process of increasing the cultural competence of staff: limits on staffing patterns, fit between staff and the organization, and barriers to organizational change. The staffing pattern includes having coverage so that there is enough time for staff to receive the education necessary to increase cultural competency. Staffing also includes having a diverse workforce as a venue for staff to learn from each culture. Individual staff beliefs, values, and goals need to be congruent with those of the organization. Fit is an appropriate criterion for hiring decisions (Bowen, Leadford, & Nathin, 1991; Cable & Judge, 1997). Taking these and similar actions to become a culturally competent organization and program may involve fundamental changes for the organization or program. And naturally, there will be barriers to making changes that address cultural issues.

Fong and Gibbs suggested that a key strategy to overcoming these barriers is developing shared goals for staff. In other words, the program staff must believe in achieving cultural competence for all program staff, not just themselves or other staff. Lientz and Rea (2002) offered realistic suggestions for addressing cultural issues in the workplace. They recommended avoiding open conflicts over cultural issues, especially since there is no one right way. They also recommended working through informal communication channels when cultural issues need to be addressed or to achieve changes in organizational culture. Another realistic suggestion is for managers to focus on reinforcing new behaviors that promote cultural competence and sensitivity. Finally, acknowledging that individuals have personalities, it may be best in some situations to rotate staff to other work units or programs. The positive aspect of this last suggestion is a recognition that when a fit between the program and staff does not exist; both parties may benefit from a change in the relationship.

Stakeholders and Coalitions

An additional, key approach to achieving requisite variety is through the inclusion of diverse stakeholders in the process of planning and evaluating the health program, which is often done through the development of coalitions. Several federal agencies, such as the Office of Minority Health and the Centers for Disease Control and Prevention (CDC), and private foundations, such as the W. K. Kellogg Foundation and the Robert Wood Johnson Foundation, have funding priorities related to health disparities that require programs to engage in coalition development, often in the form of community engagement. The emphasis on developing coalitions parallels the emphasis on health disparities and diversity. Coalitions, partnerships, alliances, consortia, and collaborative linkages are some of the structural forms that result when stakeholders, interested parties, members of the target audience, and professionals with expertise agree to work together toward the common goals of community and health improvements for common constituents. The term "coalition" is used as the umbrella term for such agreements.

Coalitions, in whatever form, can be viewed as potentially having power and being power brokers (Braithwaite, Taylor, & Austin, 2000). Underlying the emphasis on coalition initiatives is a belief that collaboration among stakeholders is key to effective community development and to decreasing health disparities (Braithwaite et al., 2000). Coalitions for health programs may be developed for various reasons. One is to create a power base from which to gain attention for the health problem or resources to address the problem. Coalitions also are established as a means toward sustainability of the health program, which requires that they be successful. Coalitions are more likely to be successful if they include stable, established organizations and not just ad hoc, newly formed groups. Program sustainability through coalitions often is accomplished by empowering individuals and organizational members of the coalition to contribute to the continued addressing of the health disparities.

The process of forming a coalition follows commonsense, deceptively simple steps. At the core of a coalition is attention to group process, as the following steps and suggestions show. The initial step in forming a coalition is to identify potential coalition members who are either individual stakeholders or representatives of organizations with a potential stake in the health care program. Naturally, the potential members ought to reflect the diversity being addressed by the health program. An early step is the task of articulating the common goal for the coalition. Coalitions are more likely to succeed if they have a defined goal with specific tasks that can be realistically accomplished with minimal expense. As coalition members change, funding priorities change, leadership changes, and time passes, the goal for which the coalition was established will need to be reiterated as a sounding board for decisions and directions. Early in the formation of the coalition, it will be essential to build credibility and trust. These take time to build, are tested, and are extremely difficult to recover if lost. The credibility and trustworthiness of the organizers are especially important when working with culturally and ethnically diverse groups that have had negative experiences with coalitions or health programs in the past.

Rose (2000) suggested two strategies for building relationships in the coalition. One is to adopt issues of the coalition members as issues for the coalition. This would be feasible when issues overlap—say, housing afford-ability and health programs for the homeless. The other strategy is to promote honest dialogue, in which members can be frank without feeling threatened by retribution for ideas. Complementing this strategy is adopting the policy of "agree to disagree." This ground rule for interactions tends to foster coopera-tion as well as trust. Rose reminds us that humor is a very effective tool for unifying members and for relieving tensions. It is always healthy to laugh at situations, to find the bright side, and to be amused. This transcends cultures, despite cultural differences in what makes something humorous.

Throughout the process of forming and working with a coalition, attention to cultural competency is crucial. One aspect of being culturally competent involves conducting a self-assessment that assesses the values and principles that govern participation in coalitions. The National Center for Cultural Com-petence developed a checklist that can be used to assess cultural competence in community engagement (Exhibit 2.7) (Goode, 2001). The health program

---

Exhibit 2.7   Checklist to Facilitate Cultural Competence in Community Engagement

Does the health care organization, primary health care system, or program have:

❑ A mission that values communities as essential allies in achieving its overall goals?

❑ A policy and structures that delineate community and consumer participation in planning, implementing, and evaluating the delivery of services and supports?

❑ A policy that facilitates employment and the exchange of goods and services from local communities?

❑ A policy and structures that provide a mechanism for the provision of fiscal resources and in-kind contributions to community partners, agencies, or organizations?

❑ A position description and personnel performance measures that include areas of knowledge and skill sets related to community engagement?

❏ A policy, structure, and resources for in-service training, continuing education, and professional development that increase capacity for collaboration
and partnerships within culturally and linguistically diverse communities?

❏ A policy that supports the use of diverse communication modalities and technologies for sharing information with communities?

❏ A policy and structures to periodically review current and emergent demographic trends to:

Identify new collaborators and potential opportunities for community engagement?

Determine whether community partners are representative of the diverse population in the geographic or service area?

❏ A policy, structures, and resources to support community engagement in languages other than English?

Source: Goode (2001).

---

planners could use this tool as a means of gauging the cultural competence of
the health program to engage the community in health program development.

ACROSS THE PYRAMID

At the direct services level of the public health pyramid, disparities are
seen as affecting individuals and their health status. As individuals from
diverse cultures, ethnicities, races, and SES backgrounds interact with
health professionals and the health program staff, the training in cultural
sensitivity and competence is put into practice. If the professionals and staff
have not received or integrated this knowledge into their practice, the potential for continued health care disparities is present. In addition, health
programs designed for the direct services level of the pyramid will need to
verify that the interventions being used in the program match the culture,
language, and norms of the program recipients. It may also be necessary for
the health program to be designed so that the intervention can be culturally,
ethnically, and linguistically tailored "on the spot" to those participating
in the program at the moment. In terms of measurement considerations at
this level of the pyramid, the direct interaction with program participants
allows for needs assessment, program process, and program effect data to
be collected from individuals, either through quantitative questionnaires or
qualitative interviews.

At the enabling services level of the pyramid, disparities are seen as they affect aggregates and families. Diversity is manifested in subcultures or enclave ethnicity, as well as in the larger cultural context. The interpersonal interaction between the program staff and the program recipients continues to be an essential element of services at this level. Therefore, the cultural competency of individual program staff also continues to be important as they put into practice the program interventions. The interventions provided as enabling services will need to be tailored to the specific sociocultural characteristics and preferences of the target aggregate. For example, an existing enabling service may be in the process of being planned for a new target audience. This would result in fairly specific changes, modifications, or additions to the existing program in order to make it culturally and linguistically acceptable to the new target audience. In terms of measurement, data are likely to be collected from individuals, allowing for tailoring the data collection to the characteristics of the aggregate.

At the population-based services level of the pyramid, disparities within a population are revealed through the data about that population, such as vital statistics and health care utilization. For all practical purposes, disparities are most easily identified by examining differences within a population, although they can also be identified within large aggregates, such as schools. Because health programs designed for the population level of the pyramid are delivered or provided to the population, interpersonal interaction between program staff and program recipients will vary from minimal, as with an immunization campaign, to none, as with a media campaign. Thus, issues of cultural competence for program staff are lessened. However, the need for the intervention to reflect cultural competence remains. Health programs targeted at populations will face the challenge of deciding whether to make the program generically acceptable for most members of the population or whether the intervention needs to have different versions tailored to known culturally distinct subpopulations or aggregates. This challenge, while similar to the need for flexibility in direct services programs, is complicated by the inability to tailor the intervention during a program encounter. Finally, with regard to measurement, most data collected will be on such a scale that simple, generic data collection methods will be needed. This will result in having data with less detail but on more program recipients. Unlike programs at the direct services or enabling services levels, a population-based program may not be able to gather data on actual program recipients. This fact of population-level programs creates a situation in which program planners may need to work more closely with the organizations and agencies responsible for collecting population-level data to ensure that the measures being used are as relevant to the program as possible.

At the infrastructure level, personnel diversity, organizational culture, and program culture play a role in program planning and delivery. Overall, diversity and disparities are visible through their effects on existing and new health policy and priorities, and on organizational processes and culture. Interpersonal interactions among program planners, staff, stakeholders, and policy makers are the focus of efforts to address health disparities and cultural issues. Programs at the infrastructure level are aimed at changing the cultural competence of the workforce and the capacity of the workforce to address health disparities and cultural diversity. As with programs for the other levels of the pyramid, the interventions need to be tailored to the sociocultural characteristics of the target audience within the infrastructure. The addition is that interventions also need to address the professional diversity that exists within the infrastructure, health care organizations or agencies, as well as within the health care system as a whole. With regard to measurement, the availability of individual versus aggregate data will depend on the nature of the health program. Health programs provided to groups of workers, such as cultural competency training, make it possible to measure specific attributes of program participants. Health program interventions designed to change health policy are not amenable to direct data collection but would rely on population-level data, especially for program effects.

One other infrastructure issue that warrants mentioning is the legal implications of diversity. For example, the Americans with Disabilities Act of 1990 means that planning for programs must take into account issues of accessibility for disabled persons. Another legal issue is antidiscrimination laws, which affect both the management of program personnel and the process by which program participants are recruited and accepted into the health program. There are also state laws and local ordinances regarding same-sex marriage; these may affect reimbursement for programs, responses to survey questions about marriage, and recruitment of family members into programs. These are all factors that influence the planning and evaluation of the health program and that therefore fall within the infrastructure level.

DISCUSSION QUESTIONS

1. Discuss the ways in which linguistic diversity within a target audience would affect programs being planned at each level of the pyramid.

2. Think of a specific health program provided by a specific health care organization with which you are familiar. Complete either of the cultural competency self-assessments included in the chapter (Exhibits 2.6 and 2.7). What surprised you about taking the self-assessment? What recommendations would you make based on the results of the assessment?

3. Identify one health-related questionnaire that has been used with more than one cultural or linguistic group. Discuss the adequacy of the linguistic and conceptual translations of the questionnaire.

4. List four health programs in your community. Do they have coalitions? What is the composition of each coalition? Does there appear to be a relationship between coalition diversity and health program success?

References

Airhihenbuwa, C. O. (1994). Health promotion and the discourse on culture: Implications for empowerment. *Health Education Quarterly, 21*, 345–353.

Akinbami, L. J., LaFleur, B. J., & Schoendorf, K. C. (2002). Racial and income disparities in children with asthma in the United States. *Ambulatory Pediatrics, 2*, 382–387.

Anderson, R. (2002). Deaths: Leading causes for 2000. *National Vital Statistics Report, 50*(16).

Bhopal, R., & Donaldson, L. (1998). White, European, Western, Caucasian, or what? Inappropriate labeling in research on race, ethnicity, and health. *American Journal of Public Health, 88*, 1303–1307.

Boekaerts, M. (1998). Do culturally rooted self-construals affect students' conceptualization of control over learning? *Educational Psychologist, 33*(2/3), 88–108.

Bowen, D. E., Leadford, G. E., & Nathin, B. R. (1991). Hiring for the organization, not the job. *Academy of Management Executive, 5*(4), 35–51.

Braithwaite, R. L., Taylor, S. E., & Austin, J. N. (2000). *Building health coalitions in the Black community*. Thousand Oaks, CA: Sage Publications.

Bureau of Primary Health Care. (2003). *Cultural competence. http://www.bphc.hrsa.gov/culturalcompetence/default.hm* (accessed 7/23/03).

Cable, D. M., & Judge, T. A. (1997). Interviewers' perceptions of person-organization fit and organizational selection. *Journal of Applied Psychology, 82*, 546–561.

Carragee, E. J., Vittum, D., Truong, T. P., & Burton, D. (1999). Pain control and cultural norms and expectations after closed femoral shaft fractures. *American Journal of Orthopedics, 28*, 97–102.

Cohen, E. & Goode, T. (1999). Policy brief 1: Rationale for cultural competence in primary health care. Washington, DC: National Center for Cultural Competence, Georgetown University Child Development Center. *http://www.georgetown.edu/research/gucdc/nccc/nccc6.html* (accessed 7/29/03).

Cox, T. (1991). The multicultural organization. *Academy of Management Executive, 5*(2), 34–47.

Cox, T. (2001). *Creating the multicultural organization*. San Francisco: Jossey-Bass.

Cross, T. L., Bazron, B. J., Dennis, K. W., & Isaacs, M. R. (1989). *Toward a culturally competent system of care*. Washington, DC: National Center for Cultural Competence, Georgetown University Child Development Center.

Dana, R. H. (1998). Cultural competence in three human service agencies. *Psychological Reports, 83,* 107–112.

Day, J. C. (1996). *Current population reports: Population projections of the United States by age, sex, race, and Hispanic origin: 1995-2050.* US Census Bureau. *http://www.census.gov/prod/1/pop/p25-1130/p251130.pdf* (accessed 8/27/03).

Deal, T. E., & Kennedy, A. A. (1982). *Corporate cultures: The rites and rituals of corporate life.* Reading, MA: Addison-Wesley.

Department of Justice. (1999). *Annual report: Legal immigration, fiscal year 1998.* Number 2. Washington, DC: Department of Justice, Office of Policy and Planning, Statistics Branch.

Ferketich, S., Phillips, L., & Verran, J. (1993). Development and administration of a survey instrument for cross-cultural research. *Research in Nursing and Health, 16,* 227–230.

Fong, L. G., & Gibbs, J. T. (1995). Facilitating services to multicultural communities in a dominant culture setting: An organizational perspective. *Administration in Social Work, 19* (2), 1–24.

Ford, E. S., & Cooper, R. S. (1995). Racial/ethnic differences in health care utilization of cardiovascular procedures: A review of the evidence. *Health Services Research, 30*(1 pt. 2), 237–252.

Gager, P. J., & Elias, M. J. (1997). Implementing prevention programs in high risk environments: Application of the resiliency paradigm. *American Journal of Orthopsychiatry, 67,* 363–373.

Goode, T. (2001). *Policy brief 4: Engaging communities to realize the vision of one hundred percent access and zero health disparities: A culturally competent approach.* Washington, DC: National Center for Cultural Competence, Georgetown University Child Development Center.

Goode, T., Jones, W., & Mason, J. (2002). *A guide to planning and implementing cultural competence organization self-assessment.* Washington, DC: National Center for Cultural Competence, Georgetown University Child Development Center.

Guranaccia, P., & Rogler, L. H. (1999). Research on culture-bound syndromes: New directions. *The American Journal of Psychiatry, 156,* 1322–1327.

Higginson, J. G. (1998). Competitive parenting: The culture of teen mothers. *Journal of Marriage and the Family, 60,* 135–149.

Hoskins, M. L. (1999). Worlds apart and lives together: Developing cultural attunement. *Child and Youth Care Forum, 28,* 73–84.

Katz, A. M., Conant, L., & Inui, T. S. (2000). A council of elders: Creating a multi-voiced dialogue in a community of care. *Social Science and Medicine, 50,* 851–860.

Khoury, M. J. (2003). Genetics and genomics in practice: The continuum from genetic disease to genetic information in health and disease. *Genetics in Medicine, 5,* 261–268.

Kim, S., McLeod, J. H., & Shantzis, C. (1992). Cultural competence for evaluators working with Asian-American communities: Some practical considerations. In M. A. Orlandi, R. Weston, & L. G. Epstein, (Eds.), *Cultural competence for evaluators: A guide for alcohol and other drug abuse prevention practitioners working with ethical/racial communities* (pp. 203–260). (DHHS Publication No. (ADM) 92–1884). Washington, DC: US Government Printing Office.

Kleinman, A. (1980). *Patients and healers in the context of culture.* Berkeley, CA: University of California Press.

Kohn, A., & Bryan, K. (1998). Ritual practice in a social model recovery home. *Contemporary Drug Problems, 25,* 711–739.

Kosa, J., & Zola, I. K. (1975). *Poverty and health: A sociological analysis* (Rev. ed.). Cambridge, MA: Harvard University Press.

Legge, C., & Sherlock, L. (1991). Perceptions of alcohol use and misuse in three ethnic communities: Implications for prevention programming. *International Journal of Addictions, 25*, 629–653.

Lew, R., Chau, J., Woo, J. M., Nguyen, K. D., Okahara, L., Min, K. J., & Lee, D. (1999). Annual walkathons as a community education strategy for the Asian American/Pacific Islander populations in Alameda County, California. *Journal of Health Education, 30*, 25–30.

Lientz, B. P., & Rea, K. P. (2002). *Project management for the 21st century* (3rd ed.). San Diego, CA: Academic Press.

Lin, S. S., & Kelsey, J. L. (2000). Use of race and ethnicity in epidemiologic research: Concepts, methodological issues, and suggestions for research. *Epidemiology Review, 22*, 187–202.

MacDorman, M. F., Minion, A. M, Strobino, D. M., & Guyer, B. (2002). Annual summary of vital statistics: 2001. *Pediatrics, 110*, 1037–1052.

Mallak, L. (2001). Understanding and changing your organization's culture. *Industrial Management, 43*(2), 18–24.

Martin, J. A., Hamilton, B. E., Ventura, S. J, Menacker, F., & Park, M. M. (2002). Births: Final data for 2002. *National Vital Statistics Report, 50*(5).

Mathews, D. A., McCullough, M. E., Larson, D. B., Koenig, H. G., Swyers, J. P., & Milano, M. G. (1998). Religious commitment and health status: A review of the research and implications for family medicine. *Archives of Family Medicine, 72*, 118–124.

McKenny, N. R., & Bennett, C. E. (1994). Issues regarding data on race and ethnicity: The Census Bureau experience. *Public Health Reports, 109*(1), 16–25.

National Cancer Institute. (2003). *Breast: U.S. racial/ethnic cancer patterns.* http://www.nci.nih.gov/statistics/cancertype/breast-racial-ethni (accessed 7/29/03).

National Diabetes Information Clearinghouse. (2003). *National Diabetes Statistics.* http://diabetes.niddk.nih.gov/dm/pubs/statistics/index.htm (accessed 7/29/03).

Navarro, J., Wilson, S., Berger, L. R., & Taylor, T. (1997). Substance abuse and spirituality: A program for Native American students. *American Journal of Health Behavior, 21*, 3–11.

Nickens, H. W. (1995). The role of race/ethnicity and social class in minority health status. *Health Services Research, 30* (1 pt. 2), 151–162.

Orlandi, M. A. (1992). Defining cultural competence: An organizing framework. In M.A. Orlandi, R. Weston, & L. G. Epstein (Eds.), *Cultural competence for evaluators: A guide for alcohol and other drug abuse prevention practitioners working with ethical/racial communities* (pp. 293–299). (DHHS Publication. No. (ADM) 92–1884). Washington, DC: US Government Printing Office.

Polednak, A. P. (1997). *Segregation, poverty, and mortality in urban African-Americans.* Oxford: Oxford University Press.

Rose, F. (2000). *Coalitions across the class divide: Lessons from the labor, peace and environmental movements.* Ithaca, NY: Cornell University Press.

Rossiter, J. C. (1994). The effect of a culture-specific education program to promote breast-feeding among Vietnamese women in Sydney. *International Journal of Nursing Studies, 31*, 369–379.

Rotheram-Borus, M. J. (2000). Variations in perceived pain associated with emotional distress and social identity in AIDS. *AIDS Patient Care and Standards, 14*, 659–665.

Sabbioni, M. E., & Eugster, S. (2001). Interactions of a history of migration with the course of pain disorder. *Journal of Psychosomatic Research, 50*, 267–269.

Schein, V. E. (1995). *Working from the margins: Voices of mothers in poverty.* Ithaca, NY: ILR Press, Cornell University Press.

Schulman, K. A., Rubenstein, L. E., Chesley, F. D., & Eisenberg, J. M. (1995). The roles of race and socioeconomic factors in health services research. *Health Services Research, 30*(1 pt. 2), 179–195.

Scott, T., Mannion, R., Davies, H., & Marshall, M. (2003). The quantitative measurement of organizational culture in health care: A review of the available instruments. *Health Services Research, 38*, 923–945.

Shakoor-Abdullah, B., Kotchen, J. M., Walker, W. E., Chelius, T. H., & Hoffman, R. G. (1997). Incorporating socio-economic and risk factor diversity into the development of an African-American community blood pressure control program. *Ethnicity and Disease, 7*, 175–183.

Smedley, B. D., Stith, A. Y., & Nelson, A. R. (2002). *Unequal treatment: Confronting racial and ethnic disparities in health care.* Washington, DC: National Academy Press.

Smith, C. S., Francovich, C. G., & Gieselman, J. (2000). Pilot test of an organizational culture model in a medical setting. *Health Care Manager, 19*, 68–77.

Spector, R. E. (1991). *Cultural diversity in health and illness* (3rd ed.). Norwalk, CT: Appleton & Lang.

Spratley, E., Johnson, A., Sochalski, J., Fritz, M., & Spence, W. (2000). *The registered nurse population: Findings from the National Sample Survey of Registered Nurses.* United States Department of Health and Human Services, Health Resources and Services Administration, Bureau of Health Profession, Division of Nursing. *http://ftp.hrsa.gov/bhpr/rnsurvey2000/rnsurvey00-1.pfd* (accessed 7/28/03).

Sue, S. (1998). In search of cultural competence in psychotherapy and counseling. *American Psychologist, 53*, 440–448.

Trofino, J., Hughes, C. B., O'Brien, B. L., Mack, J., Marrinan, M. A., & Hay, K. M. (2000). Primary care parish nursing: Academic, service and parish partnership. *Nursing Administration Quarterly, 25*, 59–74.

Weick, K. (1979). *Social psychology of organizing* (2nd ed). Reading, MA: Addison-Wesley.

Williams, D. R. (1996). Race/ethnicity and socioeconomic status: Measurement and methodological issues. *International Journal of Health Services, 26*, 483–505.

CHAPTER 3

Planning for Health Programs and Services

Planning is one of those undertakings that everyone thinks they can do. The reality is that planning is not a single task, and it can be time-intensive to do well. It is also one of those words that has a plethora of implicit meanings. Exploring the meaning and delineating the process of planning have a substantial history in public health. The pioneers of public health planning were primarily concerned with planning at the systems level—that is, with planning as it relates to the infrastructure of the health care or public health system. Planning with this more global or national focus is different from planning for more discrete and specific health programs at a local level. Nonetheless, many of the concerns and processes used in planning for the health system are applicable and adaptable to planning of local health programs.

Tension will always exist between planning on a local level—say, within one small community organization or one county—and planning at a global level, such as through national health policy or the World Health Organization. At a minimum, local planning for health programs ought to be done with an awareness of the priorities and programs established through global and national planning. In addition, the local planning process for developing health programs can be enhanced by adapting the processes used at the systems level.

The purpose of this chapter is to draw upon and adapt approaches developed for systems for use in local program planning. To this end, it identifies tools and techniques currently used in planning public health programs or projects. The focus here is not on the type of strategic planning done by health care organizations or agencies; rather, it is on tactical planning, which is the set of planning activities done to implement a broader, more global strategy. Tactical planning is more time-limited, is focused on meeting current needs and demands, incorporates current scientific knowledge in identifying viable and feasible alternatives, and progresses in stages from problem definition to implementation. Although planning is generally described as a linear process, program planning is a cyclical activity, with recursive events requiring additional or refreshed courses of action for the life of a health program.

DEFINITIONS OF PLANNING

Blum (1974) defined planning as "the deliberate introduction of desired social change in orderly and acceptable ways." Nutt (1984) identified several ways in which planning is visible: as forecasting, as problem solving, as programming, as design, as policy analysis, and as a response to a problem. He concluded that planning involves synthesis in terms of putting together plans, policy, programs, or something else that is new. In this regard he viewed planning as creating change. Hoch (1994) described good planning as the popular adoption of democratic reforms in the provision of public goods. Others have viewed planning as the effort to control social or collective uncertainty by taking action now to secure the future (Marris, 1982 cited in Hoch, 1994). These definitions have the elements of using a rational approach, making change, and using a democratic or participatory process. In terms of programs, planning is the set of activities in which key individuals define a set of desired improvements, develop a strategy to achieve those desired improvements, and establish a means to measure the attainment of those desired improvements.

HISTORICAL BACKGROUND ON PLANNING IN PUBLIC HEALTH

The planning of programs to address health problems essentially began as public health planning. The history of public health planning began in antiquity with the environmental planning of water and sewer systems in cities in the West (Rosen, 1958) and civic planning in the East (Duhl, 2000). These early forms of planning for the health and well-being of populations were not dramatically changed until the late 20th century.

Population-based planning became necessary with the advent of immunizations, including the administration of the first polio vaccine. In public health, Henrik Blum (1974) was one of several scholars to consider what public health planning is and how it ought to be done. He advocated the use of a rational approach to health planning, which included considering the problem and systematically applying a solution. The rational approach to health planning was further developed in Dever's textbook (1980), which extensively applied epidemiological techniques to the identification and prioritization of health problems.

Following more in the civic planning tradition, Duhl (1987) advocated for health planning from a social awareness perspective. Duhl was building upon the work of LaLonde (1974), who is recognized as being the first public health scholar to articulate and emphasize the interaction of social conditions and well-being. The LaLonde report had a broad range of effects, including influencing Duhl to emphasize the involvement of community members in the betterment of their lives and environment. Duhl has continued to highlight the inseparable relationship between planning from a social framework and health.

During this period, considerable work was also being done in the organizational behavioral sciences on the issue of decision making and development of business strategies. This knowledge was transferred into health care through scholars such as Nutt (1979), who developed a model of the planning process that included stages and elements that were interactive and iterative. His model included not only activities but the central notion that a problem is real and that awareness of the problem is the stimulus of the planning activities. Nutt's textbook (1984) expanded on the model for organizational planning and focused on planning as done by health care organizations. Today, his work would be considered organizational strategic planning. The extent to which organizational strategic planning has influenced planning for population health and health programs is reflected in Dever's later textbook (1997), which drew more heavily on the strategic and organizational knowledge about planning.

These academic advances in health program planning have been paralleled by practitioner-focused advances. Beginning in the mid-1980s the Centers for Disease Control and Prevention (CDC) began to develop and promote methodologies for systematic approaches to health planning for those working in public health. These models are important for their structured approach to planning health programs and for synthesizing the knowledge available at the time about health and program planning.

PATCH

The Planning Approach to Community Health (PATCH) model was based on Green's PRECEDE (Predisposing, Reinforcing, and Enabling Factors in Community Education Development and Evaluation) model of health education planning (Green, Kreuter, Deeds, & Partridge, 1980). Built into the PATCH model of planning for public health was the notion that health promotion is a process that enables people to be more in control of their health and of ways to improve their health (CDC PATCH, n.d.). The PATCH model incorporated information on each of several elements viewed as essential to the success of planning public health programs. One element was community participation in the process. Other elements were the use of data to drive the development of health and a comprehensive health promotion strategy. The PATCH model also included the element of evaluation for program improvement and had as a long-term goal increasing community capacity for health promotion. These elements were to be achieved through steps outlined in the PATCH model: mobilize the community, collect data, choose health priorities, develop a comprehensive intervention plan, and evaluate the process. Although the CDC no longer provides training on using PATCH, PATCH materials are available online through the CDC website (CDC PATCH, n.d.). PATCH was implemented as the first national attempt to standardize public health planning and to provide technical assistance to local health agencies.

APEXPH

Subsequently, the CDC, in cooperation with the National Association of City and County Health Officers (NACCHO), developed and introduced the Assessment Protocol for Excellence in Public Health (APEXPH). Although development of the APEXPH began in 1987, the manual for using the APEXPH approach was not released until 1999 (CDC PATCH, n.d.). A key feature of the APEXPH approach is its addressing of the three core competencies of public health: assessment, assurance, and policy development. These core competencies were articulated in the Institute of Medicine's (1988) report on the future of public health and have since become pivotal in thinking about assuring the health of populations.

APEXPH differs from PATCH in that it provides a framework to assess the organization and management of health departments, as well as a framework for working with community members in assessing the health of the community. The APEXPH workbook, available through the NACCHO website (National Association of City and County Health Officers [NACCHO], 2000), outlines planning in three parts: assessing internal organizational capacity, assessing and setting priorities for community health problems, and implementing the plans. In one study, 24 county health departments in Washington State used the APEXPH to assess their strengths and weaknesses in each of these functional areas (Pratt, McDonald, Libby, Oberle, & Liang, 1996). The results could then be used to identify specific areas that needed strengthening. To the extent that the APEXPH addresses organizational capacity, it draws upon the strategic planning perspective of Nutt (1984) and others.

MAPP

More recently, the CDC and NACCHO have released the MAPP (Mobilizing for Action through Planning and Partnership). MAPP is a strategic planning tool that helps public health leaders facilitate community prioritization of public health issues and identify resources for addressing them. The first phase of MAPP is to mobilize community members and organizations under the leadership of public health agencies. The second phase is to generate a shared vision and common values that provide a framework for long-range planning. The third step of MAPP involves conducting four assessments of four areas: community strengths, the local public health system, community health status, and the forces of change. The final step is implementation. MAPP materials can be ordered from the MAPP website, which can be accessed through the NACCHO website (NACCHO, n.d.).

SUMMARY

This brief overview of the models that have been used in planning public health programs highlights the ongoing evolution of thinking in this area. Evident in this evolution is the development of tools for designing health promotion programs, particularly those focused at the community or population level. Although the materials are targeted to public health agencies and leaders, the content of the materials and the underlying philosophical perspectives are applicable to other types of health agencies that provide health programs to individuals or populations.

Triggering the Cycle

Common across the planning models that have been developed is the inclusion of various feedback loops among planning processes, implementation, evaluation, and the problem. The feedback loops create a cycle (Exhibit 3.1). One mechanism that initiates the cycle occurs when an influential individual's attention is caught. A wide variety of factors act as the attention-getting event. New opportunities can stimulate planning for a health program, such as a grant announcement or the hiring of an enthusiastic, motivated, and knowledgeable employee who is passionate about a particular health problem. The trigger event might also be a mandated process, such as a five-year strategic planning process or a grant renewal, or it might be a less positive event, such as a news media exposé or local activism. For those seeking to initiate the planning process, getting the attention of influential individuals requires having access to them, packaging the message about the need for planning in ways that are immediately attractive, and demonstrating the salience of the issue. Thus, to get a specific health problem or issue "on the table," activists can use the salient events to get the attention of influential individuals. Although this may seem obvious, it is also a reminder that key individuals mentally sort and choose among competing attention getters.

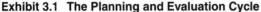

Exhibit 3.1   The Planning and Evaluation Cycle

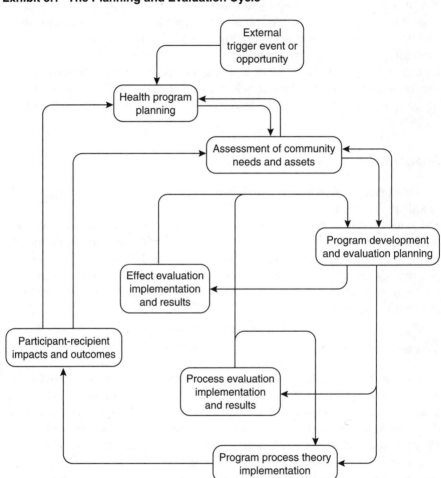

As shown in Exhibit 3.1, there are also arrows from the results of process and effect evaluations to program development. In other words, the indirect trigger for planning could be information generated from an evaluation that reveals either the failure of a health program, extraordinary success, or the need for additional programs. Although information on developing and evaluating health programs is presented in other publications, the reality is that possible feedback paths throughout the cycle make the whole process far more iterative and fluid than can be adequately portrayed in a textbook.

Once the cycle has been triggered, the early stage of planning centers on how to progress from awareness of a need or opportunity to a formal assessment and program plan. During this formative stage, thinking about developing a program often generates a disorganized set of meetings and activities that eventually fall into a more organized pattern. One reason that the early planning stage is disorganized is that several paradoxes and assumptions about planning are revealed and must be addressed, or at least acknowledged.

PLANNING PARADOXES, ASSUMPTIONS, AND ETHICS

Several paradoxes pervade health planning (Reinke & Hall, 1988), which may or may not be resolvable. Individuals involved also hold assumptions about planning that complicate the act of planning, whether for health systems or programs. Being aware of the paradoxes and assumptions can, however, help program planners understand possible sources of frustration.

Paradoxes

One paradox is that planning is shaped by the same forces that created the problems planning is supposed to correct. The health care, sociopolitical, and cultural factors that contributed to the health problem or condition are very likely to be the same factors that affect the health planning process. In other words, the intertwined relationship of health and other aspects of life affects health planning. How can health be planned if the planning, particularly for public concerns, is limited to what occurs within the health care sector? For example, given that housing, employment, and social justice affect health, then health planning is automatically flawed to the extent that the context within which individuals live is not acknowledged or addressed in the health planning.

Another paradox is that the "good" of individuals and society experiencing the prosperity associated with health and well-being is "bad" to the extent that prosperity produces ill health. Prosperity has its own associated health risks, such as higher cholesterol levels, increased stress, increased cardiovascular diseases, and increases in environmental pollutants. Also, as one group prospers, other groups become disproportionately worse off. So, to the extent that health program planning contributes to the prosperity of a society or a group of individuals, other health issues will arise that will require health program planning.

A third paradox is that what may be easier and more effective may be less acceptable. A good example of this stems from decisions about active and passive protective interventions. Active and passive protection are two approaches to risk reduction and health promotion. Active protection requires that individuals actively participate in reducing their risks—for, example, through diet changes or the use of motorcycle helmets. Passive protection occurs when individuals are protected by virtue of some factor other than their behavior—for example, water fluoridation and smoke-free workplaces. For many health programs, passive protection in the form of health policy or health regulations may be more effective and efficient. However, ethical and political issues can arise when an emphasis on passive protection, through laws and communitywide mandates, does not take into account cultural trends or preferences.

Another paradox is that planning health programs ideally is triggered by those in need, not the health professionals. This paradox addresses the issue of who knows best and has the best ideas for how to resolve the "real" problem. The perspective held by health professionals often does not reflect broader, more common health social values (Reinke & Hall, 1988), including those with the "problem." Because those in need of health programs are most likely to know what will work for them, community and stakeholder participation become not only crucial but, in many instances, mandated by funding agencies. This paradox also calls into question the role of health professionals in developing health programs. The normative perspective and scientific knowledge need to be weighed against individual choice that may have caused the health problem. A corollary to the paradox of where the best ideas come from is that politicians prefer cures that are immediate and permanent, whereas health planners prefer prevention that is long-term, strategic, and less visible (Reinke & Hall, 1988). Generally, people want to be cured of existing problems, rather than to think probabilistically about preventing problems that may or may not occur in the future. Thus, the prevention and long-term solutions that seem obvious to public health practitioners can come into conflict with the solutions identified by those with the "problem."

One possible reason that the best solutions come from those with the problem is that health professionals can be perceived as blaming those with the health problem for their problem. Blum (1982) identified blaming the victim as a threat to effective planning. When a woman who experiences domestic violence is said to be "asking for it," the victim is being blamed. During the planning process, blaming the victim can be implicitly and rather subtly manifested in group settings through interpretation of data about needs and, hence, can affect decisions. Having the attitude that the victim is to blame can also cause conflict and tension among those involved in the planning process, especially if the "victim" is included as a stakeholder. The activities for which the victim is being blamed need to be reframed in terms of the causes of those activities or behaviors.

A fifth paradox is that planning is done to be successful; no one plans in order to fail. Because of the bias throughout the program planning cycle in favor of succeeding, unanticipated consequences may not be investigated or recognized. The unanticipated consequences of one action can lead to the need for other health decisions that were in themselves unintended (Patrick & Erickson, 1993). To overcome this paradox, brainstorming and thinking creatively at key points in the planning process ought to be fostered and appreciated.

Assumptions

Assumptions as well as paradoxes influence the effectiveness of planning. The first and primary assumption underlying all planning processes is that a solution, remedy, or appropriate intervention can be identified or developed and provided. Without this assumption, planning would be pointless. It is fundamentally an optimistic assumption about the capacity of the planners, the stakeholders, and the state of the science to address the health problem.

The assumption of possibilities further presumes that the resources available, whether human or otherwise, are sufficient for the task and are suitable to address the health problem. The assumption of adequate capacity and knowledge is actually tested through the planning process. A companion assumption is that planning leads to the allocation of resources needed to address the health problem. This assumption is challenged by the reality that four groups of stakeholders have interests in the decision making regarding health resources (Sloan & Conover, 1996). One group is those with the health problem, who are members of the target audience for the health program. Another group of stakeholders is health payers, such as insurance companies and local, federal, and philanthropic funding agencies. The third group of stakeholders is individual heath care providers and health care organizations and networks. And finally, the general public is another stakeholder in the issue of how resources are allocated for health programs.

It is natural to assume that those involved in the planning process share an interest in addressing the health problem. However, stakeholders have a variety of motives for being involved in health program planning, such as personal gain, visibility for an organization, or acquisition of resources associated with the program. Other assumptions about those involved is that they have similar views on how to plan health programs. During the planning process, their points of view and cultural perspectives will likely come into contrast. Hoch (1994) suggested that planners need to know what is relevant and important for the problem at hand. Planners can believe in one set of community purposes and values and still recognize the validity and merit of competing purposes. Hoch argued that effective planning requires tolerance, freedom, and fairness and that technical and political values are two bases from which to give planning advice. In other words, stakeholders involved in the planning process need to be guided into appreciating and perhaps applying a variety of perspectives about planning.

Each stakeholder group assumes that there are limited resources to be allocated for addressing the health problem and is receptive or responsive to a different set of strategies for allocating health resources. The resulting conflicts among the stakeholders for the limited resources apply whether they are allocating resources across the health care system or among programs for specific health problems. Limited resources, whether real or not, raise ethical questions of what to do when possible gains from needed health programs or policies are likely to be small, especially when the health program addresses serious health problems.

Interestingly, within the assumption of limited resources is also the paradox that planning occurs around what is limited rather than what is abundant. Rarely is there a discussion of the abundant or unlimited resources available for health planning. Particularly in the United States, there is an amazing abundance of volunteer hours and interest, and of advocacy groups and energy. There is also an abundance of recently retired equipment that may be appropriate in some situations. Such resources, while not glamorous or constituting a substantial amount on a balance sheet, deserve to be acknowledged in the planning process.

Another assumption about the planning process is that it occurs in an orderly fashion and that a rational approach is best. To understand the implications of this assumption, it is important to first acknowledge that there are four key elements inherent in planning: ambiguity, conflict, risk, and control. The presence of each of these elements contradicts the assumption of a rational approach, and each generates its own paradoxes.

Ambiguity, Conflict, Risk, and Control

Despite the orderly approach implied in "planning," it is important to be aware of the limits of both scientific rationality and the usefulness of data to cope with the ambiguities, conflicts, and risks being addressed by the planning process.

Ambiguity is the awareness that known and unknown factors exist that decrease the possibility of certainty. In this sense, ambiguity is a result of uncertainty. Both uncertainty and ambiguity pervade the planning process because it is impossible to know and estimate the effect of all relevant factors, from possible causes of the health problem, to the range of possible health effects from program interventions, to the acts and intentions of individuals.

A rational approach to planning presumes that all relevant factors can be completely accounted for by anticipating the effect of a program. Our experiences as humans tell us otherwise.

Ambiguity is a state that tends to be uncomfortable and undesirable. Change, or the possibility of change, is a likely source of ambiguity. This may explain why change is distasteful to those affected and subsequently influences the likelihood of successfully implementing programs (Reinke & Hall, 1988). So steps are taken either to deny the ambiguity, regardless of its source, or to eliminate it. Both of these actions have the potential to lead to conflict among stakeholders and planners, among planners and those with the health problem, or among those with various health problems vying for resources. The conflict, whether subtle and friendly or openly hostile, detracts from the planning process by requiring time and personnel resources to address and resolve the conflict. Nonetheless, to the extent that the conflict is open and constructive, it can lead to innovations in the program.

Although little has been written in the health planning literature about ambiguity, much has been written about its corollary, risk. Risk is the perceived possibility or uncertain probability of an adverse outcome in a given situation (Lupton, 1999). Health planners need to be aware of the populace's perception and interpretation of probabilities as they relate to health and illness. Risk is not just about taking chances, such as bungee jumping or unsafe sex, but is about uncertainty and ambiguity, such as estimates of cure rates and projections about future health hazards. Risk is pervasive and inherent throughout the planning process in terms of who to involve and how, which planning approach to use, and which intervention to use, and in estimating which health problem deserves attention. The importance of understanding risk as an element both of the program planning process and of the target audience provides planners with a basis from which to be flexible and speculative, rather than prescriptive and authoritative.

Control, as in being in charge of or managing, is a natural reaction to the presence of ambiguity, conflict, and risk. Control can take the form of directing attention and resources or of exerting dominance over others. Although control has historically been a key element of management, advances in complexity theory highlight the detrimental effects of control in situations of uncertainty (McDaniel, 1997). In other words, addressing the ambiguity, uncertainty, and risk that might have been the trigger for the planning process requires less, not more, control. Those who preside over and influence the planning process are thought of as having control over solutions to the health problem or condition. They do not. Effective guidance of the planning process limits the amount of control exerted by any one stakeholder and addresses the anxiety that often accompanies the lack of control.

APPROACHES TO PLANNING

An awareness of the various approaches used to accomplish planning helps planners interpret events and guide others through the planning process. Each of the approaches provides a basis for assessing possible points of contention or agreement regarding health and program priorities. Six different perspectives on planning are offered here as different lenses through which the program planning process can be viewed, understood, and used to address the health problem. They are based on the processes identified by Beneviste (1989), whose international work on planning includes a broader set of approaches than those described by Blum (1974) or Nutt (1984). Each approach is typified by various planning activities (Exhibit 3.2). None of the approaches is inherently better or worse than another. Rather, the purpose for being aware of the six approaches is so that one can select an approach that matches the situation, and so that the strengths of the approaches can be used to arrive at an optimal process for developing a health program and its evaluation.

Incremental Approach

The incremental approach to planning does not attempt to address the problem in any context or across any time span. The approach is one of addressing immediate concerns and, to some extent, having faith that the small, rather disconnected plans and actions will have a cumulative effect on the problem. Incrementalism, by its nature, focuses only on the immediate, without having a big picture or long-term plan.

In the very early days of the AIDS epidemic, before the virus had been identified or named, the only health planning options were incremental: shut down bath houses, use infectious disease precautions, and seek funding to study the health problem. These actions were isolated, disjointed efforts, but under the circumstances, the incremental approach was the only available option. There were not yet advocates for infected individuals, nor was there a scientific basis for making rational, apolitical decisions. As this example points out, incrementalism, while not the most effective planning approach, may be the only option in some circumstances. In addition, when resources are limited, incrementalism can lead to small gains to immediate problems. The major disadvantage of incrementalism is that the small planning efforts may lead to conflicting plans, confusing programs, programs or services that are not integrated, or personnel redundancy or mismatch with the "new" program.

Exhibit 3.2 Summary of the Six Approaches to Planning, with Public Health Examples

Approach	Underlying Assumptions	Consequences of Use	Public Health Example
Incremental	Not feasible to do more than small portions at a time; the parts are greater than the whole	Can be done quickly; results in plans that may be redundant or leave gaps; no guarantee that the parts will build upon each other	Specific programs implemented that reflect discrete, categorical funding, despite potential overlap or existing similar programs
Apolitical	Options are known; technicalizes the problem; the means to the ends are known; can anticipate all caveats	Plans may fail because of unforseen of unaccounted-for factors	Evidence-based practice
Advocacy	An external expert can accurately speak for those with less political power	Experts many not accurately speak for others; media attention is likely to focus on the spokesperson rather than the issue	Environmental activists
Communicative action	Language is powerful; those with the problem have the capability to enact a solution	An increased sense of confidence and an increased ability to solve one's own problems; potential for conflict	Community coalitions that take on a program or become not-for-profit organizations
Comprehensive rational	System feedback loops are contextual and can be known; rational choices are preferred	Takes considerable time and effort to do; more likely to have more dissent to overcome; results in an encompassing, intertwined set of actions	Community-focused initiatives
Strategic planning	Can anticipate and predict the future; stability is more pervasive than change	Lacks flexibility to respond to emerging issues; a costly process to arrive at a plan	Healthy People series; state 2- to 5-year plans, Title V 2-year plans

Apolitical Approach

The apolitical approach to planning relies solely on technical knowledge to arrive at a solution and assumes that technical knowledge makes it possible to achieve compromises among those involved in the health problem and the planning process. In a sense the apolitical approach is fundamentally a problem-solving approach that relies on current knowledge about the problem and known alternatives to addressing the problem. The apolitical approach is so called because its focus on the technical aspects and ignores the political aspects inherent in any problem. This approach is implicitly a gold standard of planning, particularly when those involved in the planning process are more technically inclined and focused.

To the extent that the apolitical approach relies on objective information for decision making, the application of evidence-based medicine (EBM) and evidence-based practice (EBP) guidelines can be viewed as essentially apolitical approaches to planning. In EBP, guidelines for practice by individual practitioners and complex health promotion programs are developed solely on the best available scientific knowledge, without consideration of the context of the practice or the preferences of those experiencing the health problem. When planners use EBP guidelines as the basis for health program planning without taking other factors into account, they are engaged in apolitical planning.

One of the criticisms of the apolitical problem-solving approach is that it does not account for interpersonal dynamics and possible struggles for control (Forester, 1993). It also neglects cultural issues involving the potential program participants and program staff. These can be substantial stumbling blocks in applying the apolitical approach to planning health programs. Nonetheless, this approach has the advantage of being, or at least providing, the appearance of being logical and rational, and of specifying solutions with the highest efficacy.

Advocacy Approach

The advocacy perspective on planning is client focused and includes mandated citizen participation in planning activities. Beneviste (1989) described advocacy planning as a bottom-up form of comprehensive rational planning. Planners using the advocacy approach, however, would be likely to speak for or on behalf of those with the health problem.

There are times when experts in environmental hazards testify before city or county elected officials to plead the case for people living in a hazardous waste area. When those who live in the area are unaware of a problem but their best interest is being safeguarded by an expert, advocacy planning is occurring. Another example is the trend of many federal granting agencies, such as the CDC, to mandate participation of community members in health planning activities. These federal agencies now regularly require that, during a year of program planning, representatives from the community be included in the development of the priorities and the action plan for addressing those health priorities. In this instance, the federal agencies are advocating for the communities that will be affected by the grant they are about to fund.

The advantages of the advocacy approach are most evident in situations in which clients or citizens are, for whatever reasons, not empowered to convey their own preferences or concerns. In such situations, having an advocate may be the only option for planning a needed health program. The disadvantages are that the clients or citizens may not agree with the opinions or views of the advocate. In fact, their advocate may not even be actually representing those he or she claims to speak for. The advocate implicitly holds a normative view of the needs of the clients or citizens. The advocacy approach also implicitly entails some degree of conflict or confrontation, which may have negative repercussions in the long term. Social irresponsibility occurs when the solution ignores important social or cultural factors (Blum, 1982). Strong advocates and users of the apolitical approach to planning may be prone to this factor simply because a scientific basis may not take into account social realities and needs.

Communicative Action Approach

Communicative action, or critical planning theory, is concerned with the distribution of power and communication. From this perspective, those involved in the planning make efforts to empower those with the problem through communication and the sharing of information. Whereas the advocacy approach does not enable those with the problem to participate as equals with the "experts" in the planning process, the critical or communicative action approach is predicated on making those with the problem equals in the planning process. According to Forester (1993), this perspective leads planners to think of planning as shaping the attention, changing beliefs, gaining consent, and engendering trust and understanding among those involved. This approach to planning is gaining in favor, as reflected in reports of its use in health program planning (cf. Bogue, Antia, Harmata, & Hall, 1997; Bond, Belensky, & Winstock, 2000; Hancock et al., 2001; Quigley, Handy, Goble, Sanchez, & George, 2000).

One example of this approach to planning is evident in mental health. The National Alliance for the Mentally Ill (NAMI) is a not-for-profit organization whose purpose is to support those with mental illness, and it is run by individuals with mental illness. Individuals with mental health problems are taught and guided in the process of developing small-scale, community-based programs and services for those with mental illnesses. This approach, used implicitly by NAMI, exemplifies the communicative action approach.

A major advantage of the communicative action approach is that members of the target audience gain skill, knowledge, and confidence in addressing their own problems. However, the health planner who is involved in critical planning needs to have a different set of skills from those needed to do rational or incremental planning. Also, because time and effort are needed to enable those with the problem to participate fully in the planning process, it can be a slower approach to planning. The time needed to fully implement communicative action also affects any timeline or meeting deadlines.

Comprehensive Rational Approach

The comprehensive rational perspective on planning is fundamentally a systems approach. This approach involves analyzing the problem by drawing upon ideas from systems theory—namely feedback loops, input and output, systems, and subsystems. This systematic, logical sequence of thought processes and actions is the basis for calling it rational. It assumes that the factors affecting the problem (the elements of the systems that contribute to the goals) are knowable and that virtually all contingencies can be anticipated. In this sense it is rational and logical. It is comprehensive in the sense that planners can take into account those contingencies and peripheral influences. In the comprehensive rational approach, the planners set goals, identify alternatives, implement programs, and monitor results. This approach is clearly the dominant perspective of this textbook and of most courses in planning and evaluation. Health program planning, particularly of national initiatives, reflects the efforts to use a comprehensive rational approach. In fact, one of the planning principles outlined by Reinke and Hall (1988) is to be as objective as possible, given the context, and to use rationality rather than status or position as much as possible as a basis for power.

One benefit of this approach is that it facilitates obtaining information from stakeholders who might otherwise be reluctant to share information, because it diffuses power from an authority base to an information and rational base. The comprehensive rational approach allows planners to address issues faced by the entire system rather than just by subsystems; in this respect it resembles quality improvement methodologies. Another benefit of the comprehensive rational approach is that it yields more information for decision making than does an incremental approach.

The comprehensive rational approach is not without its flaws. Forester (1993) critiqued the cybernetic (systems) perspective that underlies this approach for its failure to take into account the norms and values of individuals either involved in the planning process or affected by the planning process. Beveniste (1989) acknowledged that the comprehensive rational approach separates planners from the political realities of the health situation. Forester (1993) also pointed out that this approach assumes that the means and ends are known, which may not be the case. Claims of professional expertise about the relationship of the means to the ends, may be dysfunctional when the claims cannot be substantiated, according to Forester. The claim that the means and ends are understood leads to a choice that also takes into account other system constraints. When planners choose an option that satisfies the need—in other words, when they take the path of least effort that will meet minimum requirements—"satisficing" has occurred. While satisficing is rational and often a reality, inherent in a satisficing decision is the assumption that the decision is rational and based on a comprehensive understanding of the consequences. This may not be the case. Finally, the idea that planners know best, in terms of which means are optimal, reveals a normative perspective on planning that may be unacceptable to stakeholders with less expertise.

Strategic Planning Approach

The strategic planning perspective focuses on the organization and its ability to accomplish its mission in a fiscally responsible manner. While this approach is rarely used to address specific health conditions, it is particularly applicable to the infrastructure level of the public health pyramid. Through strategic planning, resources needed to address the health problem are identified and considered in terms of the mission of the organization. The strategic planning approach is widely used. It can be seen to affect program choices, as in health care organizations whose services are centered on one disease entity, such as Planned Parenthood or the March of Dimes, or on one aggregate, such as the Boys and Girls Club or the American Association of Retired Persons. Strategic planning is also used in community health centers (Clark & Boissoneau, 1999) to identify future directions for services. To some extent, the national goals and objectives set forth in *Healthy People 2010* is an example of strategic planning.

This approach, used by one member of a planning team, can affect the planning of the whole team. For example, the CDC awarded a large urban city a grant for a one-year planning phase of a major community-based health promotion initiative. The funded agency involved numerous local community agencies in the planning process. The chief executive officer of one of the community health agencies asked at a planning meeting what his organization could do, what was being asked of his organization, and how his organization would benefit from participating in the health programs that would result from the planning process. His questions reflect implicit thinking about how to strategically place his organization within the field of contenders for grant money. His participation in the planning process also implied that his organization's mission was compatible with the general direction of how the health problem was being addressed.

The advantages of a strategic planning approach are that it takes into account the context, whether competition or policy, as well as having a slightly longer-term focus. Most strategic planning scholars recommend approximately a five-year time frame, as it takes that long to make strategic changes in programs and services. Because strategic planning is a rational model or systematic approach to decision making, decision points can be quantified, weighted, and sequenced, and hence programmed into computer software that then shows which is the "best" option.

Despite the capability to mathematically quantify the decision-making process, knowing which is the best option does not guarantee that the best decision, or option, or program plan, will be adopted. One of the reasons that a quantitative decision might not become an implemented decision is that human beings are irrational (March, 1988), with biases in how they think about probabilities and possibilities (Tversky & Kahneman, 1974). These human characteristics are usually not quantified in the decision models, but they are powerful shapers of the actions taken. This leads to situations in which the broad goals developed during the process are not acted upon. Another disadvantage of the strategic planning approach is the subsequent lack of flexibility to respond to new environmental opportunities or threats (Egger, 1999). In addition, strategic planning, if properly done, is time and resource intensive.

Summary of Approaches

To some extent, all of the approaches to health planning discussed here are likely to occur during the planning phase of addressing a health problem. One example is the effort to increase childhood immunization in one community. The need to track immunizations necessitated the involvement of state health officials, as well as representatives from large health maintenance organizations, in the planning process. A lobbyist used advocacy to gain passage of state legislation supportive of mandatory childhood immunizations, particularly for underinsured children of color. The choice of vaccines was an apolitical decision, based on the science of what combinations were likely to result in the highest levels of protection for the children. To the extent that parents were involved as informed consumers in shaping policy and tracking procedures, communicative action was a part of the planning process. It is quite unlikely that individuals involved in the immunization planning efforts were aware of the mixture of approaches being used in this community-based effort. Had they been aware of the approaches being used by various constituents, additional strategies could have been developed that would have made the planning process more effective, efficient, and palatable to parents, providers, and policy makers. Undeniably, a blend of approaches is needed, particularly in health program planning that aims to address more recalcitrant or population-based health problems.

Each of the six approaches to health planning represents a way to identify a problem, identify options, and make a choice. This is the classic definition of decision making. In other words, planning is decision making (Veany & Kaluzny, 1998). From the perspective of an organization or agency engaged in health planning, health planning activities can be framed in terms of managerial and organizational decision making. This fact is important when assessing and developing the organizational resources and constraints for implementing the health program.

PLANNING STEPS AND STAGES

The steps or sequence of considerations that are common across the planning models are essentially a form of problem solving, with a mixture of empowerment. Planning rarely occurs step by step, in a linear fashion; rather, it is an iterative process, particularly with data from the community needs assessment and the previous program evaluations, as is shown by the feedback arrows in Exhibit 3.1. For the sake of simplicity, the diagram shows only the key planning steps. The steps are revised, expanded, and adapted to the particular situation, using the community needs assessment data and resulting in a priority given to a health problem. To the extent that cost considerations are included in the steps, they can apply to making decisions about health resource allocation (Patrick & Erickson, 1993).

Planning also tends to evolve as a process though stages that are common to work groups, beginning with formation. This stage ought to be viewed as the groundwork that lays out the processes and oversees the cycle, from assessment through program and evaluation development to implementation and evaluation.

Formation Stage and Team Development

Planning is a collective activity. The individuals involved at the various stages of the planning cycle easily influence the directions and decisions made. A key strategy for achieving successful planning is to have a visible, powerful sponsor. Given that politics of one form or another are inherently a part of the planning process, having a backer who is recognized, respected, and influential becomes an essential element to successfully planning and implementing a health program.

Member selection is influenced by legal considerations (such as antidiscrimination laws and municipal mandates for advisory boards), the reasons for wanting to participate, the level and type of expertise that an individual can contribute to the process, the amount and type of resources that an individual can contribute to the process, whether the person is or will be a user or client of the health program, and whether the person is an advocate for a group likely to be affected by the health program. Group size is another consideration, with groups of 10 to 15 being acceptable for the planning process, recognizing that an optimal size for a task force or work group is 5 to 7 persons. One "law" of groups is that there will always be one person who is not a team player. Therefore it is crucial to know the strengths and weaknesses of the individuals involved and why each individual is being selected. Having such information helps assure that a planning group has a balance of strengths that will contribute to an efficient and effectively functioning group. Attention to the composition of the planning group also ensures that a breadth of knowledge and concerns are represented, without having disruptive individuals. Reinke and Hall (1988) also remind us that it is critical to have trained, skilled, and knowledgeable planning staff. Similarly, Goodman, Steckler, Hoover, & Schwartz (1993) found that to have successful planning using the APEXPH approach, the planning group needed to have awareness, concern, and skills to address the problem.

Different types of planning groups exist (Nutt, 1984), but the most common type is a consortium. A consortium is a quasi-temporary body constituted for a specific programmatic purpose and has an independent sponsor, broad representation, and experts. Consortia have become widely used in public health program planning as a means to increase involvement of community members and to address (implicitly) the paradox of professionals not having the "right" solution. Constituting a planning board is one way to assure the involvement of both professionals and those affected by the planning. Participation of those affected by a decision in the actual decision-making process tends to enhance the strategic ability of organizations (Issel & Anderson, 2001). It follows, then, that involving stakeholders in decisions involving program planning and implementation will enhance the plan for the program. Also, participation in the decision-making process by those who will do the work increases worker satisfaction (Coopman, 2001; Wagner, 1994). Similarly, involving the future program employees, if possible, will increase their commitment to the program. Overall, the literature on participation in decision making reveals a pattern in favor of involving those affected by the decision in the decision-making process. For this reason, the involvement of stakeholders throughout the planning, implementation, and evaluation cycle is stressed. It is also important to educate those involved in the planning process, using a communicative action approach as was discussed earlier. When those affected are involved, their resistance to the change is likely to be diminished and they will begin to "own" the program or plan, although participation does not guarantee ownership (Goodman et al., 1993).

The last consideration is the selection of a leader for the planning group. Duhl (2000) argued that many types of leaders may be necessary for an effective planning process. A leader can emerge or be appointed for his or her capability to function as an educator, a doer, or even a social entrepreneur. At any point in the planning process, or even during oversight of the program implementation, different individuals may be better suited to play a leadership role. Recognizing this and acting upon that recognition is healthy and useful. What may be less articulate, especially during the earliest stages, is the degree of formalization of leader selection. In other words, does the planning group have an acknowledged and standard process for designating a legitimate leader? The process can and does vary, from the ad hoc emergence of a natural leader to the election of an individual from a slate of candidates according to formalized bylaws. Regardless of where along that continuum of formalized process the group wants to be, the key will be to have an articulated and accepted process that facilitates the planning process, rather than hindering the creativity and commitment. Ideally, each member of the planning group needs to be actively involved in assuring that the process is open and agreed upon.

Create a Vision

The first step in planning, according to the American Planning Association, is to create a vision. This step is rarely mentioned in health planning, yet vision and mission creation is the first step in strategic planning (Van Wart, 1995). Specific elements of the mission statement appear to be related to the success of health care organizations (Bart, 1999). For example, *Healthy People 2010* provides a national vision of eliminating racial and ethnic disparities in health and increasing the quality of life. Whatever the trigger event, health program planners must create a vision with which existing and future stakeholders can identify and to which they can devote attention and energy. Patrick and Erickson (1993), in their discussion of health resource planning, start with specifying the health decision. A vision frames information for stakeholders and helps identify economic assumptions that may affect the overall health program.

Part of creating a vision of the final "product" is the creation of a consensus on how to arrive at that final ideal. In this regard, an element of creating a vision is deciding upon a system for prioritizing among problems and among possible solutions to the highest-priority problems. How decisions are made—whether by voting, consensus, or complex algorithm—is one of the first decisions of the planning group.

Investigation Stage

The investigation phase of planning is the time during which data are gathered that will be used to first prioritize health problems and then prioritize possible programmatic solutions. Generally, data relevant to planning health programs comes from community assessment, population preferences, previous program evaluations, and EBP information. The importance and possible scope of collecting relevant data through community assessment is so substantial that the next chapter is entirely devoted to community assessment. Two elements of the nonlinear nature of health program planning are worth introducing during this stage of planning. One is the need to focus on future considerations, specifically interventions, even before the program direction has been decided. The other is the need to be aware of the willingness of key individuals to support the planning and program process, and to understand the quantification of health problems in terms of quality of life.

Focus on Interventions

Interventions are actions that are done intentionally to have a direct effect on the health problem or condition. This broad definition of intervention thus includes medical treatment, pharmacological treatment, behavioral treatment, and health policy development, as well as education and skill enhancement, social support, and financial aid. EBM and EBP can be used to determine the effectiveness of potential interventions. Of particular concern is the sensitivity of the health problem to the intervention and the specificity of the intervention with regard to the health problems it is effective in addressing. Another consideration in determining the effectiveness of an intervention is the theoretical or conceptual logic underlying the way in which the intervention alters the health problem or condition. Chapter 5 discusses this consideration.

Solutions, whether programmatic interventions or other ideas, exist, and they exist before the problem is recognized as such. Proponents of the solution can be waiting for a window of opportunity for "their" idea to be applied. Although having solutions can be helpful, the inclination of many individuals is to jump to a solution before fully understanding the problem. To the extent that any intervention or solution is well suited to a clearly defined problem, the planning process is effective.

A factor adversely affecting planning is wishful thinking, according to Blum (1982), by which he meant that solutions are sometimes based on idealistic and overly optimistic hopes rather than on scientific knowledge. This factor leads to the failure to examine the range of possible effective interventions or solutions to the problem. A key to avoiding this pitfall is the use of EBM and EBP, even though facts may not convince individuals with strongly held beliefs about what is scientifically the right thing to do.

An additional benefit of focusing on interventions is that it helps avoid an undue emphasis on needs assessment and data collection. Goodman et al. (1993) found that planning groups have a tendency to "front load" the planning cycle, with considerable time and effort devoted to collecting risk and health problem data and data analysis. Focusing on identifying realistic interventions balances the early planning stages with the later stages of implementation.

Determine Willingness and Preferences

Policy makers, health providers, and other stakeholders need to be willing to do more than support a program aimed at addressing a large, serious health problem for which there is an effective intervention. They need to be willing to make a commitment to address whichever health problem is chosen in a manner determined to be effective. Several factors influence willingness: availability of existing or obtainable resources, political or ideological constraints, differences in perceived and normative needs, and the timing of the planning process or the health program (i.e., postponing chronic issues in favor of current epidemics). In addition, planning health programs from the perspective of public health entails consideration of the preferences of the population for one health state over another, the quality of life in relationship to the lifespan in view of disabilities and death, and the existing methodologies that have been developed for public health planning.

Years and Quality of Life. A number of measures have been developed to account for not only deaths but also the quality of years lived with an illness. Exhibit 3.3 is a summary of these measures, with definitions drawn from a variety of sources. Each of these measures can be used in health program planning. These are the same measures that can and are used in the economic evaluations of programs, particularly in cost-benefit analyses (see Chapter 13). Understanding the ways in which the negative effects of health problems are quantified, besides mortality and morbidity rates, can be useful during the planning and prioritization processes.

Quality of life, particularly health-related quality of life (HRQOL), is a major consideration in public health planning. HRQOL measures have been found to correlate significantly with utility scores and general ratings of health (Lee, Fos, Zuniga, Kastl, & Sung, 2000). Although each person has a sense of what constitutes quality of life, its measurement is complex; hence the plethora of quality-of-life measures that are available (Dijkers, 1999). From an epidemiological

Exhibit 3.3   Quality-of-life Acronyms and Definitions

Acronym	Spelled-Out Form	Definition
QALYs	Quality-adjusted life years	Number of years of life expected at a given level of health and well-being.
DALYs	Disability-adjusted life years	Number of years of life lost from living with a level of morbidity or disability.
YLL	Years of life lost	Number of years a person is estimated to have remained alive if the disease experienced had not occurred.
YPLL	Years of potential life lost	A measure of the impact of disease or injury in a population that calculates years of life lost before a specific age (often age 65 or age 75). This approach places additional value on deaths that occur at earlier ages.
HYE	Healthy years equivalent	Number of years in perfect health that are considered equivalent to a particular health state or health profile.
YHL	Years of healthy life	Number of healthy years of life lived or achieved, adjusted for level of health status.

perspective or an actuarial stance, the length of life is as important as its quality. Since it is possible to live with a health condition for varying lengths of time, the length of life as affected by that health condition is what becomes important. In other words, it is important to take into consideration the quality of the life as lived with the health condition. Quality-adjusted life years (QALYs) and disability-adjusted life years (DALYs) were developed specifically to give a numeric value to the quality of years of life. They are composite scores that are used with populations and thus have the advantage of being indifferent to individual preferences. However, because the number of years for which quality can be adjusted is naturally shorter for older persons, QALYs and DALYs mathematically discriminate against the elderly. Nonetheless, the use of DALYs reveals the extent to which diseases affect the years of life (Exhibit 3.4). For example, internationally, lower respiratory tract infections account for not only almost 4 million deaths but nearly 97 million years of disability from the disease (Michaud, Murray, & Bloom, 2001).

Exhibit 3.4 Leading Causes of Disability-Adjusted Life Years (DALYs)

	World 1999					United States, Men, 1996					United States, Women, 1996			
Rank	Cause	DALYs	% of Total DALYs	Deaths	Rank	Cause	DALYs	% of Total DALYs	Deaths	Rank	Cause	DALYs	% of Total DALYs	Deaths
1	Lower respiratory tract infections	96,682,000	6.72	3,963,000	1	Ischemic heart disease	1,969,256	10.75	286,999	1	Ischemic heart disease	1,181,298	7.45	249,315
2	HIV/AIDS	89,819,000	6.25	2,673,000	2	Road traffic collisions	933,953	5.10	29,105	2	Unipolar major depression	1,073,911	6.77	25
3	Conditions arising during perinatal period	89,508,000	6.22	2,356,000	3	Lung, trachea, and bronchus cancers	812,675	4.44	102,071	3	Cerebro-vascular disease	836,345	5.27	98,551
4	Diarrheal diseases	72,063,000	5.01	2,213,000	4	HIV/AIDS	773,640	4.22	25,307	4	Lung, trachea, and bronchus cancers	549,963	3.47	66,134
5	Unipolar major depression	59,030,000	4.10	1000	5	Alcohol abuse and dependence	736,572	4.02	5231	5	Osteo-arthritis	521,443	3.24	508

Adapted from Michaud, C. M., Murray, C. J. L., & Bloom, B. R. (2001). Burden of disease—Implications for future research. *Journal of the American Medical Association, 285*(5); 535–539.

Another issue with quality-of-life measures, as Kaplan (1996) stressed, is that quality of life is multidimensional, and the measures must address the relative importance of the many dimensions of quality of life. One approach to measuring such complexities is to use an overall index of years of healthy life (YHL). Doctor, Chan, MacLehose, and Patrick (2001) found YHL to be a stable overall index of health within the Medicare population. The choice of which measure to use in health program planning will depend upon the resources available, the sophistication of the planning team, and whether a rational approach dominates in the planning process.

A slightly different perspective is to consider the number of years of life that are lost due to a health condition. Years of life lost (YLL) reveals the years lost at the end of life, such as the shortening of life due to lung cancer or prostate cancer. The years of potential life lost (YPLL) is a similar measure but indicates the number of years of life lost at the beginning of life, such as the shortening of life due to neonatal sepsis or childhood drowning. All of these quality-of-life and life-year measures are particularly useful, as health planners must choose and decide which health condition warrants health promotion or disease prevention programs, particularly when resources are severely limited.

Population Preferences. Fitch et al. (1997), in conducting a community needs assessment, found that older community members were concerned about how cancer would affect their ability to do what they wanted to do. Their perception about the consequences of an illness and their preferences about being healthy are precisely what a genre of health measures called utility measures are intended to uncover and quantify A trade-off exists between how an illness or health condition affects an individual and the consequences of the treatment (Donald-Sherbourne, et al., 2001); this trade-off is often overlooked when planning health programs. Yet the preferences held by a population for health versus treatment influence the rational approach to prioritizing health care resources and form a foundation of policy positions taken by active citizens.

Population preferences are identified through the use of utility measures that are a set of established techniques to quantify perceptions and preferences about illness and health states. Preference or utility assessment provides a way to integrate the preferences or values attributed to the worth of life at a given point in time with the quality of life spent in various health states (Patrick & Erickson, 1993). Utility measures are used to arrive at the *perceived* seriousness of an illness or health condition (Veany & Kaluzny, 1998), and they roughly equate to population preferences with regard to treatment. These measures are helpful in assessing the worth or value of small changes in a health state, whether those changes are a result of medical treatment or programmatic interventions. The measures are specifically designed to be used across different conditions and health states, thus allowing comparison of preferences between health states or conditions, making them quite useful during the prioritization phase of planning. Fundamentally, utility measures are based on preferences and subjective assessments, and therefore they diminish the guesswork on the part of health program planners or providers about the population's preferences. Lastly, utility measures are designed to take into account states of health that people may view as worse than death. This can be done, for example, by comparing a specific chronic condition or a temporary or episodic condition with death. For example, some individuals may view the loss of vision as worse than death or may feel that having a child with a severe developmental disability is worse than losing the child.

There are different types of utility measures: rating scales, paired comparisons, standard gambles, and time trade-offs. Utility measures are predicated on the assumption that individuals prefer healthy states. Being completely healthy with no disabilities is scored 1.0, and death is scored as 0. Each of the different methods arrives at a score of 0 to 1.0 for the health states being compared, with regard to the preferences people hold about those states. In addition, each type of utility measure yields slightly different utility scores, although they are generally quite similar (Post, Stiggelbout, & Wakker, 2001). Voruganti and associates (2000) found that rating scales, time trade-offs, and willingness-to-pay methods to assign utilities were used with reliability and validity with mental health patients. This suggests that these techniques may be potentially useful tools with other populations.

Rating scales, such as the familiar Lickert scale, or an analog scale can be used to determine the relative strength of preferences for various health states. For example, categorical rating scales were used by Revicki, Wu, and Murray (1995). Using those scales, they found that preferences changed as the symptoms of patients increased. A paired comparison, another type of utility measure, is a simple procedure in which the two states of health are presented in pairs and one state is selected as preferable over the other. The paired comparison essentially results in a ranking of preferred heath states.

The standard gamble compares two or more alternatives, and one of the alternatives can have an adverse outcome or an outcome generally considered very undesirable. Utility scores derived from the standard gamble can be sensitive to both gender and race differences, as Cykert, Joines, Kissling, and Hansen (1999) found in a study of limited functioning. Saigal, Stoskopf, et al.

(2000) used a standard gamble method to compare the preferences of neona-
tologists, neonatal nurses, adolescents who were normal birth weight, parents
of normal birth weight infants, and parents of extremely low birth weight
infants. They found that the health providers provided lower utility scores for
selected health states than did parents or adolescents. This difference
between providers and members of the target audience reinforces the idea
that health planners are well advised to consider the values and preferences
of non-health professionals when planning heath programs.

A timed trade-off is a bit more complex and sophisticated in what is
learned about preferences. The element of time is added, so that a health state
is considered within the context of a period of time. This method takes into
account the amount of time spent in a less desirable health condition compared to spending an uncertain amount of time in a more desirable health condition. The use of timed trade-off is supported by the findings of Ganiats et al.
(2000) that patients have different preferences for future health states,
depending on the disease.

Each type of utility measure has been developed with sophisticated techniques and analytic procedures and has resulted in weighted choices based on
data from individuals regarding their health state preferences. Health program
planners can review the literature for utility studies that will inform the planning
process and program development. Be aware, however, that Bastian (2000) crit-
icized the valuation of alternative health states as favoring short-term interventions over long-term strategies. While much of the research into health utilities
has focused on acute illness, researchers increasingly are using both health utilities measures and measures of quality of life, which account for more long-term
effects. For example, Saigal, Rosenbaum, et al. (2000) found that, although the
quality-of-life scores were very similar among parents of extremely low birth
weight infants and parents of normal birth weight infants, the parents differed
with respect to their preferences regarding their infants.

Prioritization Stage

During the prioritization stage, data and information gained during the
community health assessment (Chapter 4), along with the information on preferences and interventions, is integrated into a decision about what to address
and how.

A prerequisite for planning the community health or needs assessment is
having a framework for guiding what data need to be collected and, thus, for
understanding the causes and various pathways leading to the health problem.
Each health state or problem is a result of direct causes or determinants of the

health problem, as well as factors existing before the health problem that indirectly influence the direct causes and a vast set of secondary indirect contributing factors leading to the health problem. The relationship of these factors to the health problem is illustrated in a diagram that shows the most rudimentary and basic set of relationships (Exhibit 3.5).

A commonly used approach to understanding the parameters of a health problem focuses on direct and indirect causes. While this terminology is useful during the planning and assessment stages of the overall program planning cycle, it does not denote the subsequent attention given to the smaller set of factors selected as the focus of the program. Throughout this text, those factors of programmatic concern are called the determinants. The indirect causes are grouped as direct antecedents to the health problem, and the secondary indirect causes are called contributing factors. The diagram in Exhibit 3.5 provides a visual representation and is *not* intended to be the only way the factors are related. It is simply intended as a starting point that evolves during the planning cycle, and it is used throughout this text to demonstrate how the "picture" of a health problem developed early in the planning cycle guides and frames subsequent program activities. At a minimum, during the prioritization stage of planning, some agreement is needed on how the parameters of the final health problem will be developed and represented.

Exhibit 3.5   Simplified Model of the Relationship of Antecedent, Determinant, and Contributing Factors and Interventions to the BPRS Score for a Health Problem

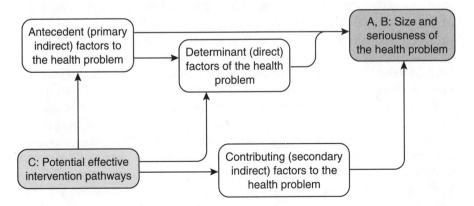

The final health problem is the one selected from among the many health concerns for programmatic attention. One approach to prioritizing which health problem ought to be addressed is the Hanlon method (1973). An overview of this process will provide some initial insight into the depth and breadth of the data that will be needed for making decisions about program directions. Hanlon's approach to planning public health programs has been codified into a deceptively simple formula known as the basic priority rating system (BPRS), which is being used in the CDC's Sustainable Management Development Program (CDC Sustainable Management Development Program, n.d.). This method entails prioritizing health problems based on the size of the problem, the severity or importance of the health problem, and the potential effectiveness of interventions. The process involves assigning values to each of these three factors. The formula is

Basic priority rating system $= (A + 2B) \times C,$

where A is the score of the size of the problem, B is the score for the seriousness of the health problem, and C is the score for the potential effectiveness of the intervention.

The scores assigned to the problem size, seriousness, and intervention effectiveness can be biased by the personal preferences of those involved in the planning process. By going through the process described to arrive at a score for each factor, members of the planning group are forced to become explicit about the assumptions underlying their assignment of values. This, in turn, helps establish consensus and consistency within the group.

The first factor to determine is the size of the health problem (A). Typically, size is measured as expressed need—that is, the demand for and utilization of services. Size can also be demonstrated through normative needs, namely what health professionals view as a deviation from a baseline or normally acceptable level. Normative need is reflected in epidemiological measures, such as mortality and morbidity rates, incidence, prevalence, and relative risk. An issue with using such epidemiological measures is that the numbers do not provide information on the factors leading to the health problem. The extent to which antecedent and contributing factors exist is more appropriately derived from individual surveys, whether national surveys, local needs surveys, or surveys conducted for research. Another difficulty with using mortality rates as the sole criterion for determining the size of a health problem is that mortality data are medical, making them less helpful in planning that is focused on behavioral or mental health problems. In addition, disability, pain, and quality of life are as important as death, as we have seen with regard to QALYs and DALYs. Thus, the size of a health problem and the factors leading to it ought to be viewed from various angles and should incorporate a diversity of measures or indicators. Some ways to do this are discussed in the next chapter, but the issue is mentioned here as a way to reinforce the iterative nature of planning health programs.

Not all health problems are equal in terms of seriousness (B), which encompasses the degree of urgency for addressing the problem, the degree of severity of the health problem, the degree of economic losses possible from the health problem, and the degree to which others can be motivated to become involved. Each of these four elements of seriousness can be rated on a scale of 1 at the lowest end to 10 on the highest end. Again, the specific data derived from the community assessment can be used to score each. The severity of a health problem or condition is also related to its virulence. Seriousness is best determined through contact with experts, as well as through input from key stakeholders on the long-term consequences of the health problem. The degree of economic loss is focused on individual loss due to disability and death, but it also might include the societal costs of providing care and the loss of revenue from disabled individuals.

Intervention effectiveness (C) is the third element in the BPRS. Scoring the effectiveness of the interventions that can be used to address a health problem also takes place on a scale of 1 to 10. Interventions for which there is considerable favorable evidence would be rated highest, where "favorable" means having a clinically and practically significant effect on the health problem. The choice of an intervention deserves considerable attention, in terms of whether and how it has the potential to affect the determinants or the antecedent and contributing factors (Exhibit 3.5). The availability of effective and efficient (lower-cost) interventions can be viewed as contributing to the extent to which it is possible to change the health problem.

Decision Stage

Competing health problems are prioritized based on the rank scores derived from the BPRS, after considering numerous factors for each aspect of the rating system (Exhibit 3.6). Inevitably, the scores and subsequent priority ranking of health problems will not be acceptable to some stakeholders. The rankings may need to be revised with stakeholder input or until a consensus is gained. Such an activity reflects the reality of blending the rational and political approaches to program planning. The decisions regarding which health problems to address are the starting point for program development and then implementation.

The severity of a health problem refers to its potential to cause disability or death, whereas a health problem's importance is the relative or subjective value assigned to it. The importance of a health problem can be assessed through the

Exhibit 3.6   Criteria for Rating Problems According to the Basic Priority Rating System (BPRS)

BPRS Factor	A	B					C
	Size	Urgency	Severity	Economic Consequences	Willingness or Involvement of Others	Intervention Effectiveness	
Rating Scale	1 (small) to 10 (endemic)	1 (not at all) to 10 (extremely urgent)	1 (low) to 10 (high)	1 (low) to 10 (high)	1 (low) to 5 (high)	1 (low) to 5 (high)	
Factors to Consider in the Rating	Stability of incidence or prevalence over time	Rate of spread	Extent to which QALYs and DALYs are affected; virulence of health problem	Health care costs; extent to which YLL and YPLL are affected	Political support for addressing the problem; popular awareness of the health problem	Recalcitrance to change; entrenchment of contributing factors	

use of utility measures, as discussed earlier, or through reliance on *Healthy People 2010* for whether the health condition is sufficiently important to warrant national attention. One other characteristic of health problems or conditions is their changeability or the degree to which any intervention has the potential to alter their course. When many health problems or conditions are being considered for an intervention or health program, each of the health problems can be rated with regard to the degree of seriousness, importance, and changeability. In short, ranking health problems retains an element of subjectivity and hence susceptibility to political forces. A simplified approach to understanding the priority of a health problem is to consider only whether an intervention can make a change in the health problem and whether the health problem is important or worth addressing. High and low changeability and high and low importance form four quadrants of program priority (Exhibit 3.7). Health problems falling into high changeability and high importance ought to be addressed first. In contrast, health problems in the low changeability and low importance quadrant are either at the bottom or off the list.

A more complex approach to deciding which health problems are appropriately addressed by the planning body is to use the PEARL system, short

Exhibit 3.7   Program Prioritization Based on the Importance and Changeability of the Health Problem

	Highly Important Health Problem	**Less Important** Health Problem
Highly Changeable Health Problem, More Effective Intervention	High priority for developing a program	Low priority, unless resources are available for developing a program
Less Changeable Health Problem, Less Effective Intervention	High priority if an innovative program can be developed	No program development is warranted

for Propriety, Economic, Acceptability, Resources, Legality (Healthy Plan-it). Each health problem being considered for further program planning is evaluated on these five dimensions, scored yes (1) or no (0). Propriety refers to whether addressing the health problem is the responsibility of those represented by the planning group. The economic feasibility of addressing the problem is also scored. Acceptability in terms of culture and population preference for the potential intervention is a further consideration to be scored. Availability of resources is, of course, a concern that needs to be factored into the score. Legality of the program is the final dimension of the selection process. Applying the PEARL approach to prioritizing among health problems may not be possible until sufficient data about the health problem, its causes, and the availability of effective interventions are known. In other words, it may not be possible to apply the PEARL scoring until a substantial amount of information has been collected about the problem. The need to revisit priorities based on new information is likely to be frustrating, but it is the reality of program planning.

Decisions about which health problems to address can fail for two major reasons. One is that the organizational norms and institutionalized objectives can have conflicting priorities regarding health problems, thus limiting which interventions are acceptable. For this reason, the organizational assessment discussed in the next chapter is critical. The other reason for decision failure is that the experts conducting the community health assessment can be biased, which will limit their findings. In other words, data from the community health assessment that are made available for planning can be a reflection of the views of those who conducted the assessment, rather than the full scope of what exists as both strengths and problems in the community.

Once a health problem or condition has been chosen as the focus of a health program or service, a detailed implementation plan needs to be developed, along with a plan for conducting the evaluation. Planners should be aware that once a health problem has been identified, the composition of the planning group is likely to change; those with vested interests will remain, and those with little expertise or interest in the chosen priority will fade away. At this point in the cycle, it may be important to revisit the group's composition and address why potential key stakeholders should become involved.

Implementation and Continuation Stage

The planning cycle, at least one iteration, is not complete until the program is implemented, monitored for the extent of the implementation, and assessed for its effectiveness. For some health programs, implementation includes a termination phase or phase-out period, as happens with health programs funded for a limited time. Evaluation, whether of immediate impacts or long-term outcomes, provides a basis for further program planning and completes one cycle. Throughout the planning process, multiple foci are useful: an epidemiological focus on the characteristics of the health problem; a scientific focus on identifying the best possible, feasible programmatic interventions; and a managerial focus on the planning cycle and program implementation. If these foci are maintained, then feedback loops will develop more quickly, new triggers to additional planning activities will be perceived, and the evolution of involvement of stakeholders will be more rapid.

ACROSS THE PYRAMID

At the direct services level of the public health pyramid, planning is focused on individual health problems and the most prevalent or most costly health problems addressed by direct services. Planning, therefore, can be rather clinical in nature, involving only those individuals affected by the clinical decisions. It can also be focused on addressing issues of small aggregates, such that the planning results in the development of health educational offerings to the clinic patients, as an example. Nonetheless, the data source for the seriousness, size, and importance of a health problem must be selected to provide information relevant to planning direct services (Exhibit 3.8).

At the enabling services level of the pyramid, planning is more focused on aggregates and prioritizing among available or potentially available enabling services. The planning may also focus on the creation of enabling services to address the highly prioritized problems. In contrast to direct services planning occurring within the boundaries of a clinic, planning at the enabling services level requires more involvement of a wider body of constituents. This is

Exhibit 3.8   Sources of Data for Prioritizing Health Problems at Each Level of the Public Health Pyramid

Level	Examples of Health Problem	Data Sources for *A*, Size	Data Sources for *B*, Seriousness	Data Sources for *C*, Intervention
Direct services	Cholesterol level; dental caries; underimmunization	Variety of sources, including epidemiological data, clinic or service provider data on rates and wait lists	Individual patient diagnostic and prognosis data; scientific literature on the nature and course of the health problem; utility measures	Scientific community; other program evaluations
Enabling services	Lack of accessibility to services	Epidemiological data; wait lists; human services sources of data	Demand data used to infer seriousness; advocacy group pressure	Translation of effectiveness across related problems
Population-based services	Nutritional knowledge; use of sealants; immunization status	Epidemiological data; acute care and outpatient data; estimation procedures	Normative perspective; extrapolation based on individual data; trends data relative to *Healthy People 2010* objectives; mandates and regulatory requirements	Availability of health program evaluations; cultural implications of application across a population
Infrastructure	Employee turnover; decreasing immunization rates; inadequate management or data information systems	Aggregated rates and incidence of infrastructure problems	Degree of impact on managerial objectives; political perspective; effects on capacity requirements	Capacity requirements if selected

because the nature of the health problems that get addressed at the enabling services level is likely to lead to plans that require a broader base of support and cooperation. For example, if health planning includes a focus on accessibility of primary health care, and transportation becomes an element in the planning, the transportation authority needs to be included in the planning activities. Again, data sources for the seriousness, size, and importance of a health problem at the enabling services level need to be applicable to the aggregate of concern.

At the population-based services level, health planning is most evident in state health plans, although health systems and networks have begun to use a population-focused approach as well. State health agencies regularly conduct assessment and planning activities as the basis for developing state-supported or state-implemented health programs. As with planning for enabling services, planning of population-based services is likely to require involvement of a wider array of stakeholders. In addition, there may be time-specific population data sources on the seriousness, size, and importance of population health problems.

At the infrastructure level, planning is an activity of the infrastructure. Therefore, the issues of resource allocation, planning for the planning, and collection of the planning data are relevant. One area that is likely to be addressed through health planning at the infrastructure level is determining the qualifications and adequate numbers of health personnel needed. Health personnel and resource planning (Reinke & Hall, 1988; Blum, 1982) are appropriate planning foci and are needed to sustain the infrastructure. At the infrastructure level, the data sources on the size, seriousness, and importance of a health problem are likely to be quite specific to infrastructure characteristics.

DISCUSSION QUESTIONS

1. Given the different ways that planning bodies can accomplish their tasks and the diverse backgrounds of those involved, planners take on different roles in various situations. For example, planners can be facilitators and educators. What other roles might planners take on in order to be effective at planning?

2. In what ways, if any, would you modify the planning steps for developing programs at each level of the pyramid?

3. Access the CDC website (CDC PATCH, n.d.) and the NAACHO website (NACCHO, 2000). Compare the planning models available through those sites, with particular attention to the manner in which health problems are prioritized.

4. Part of being effective in participation in program planning is being comfortable with using different approaches in different situations. Choose a planning approach and describe an ideal situation and a least ideal situation for its use.

REFERENCES

Bart, C. K. (1999). Mission statement content and hospital performance in the Canadian not-for-profit health care sector. *Health Care Management Review, 24*(3), 18–29.

Bastian, H. (2000). A consumer trip into the world of the DALY calculations: An Alice-in-Wonderland experience. *Reproductive Health Matters, 8*(15), 113–116.

Beneviste, G. (1989). *Mastering the politics of planning: Crafting credible plans and policies that make a difference.* San Francisco: Jossey-Bass.

Blum, H. L. (1974). *Planning for health.* New York: Human Sciences Press.

Blum, H. L. (1982). Social perspective on risk reduction. In M. M. Faber, & A. M. Reinhart (Eds.), *Promoting health through risk reduction* (pp. 19–36). New York: Macmillan.

Bogue, R. J., Antia, M., Harmata, R., & Hall, C.H., Jr. (1997). Community experiments in action: Developing community-defined models for reconfiguring health care delivery. *Journal of Health Politics, Policy & Law, 22,* 1051–1076.

Bond, L. A., Belenky, M. F., & Winstock, J. S. (2000). The listening partners program: An initiative toward feminist community psychology in action. *American Journal of Community Psychology, 28,* 697–730.

CDC PATCH. (n.d.). *http://www.cdc.org/nccdphp* (accessed 8/12/01).

CDC Sustainable Management Development Programs. (n.d.). http://www.phppo.cdc.gov/od/smdp/Healthyplanit.asp (accessed 8/12/03).

Clark, B., & Boissoneau, R. (1999). Strategic planning in community mental health centers. *Health Marketing Quarterly, 16*(3), 55–64.

Coopman, S. J. (2001). Democracy, performance, and outcomes in interdisciplinary health care teams. *Journal of Business Communication, 38,* 261–284.

Cykert, S., Joines, J. D., Kissling, G., & Hansen, C. J. (1999). Racial differences in patients' perceptions of debilitated health states. *Journal of General Internal Medicine, 14:* 217–222.

Dever, G. E. (1980). *Community health analysis: A holistic approach.* Germantown, MD: Aspen Systems.

Dever, G. E. (1997). *Improving outcomes in public health practice: Strategy and methods.* Gaithersburg, MD: Aspen Publishers.

Dijkers, M. (1999). Measuring quality of life: Methodological issues. *American Journal of Physical Medicine and Rehabilitation, 78,* 286–300.

Doctor, J. N., Chan, L., MacLehose, R. F., & Patrick, D. L. (2001). Weighted health status in the Medicare population: Development of the Weighted Health Index for the Medicare Current Beneficiary Survey (WHIMCBS). *Journal of Outcome Measurement, 4*, 721–739.

Donald-Sherbourne, C., Unutzer, J., Schoenbaum, M., Duan, N., Lenert, L., Sturm, R., & Wells, K. (2001). Can utility-weighted health-related quality-of-life estimates capture health effects of quality improvement for depression? *Medical Care, 39*, 1246–1259.

Duhl, L. S. (1987). *Health planning and social change.* New York: Human Science Press.

Duhl, L. S. (2000). A short history and some acknowledgements. *Public Health Reports,* 115, 116–117.

Egger, E. (1999). Old ways of planning, thinking won't work in today's volatile health care industry. *Health Care Strategic Management, 17*(9), 18–19.

Fitch, M. I., Greenberg, M., Levstein, L., Muir, M., Plante, S., & King, E. (1997). Health promotion and early detection of cancer in older adults: Needs assessment for program development. *Cancer Nursing, 20*, 381–388.

Forester, J. (1993). *Critical theory, public policy and planning practice: Toward a critical pragmatism.* New York: State University of New York Press.

Ganiats, T. G., Carson, R. T., Hamm, R. M., Cantor, S. B., Sumner, W., Spann, S. J., Hagen, M. D., & Miller, C. (2000). Population-based time preferences for future health outcomes. *Medical Decision Making, 20*, 263–270.

Goodman, R. M., Steckler, A., Hoover, S., & Schwartz, R. (1993). A critique of contemporary community health promotion approaches: Based on a qualitative review of six programs in Maine. *American Journal of Health Promotion, 7*, 208–220.

Green, L. W., Kreuter, M. W., Deeds, S. G., & Partridge, K. B. (1980). *Health education planning: A diagnostic approach.* Palo Alto, CA: Mayfield Publishing.

Hancock, L., Sanson-Fisher, R., Perkins, J., McClintock, A., Howley, P., & Gibberd, R. (2001). Effect of a community action program on adult quit smoking rates in rural Australian towns: The CART project. *Preventive Medicine, 32* (2), 118-127.

Hanlon, J. J. (1973). Is there a future for local health departments? *Health Services Report, 88*, 898-901.

Hoch, C. (1994). *What planners do: Power, politics and persuasion.* Chicago: Planners Press.

Institute of Medicine. (1988). *The future of public health.* Washington: DC, National Academy Press.

Issel, L. M., & Anderson, R. A. (2001). Intensity of case managers' participation in organizational decision making. *Research in Nursing and Health, 24*, 361–372.

Kaplan, R. M. (1996). Utility assessment for estimating quality-adjusted life years. In F. A. Sloan (Ed.), *Valuing health care: Costs, benefits, and effectiveness of pharmaceuticals and other medical technologies* (pp. 32–60). Cambridge, UK: Cambridge University Press.

LaLonde, M. (1974). *A new perspective on the health of Canadians.* Ottawa, Canada: Government of Canada. Ottawa Catalog No. H311–374.

Lee, J. E., Fos, P. J., Zuniga, M. A., Kastl, P. R., & Sung, J. H. (2000). Assessing health-related quality of life in cataract patients: The relationship between utility and health-related quality of life measurement. *Quality of Life Research, 9*, 1127–1135.

Lupton, D. (1999). *Risk.* London: Routledge.

March, J. G. (1988). *Decisions and organizations.* New York: Basil Blackwell.

Marris, P. (1982). *Community planning and conceptions of change.* New York: Routledge and Kegan Paul.

McDaniel, R. R. (1997). Strategic leadership: A new view from quantum and chaos theory. *Health Care Management Review, 22*(1), 21–37.

Michaud, C. M., Murray, C. J. L., & Bloom, B. R. (2001). Burden of disease—Implications for future research. *Journal of the American Medical Association, 285*, 535–539.

National Association of City and County Health Officers. (2000). Research and development: Assessment Protocol for Excellence in Public Health (APEXPH). *http://www.naccho.org/project47.cfm* (accessed 8/12/03).

Nutt, P. C. (1979). Calling out and calling off the dogs: Managerial diagnosis in public service organizations. *Academy of Management Review, 4*, 203–214.

Nutt, P. C. (1984). *Planning methods for health and related organizations.* New York: John Wiley.

Patrick, D. L., & Erickson, P. (1993). *Health status and health policy: Allocating resources to health care.* Oxford, England: Oxford University Press.

Post, P. N., Stiggelbout, A. M., & Wakker, P. P. (2001). The utility of health states after stroke: A systematic review of the literature. *Stroke, 32*, 1425–1429.

Pratt, M., McDonald, S., Libby, P., Oberle, M. & Liang, A. (1996). Local health departments in Washington State use APEX to assess capacity. *Public Health Reports, 111*, 87–91.

Quigley, D., Handy, D., Goble, R., Sanchez, V., & George, P. (2000). Participatory research strategies in nuclear risk management for native communities. *Journal of Health Communication, 5*, 305–331.

Reinke, W. A., & Hall, T. L. (1988). Political aspects of planning. In W. A. Reinke (Ed.), *Health planning for effective management.* New York: Oxford University Press.

Revicki, D. A., Wu, A. W., & Murray, M. I. (1995). Change in clinical status, health status, and health utility outcomes in HIV-infected patients. *Medical Care, 33* (Suppl. 4), 173–182.

Rosen, G. (1958). *A history of public health.* Baltimore: Johns Hopkins University Press.

Saigal, S., Rosenbaum, P. L., Feeny, D., Burrows, E., Furlong, W., Stoskopf, B. L., & Hoult, L. (2000). Parental perspectives of the health status and health-related quality of life of teen-aged children who were extremely low birth weight and term controls. *Pediatrics, 105*, 569–574.

Saigal, S., Stoskopf, B. L., Feeny, D., Furlong, W., Burrows, E., Rosenbaum, P. L., & Hoult, L. (2000). Differences in preferences for neonatal outcomes among health care professionals, parents, and adolescents. *Journal of American Medical Association, 281*, 1991–1997.

Sloan, F. A., & Conover, C. J. (1996). The use of cost-effectivness/cost-benefit analysis in actual decision making: Current status and prospects. In F. A. Sloan (Ed.), *Valuing health care: Costs, benefits, and effectiveness of pharmaceuticals and other medical technologies* (pp. 207–232). Cambridge, UK: Cambridge University Press.

Tversky, A., & Kahneman, D. (1974). Judgment under uncertainty: Heuristics and biases. *Science, 185*(4157), 1124–1131.

Van Wart, M. (1995). The first step in the reinvention process: Assessment. *Public Administration Review, 55*, 429–438.

Veany, J. E., & Kaluzny, A. D. (1998). *Evaluation and decision making for health services.* Chicago: Health Administration Press.

Voruganti, L. N., Awad, G., Oyewumi, K., Cortese, L., Zirul, S., & Dhawan, R. (2000). Assessing health utilities in schizophrenia: A feasibility study. *Pharmacoeconomics, 17*, 273–286.

Wagner, J. A. (1994). Participation's effects on performance and satisfaction: A reconsideration of research evidence. *Academy of Management Review, 19*, 312–330.

Section 2

Developing Health Programs

CHAPTER 4

Community Health Assessment for Program Planning

This chapter provides an overview of needs assessment with full acknowledgment that, as with many aspects of program planning and evaluation, it is an area of specialization.

The goal of a needs assessment is to guide and inform decisions related to program prioritization and development. Basically, a needs assessment is a procedure used to collect data that describe the needs and strengths of a specific group, community, or population. To simplify the language, "needs assessment" is used in this chapter as a broad term that encompasses both the deficit and asset perspectives. Also, the term "target audience" is used rather than "target population" as a way to denote that those for whom a program is intended audience may be a unit other than a true population. The intended audiences can be a group (a relatively small set of individuals who interact), a community, a neighborhood, an aggregate (a set of individuals who share one characteristic in common, such as a school or a health condition), or a complete population. One of the first tasks in planning and conducting a needs assessment is to determine who is likely to make up the target audience and in what larger unit they are situated. As a basis for planning the needs assessment, it is first important to have a solid understanding of "needs."

TYPES OF NEEDS

There are four types of needs (Bradshaw, 1972) that ought to be considered in a needs assessment. Understanding the characteristics of each type of need as it relates to the population of interest is critical to successful health program planning. One type of need is the *expressed* need—that is, the need expressed by behavior. Expressed need is manifested as the demand for services and the market behavior of the target audience. It is measured as the number of people who show up for services as well as in utilization rates. *Normative* need is a lack, deficit, or inadequacy as defined by experts and health professionals, usually based on some scientific notion of what ought to be or what the ideal is from a health perspective. The normative need can be viewed as similar to an etic perspective, or the view through the eyes of an observer. The third type of need is the need as felt or *perceived* by the target audience. Perceived needs include their wants, what they say they want, and their preferences. The perceived need is similar to an emic perspective, or the view through the eyes of the one having the experience. Finally, there is the comparative or *relative* need, which is the identified gap between advantaged and disadvantaged groups. Relative need entails a comparison that demonstrates a difference that is interpreted as one group having a need relative to the other group.

The ways in which the interaction of these needs plays out in day-to-day situations are seen in the experiences of one group that conducted a community needs assessment in a fictitious town called Layetteville. In conducting their assessment, they identified a neighborhood as having a relative need. They found that the neighborhood had higher rates of adolescent pregnancy, deaths due to gunshot injuries, birth defects, and diabetes than other neighborhoods in the city, and that these rates were two to three times greater than those set out in *Healthy People 2000*. When the group explored the health care utilization patterns of the residents of the neighborhood, they found that the residents rarely used a primary health care clinic; instead they used the local emergency department. Confident in their understanding of what was needed to improve the health of the neighborhood, the group approached the residents with a plan to establish a primary care clinic in the neighborhood that would provide prenatal care and diabetes management. Bluntly, the residents indicated that they were not interested. They wanted a community swimming pool in their neighborhood. They felt a strong need for recreation, a community meeting place, and an equal opportunity to engage in the healthy behavior of swimming as an alternative to the gang activities that were contributing to the shootings. Only after those conducting the assessment agreed to address the community's perceived need for a community swimming pool did the residents then consider how to address the normative, comparative, and relative needs that had been identified.

PERSPECTIVES ON ASSESSMENT

Four different types of models exist for conducting a needs assessment: the epidemiological model, the public health model, the social model, and the asset model. Each has its intellectual perspective, as well as advantages and disadvantages (Exhibit 4.1). Nonetheless, each model has a role in health needs assessment.

Exhibit 4.1   A Comparison of the Four Dominant Models of Community Needs Assessment.

	Epidemiological Models	Public Health Models	Social Models	Asset Models
Population Assessed	Populations	States and communities	Populations, selected aggregates	Community, neighborhoods
Data Sources	Registries, national probability sample surveys, existing national databases	State and local agencies, vital records	Individual surveys, national surveys	Rosters of agencies, focus groups, maps
Examples	National Health Interview Survey (NHIS), Health Care Utilization Profile (HCUP)	APEXPH, PATCH, MAPP	US Census	The Assets-Based Community Development Institute [http://www.northwestern.edu/ipr/abcd.html (accessed 8/15/03)]
Types of Needs Assessed	Normative, expressed, and relative needs can be estimated	Normative and relative needs can be estimated	Relative need can be estimated, perceived need is directly determined	Perceived need, perceived strengths
Advantages	Statistically sound and generalizable findings	Administratively sound; includes focus on constituent concerns	Statistically sound; provides information on factors contributing to health problem	Existing resources are identified
Disadvantages	No information on perceived needs; local variations may not be captured or described	Relies on other data sources; perceived needs not directly determined	Does not directly measure extent of health problem	Does not measure extent of health problem

Epidemiological Model

Epidemiological models of needs assessment focus on quantifying health problems, using national data sets and applying epidemiological methods and statistics. These models seek to answer the questions: What is the magnitude of the problem? What trends are evident? What patterns of selectivity are exhibited in the distribution of the problem? Is the problem preventable? How treatable is the problem? and What is currently being done? Epidemiological models often include a focus on identifying hazards, risks, and precursors to the health problem.

Examples of tools used in epidemiological models are disease and death registries and national probability sample surveys such as the National Health Information Survey (NHIS) and the National Health and Nutritional Examination Survey (NHANES). The advantage of the epidemiological models is that they provide data for assigning relative weights to the seriousness of a health problem, the importance of that health problem, and its prevalence. However, the epidemiological models do not provide a breadth of data that might also be key in prioritizing health problems.

Public Health Model

Public health models are focused on quantifying health problems for the purpose of prioritizing the identified health problems being addressed with limited resources. Public health models seek to answer the questions, What is the seriousness of the problem? What is the distribution of the problem? What is the perceived importance of the problem? and What resources are available to address the problem?

Public health approaches to needs assessment typically rely on existing data and epidemiological data. In addition, specific tools or models used in the public health approach to needs assessment are the APEXPH, PATCH, and MAPP. These models, reviewed in Chapter 3 as planning tools, provide a framework for determining what types of data ought to be collected as part of the needs assessment. There is considerable overlap between these models and the epidemiological approach to needs assessment. While these models are fairly comprehensive, they are weak in their consideration of the sociocultural aspects of health.

Social Model

Social models of needs assessment focus on quantifying characteristics that contribute to the socioeconomic and political context that may affect the health of individuals. Social models seek to answer the questions, What is the relationship among health problems and social characteristics? What social trends are evident? What is the relationship between the use of social and health resources and the problem? and How have social and health policies affected the magnitude, distribution, or trends of the problem?

Key characteristics of a social model needs assessment are a focus on collecting data regarding social characteristics, such as income, and on collecting data from specific aggregates about specific social and economic topics. The collection of specific information is done through national household surveys, such as the US Census. The value of a social model approach has been reflected in various studies. For example, Sherman, Gillespie, and Diaz (1996) looked at a set of social indicators in terms of their ability to predict resident use of treatment programs. They found that they were able to accurately predict the level of use based on the social indicators. Such studies reinforce the value of having data social indicators as part of a needs assessment. In health care, reliance on social indicators alone as a sole basis for program planning is not acceptable. However, the social models of assessment do generate crucial information that might help identify determinants or prior conditions leading to the health problems.

Asset Model

A fourth perspective on needs assessment is the asset model, which focuses on the strengths, assets, abilities, and resources that exist and are available, rather than focusing on the needs, deficits, lacks, and gaps between the healthy and the ill. Asset models seek to answer the questions, What social and health resources exist within the community experiencing the health problem? What do community members view as strengths and resources within their community? and To what extent are the resources mobilized or mobilizable to address health problems? The resources that individuals collectively have in the form of their social networks are called social capital. An asset model assessment would include an inventory of the social capital within the community experiencing the health problem. This perspective is aligned with the older view of health in which environment is one of four forces either fostering health or leading to illnesses (Blum, 1981; Dever, 1980). Blum (1982), in discussing considerations related to risk reduction, used the force field perspective to suggest that both forces that lead to risk conditions and forces that lead to risk minimization need to be considered. He suggested it as a way to organize areas to be assessed.

The asset models also incorporate the older concept of community competence (Cottrell, 1976; Goeppinger, Lassiter, & Wilcox, 1982). Community competence is the process whereby a community is able to identify problems and take actions to address those problems, and it is increased by community organizing (Denham, Quinn, & Gamble, 1998). Community competence has been associated with the health of the community as well as with social capital (Lochner, Kawachi, & Kennedy, 1999).

The asset perspective on community assessment seeks to identify and then build on the capabilities of a community in order to resolve health issues. Although the asset models have some appeal, especially to community stakeholders, gathering asset data can be problematic and challenging. There is no generally accepted set of asset indicators that can be used. Also, rarely does asset information exist at the time of the assessment, making data collection necessary. These disadvantages contribute to the asset models being less widely used as a sole approach to needs assessment, and they are poorly integrated into the more widely used models of needs assessment.

TYPES OF ASSESSMENTS

Before initiating a full-scale needs assessment, planners and planning groups need to be familiar with assessment as a process. This process begins by studying available data in order to gain a working knowledge of the community and the prevalent health problems. The familiarization assessment, as it is called, is a starting point from which to consider whether more data are needed and whether to proceed with conducting a larger-scale needs assessment. It is possible that a local agency has already done a needs assessment that might be adequate for the task at hand. Thus, becoming familiar with the community, the health problem, and existing assessments can save time and efforts. If it appears that an assessment is needed, there are four generic types of assessments that may need to be done: an organizational assessment, a marketing assessment, a needs assessment, and a community health assessment.

Organizational Assessment

An organizational assessment is done to determine the strengths, weaknesses, opportunities, and threats to the organization providing the health program. In the PRECEDE-PROCEED model (Green & Kreuter, 1991), widely used by health educators, an organizational assessment is viewed as a key component in planning health educational interventions. While an organizational assessment can be thought of as part of the logistics planning for a health program, it is critical to have a good sense of the organizational willingness and capabilities to provide a program for the health problem under consideration *before* planning proceeds. Thus, this type of assessment seeks to answer the question, What is the capability and willingness of the organization to provide the health program?

Data for an organizational assessment are gathered from members of the organization, as well as from existing organizational records and documents. The data help determine the organizational feasibility of providing the health program—that is, whether there are adequate and appropriate resources and whether the health program fits with the organization's mission and goals. One aspect of the organizational assessment is the assessment of human resources within the organization, with particular regard to meeting the needs identified in the community needs assessment. The organizational assessment can also identify changes needed within the organization as a prerequisite to providing the health program. In this way, the organizational assessment provides critical information for developing internal strategies to assure the success of the health program.

Marketing Assessment

Just as understanding the needs and assets of a target audience is key in program planning, it is equally important to understand the extent to which the target audience would be interested in the health program. Although market assessment is usually considered a part of actual program planning, marketing assessment data can be collected at the same time as the needs assessment data. This type of assessment seeks to answer the question, What will draw the target audience into the program? Typical market analyses, such as those conducted in businesses, differ from marketing assessments for health programs in several ways. As will be discussed in Chapter 7, in health programs, basic marketing concepts are adapted to reflect the social and behavioral focus of the programs. In addition, the price and packaging aspects that are addressed in marketing assessments play different roles in health programs. The key data that need to be collected in a marketing assessment are about competitive programs (available community resources) and overall interest in the intended program. Incorporating the marketing assessment into any early assessment activities minimizes lost opportunities to collect key data and helps to provide a more complete assessment of the conditions that are affecting both services utilization and health outcomes.

Needs Assessment

A needs assessment, in the more narrowly defined, traditional sense, is the means by which to determine the gaps, lacks, and wants relative to a defined population and a defined, specific health problem. Data from a needs assessments help to identify goals, products, problems, or conditions that the health program should address (Herman, Morris, & Fitz-Gibbon, 1987). In this way, it is a starting point for planning, implementing, and evaluating a program (Scriven & Roth, 1990). A needs assessment provides health-related information necessary to gauge priorities to be given to health problems, and helps identify the trade-offs of addressing one health problem over another. Often a needs assessment is done in order to answer the question, What health problems exist, and to what extent? Findings from the needs assessment help identify health problems or conditions that should be addressed in future health programs. In other words, it provides data necessary for program development, specifically what health interventions are needed, where, and with what target audience. A needs assessment helps make decisions more defendable and acceptable to the stakeholders. It results in the flow of money and effort to meet the needs of the target audience.

Typically, a needs assessment is problem oriented and begins with a stated health problem about which more information is wanted or needed. Also falling into the category of needs assessment is the community as a subsystem deserving of specific assessment. Sometimes more detailed information is needed about one aspect of a community. A needs assessment focused on one community can provide such information.

Community Health Assessment

A community health assessment is used to establish the magnitude of selected health problems in a selected community, neighborhood, or other designated locality relative to the strengths and resources within that community, and to determine the priority the community gives to addressing the health problem. A community health assessment casts a broad net, encompassing all aspects of the community. It includes assessing health and human service resources and assets, as well as the health problem and other community weaknesses. This type of assessment seeks to answer the question, What are the health problems, and what resources are available to address those health problems? In this sense, a community health assessment encompasses and integrates each of the four assessment models described here. From this integrative perspective, the remainder of the chapter focuses on conducting a community health assessment.

STEPS IN CONDUCTING THE ASSESSMENT

There is no one way to conduct nor is there one right way to conduct a community health assessment. There are, however, basic steps that are included in any approach to a community health assessment, including involving community members in the development and execution of the community assessment. The first step is to define the community or population to be assessed, followed by making decisions about what data to collect regarding the nature of the health problem, such as the magnitude of the problem, precursors to the health problem, and demographic and behavioral characteristics. The next step is to collect the data, using a variety of data sources and approaches. Once the data have been collected, the next step is to analyze the data using statistical procedures to arrive at statistical statements about the health problems in the population. Based on the data and the statistics, the final stage is to develop a summary statement of the need or the problem that ties together the contributing, antecedent, and determinant factors of the health problem with the hampering and asset factors that counter the existence of the health problem.

Involve Community Members

Ideally, before starting a community health assessment, the planners will devote time to developing a strategy for involving members of the community to be assessed. The involvement of those likely to be targeted by a program stems from a philosophy of empowerment as well as a practical concern with stakeholder and consumer reactions to the data. From the philosophical perspective of empowerment, involvement by community members enhances their capacity as well as their ownership of the data and results. This theme of involvement is carried throughout the phases of planning and evaluating a health program.

From a practical perspective, involving those likely to be affected by the assessment has immediate and direct consequences for how the community health assessment evolves. For example, the strong views and bias of any one group can become evident during the planning of the assessment. Program planners can then begin to anticipate how those views will influence the interpretation of the data. By involving the groups in the community health assessment, planners can uncover, acknowledge, and, hopefully, address their concerns.

Involving community members is rarely easy. Barriers to involvement must be overcome. These barriers are varied: time constraints on busy individuals, competing interests for available time, parking problems, limited accessibility of the meeting location, lack of awareness of the opportunity for involvement, feelings of inadequacy or insecurity about being involved, or lack of day care. There is no one best way to increase involvement by community members. Multiple strategies are needed, and these are likely to evolve as the community health assessment proceeds. In addition to strategies that specifically address various barriers, other strategies to increase involvement can include obtaining names of key individuals from agency personnel, providing food as an incentive, providing informal training or skills related to being involved, having specific tasks in which individuals can be involved, or having regularly scheduled meeting dates and times.

There are, however, times when it may not be wise to focus on involving community members: when there are severe time constraints on completing the community health assessment, when there are severe fiscal constraints, when profound allegiances exist that would affect the quality of interactions among community members, or when insufficient leadership skills exist to initiate and sustain community involvement. There are also times when community members must be involved in the community health assessment: when there is a mandate from a funding agency for community involvement, when doing so will reduce the perception of being excluded, when insiders' connections and perceptions are needed in order to have a complete community health assessment, or when the goal is to have the community be responsible for sustained implementation of the health program.

Define the Population

Delineating who is to be assessed is a first step in conducting a community health assessment. The question of who to assess is often influenced by who is doing the assessment. The who can be delineated geographically, enabling the population of interest to be defined by a site, such as workplace, location of residence, or school. Locality as the defining characteristic is common, and often zip code areas, census tracts, community areas, or legal boundaries are used to define who is assessed. A state health department or a state health program will focus on the state population, whereas a small, local, not-for-profit agency is likely to focus only on individuals who are potential customers. For example, the Traditional Indian Alliance in Tucson serves only Tucson's American Indian population. Not surprisingly, its needs assessment was very limited both in terms of geography and population segment (Evaneshko, 1999). In contrast, a United Way organization in a large metropolitan area will assess the health and social needs of the population in its catchment area.

Using highly specific parameters to define who allows the assessment to be more encompassing and detailed. For example, work-site needs assessments, such as that done by Phillips and Belcher (1999), yield data on a range of employee risk factors for health conditions, some of which are not related to the workplace. The data from their work-site assessment enabled them to develop work-site health promotion programs that addressed both work-site and other health risks. This example shows that defining who by a narrowly defined location may be a convenient means to access a population, obtain detailed information, and very specifically tailor a health program.

In program planning and evaluation, those for whom the program or intervention is designed and intended—in other words, those who are targeted by the program—are referred to as the *target audience. Target population* is used if the program is intended for an entire population, rather than a subpopulation. The target audience thus includes all potential participants. Those who actually receive the program or intervention are referred to as the *recipient audience.* Thinking about this distinction between target and recipients helps clarify who ought to be included in the community health assessment: basically, both groups should be included, and the target audience encompasses the potential recipients. The parameters used to distinguish individuals for whom the program or intervention is intended from individuals for whom it is not intended become the *boundaries of the target population.* The target audience is usually some portion of the *population at risk*—in other words, individuals who have some social, physical, or other condition that increases their likelihood of an undesirable health problem or state. The term "at high risk" is usually reserved for those individuals with the highest probability of having an undesirable heath state or outcome.

One aspect of conducting a community health assessment is that the boundaries of the target audience are likely to change with the collection and analysis of the data. For example, when the assessment is begun, an entire neighborhood or community area is viewed as the target audience. As epidemiological data and asset data are analyzed and interpreted, the planners may realize that only the black elderly, or white adolescents, or working mothers are at high risk for a health problem that can be addressed by the organization. This evolution of who from the broad boundaries to a refined definition of the target audience is what ought to occur as a result of the community health assessment.

Define the Problem(s) to be Assessed

Just as the who of a community health assessment evolves with the collection of information, the what is also likely to evolve. It may be that the purpose of the community health assessment is to identify the breadth of the health problems that exist within a community, as is likely with an agency such as United Way. The purpose of a community health assessment might also be to identify particular aspects of a health problem or condition that already has a high priority for being addressed. For example, the Centers for Disease Control and Prevention (CDC) funds health promotion programs designed to reduce racial and ethnic disparities with regard to diabetes, cardiovascular diseases, infant mortality, HIV/AIDS, and immunizations. An agency wishing to compete for CDC funds would need to identify, within a community with racial or ethnic disparities, specific needs and assets relative to one of those five health problems.

To understand the health problem and come to a definition of the health problem or condition, it is necessary to collect data. Baker and Reinke (1988) suggest that from an epidemiological perspective, four categories of information need to be collected as a prelude to health planning: the magnitude of the problem, the precursors of the problem, population characteristics, and attitudes and behaviors. These four categories are used in community health assessment, albeit expanded to include considerations from the public health, social, and asset perspectives.

Magnitude of the Problem

One category of information needed is the magnitude of the problem. The magnitude can be described in terms of the extent of the disease or health condition, whether the problem is acute or chronic, and the intensity of the problem. The extent of the health problem is described in terms of incidence and prevalence. The *incidence* is the rate at which new cases occur. The *prevalence* is the extent to which cases currently exist in a population. Incidence and prevalence, while usually used in reference to disease conditions, can be used to think about behaviors as well. For example, the number of new smokers among a defined group of adolescents (incidence) and the percentage of that same adolescent population that is currently smoking (prevalence) provide information that can be used to determine whether smoking is a problem of sufficient magnitude to warrant attention. The ability to obtain accurate rates and proportions depends, in part, on the quality of the tests used to identify cases. Ideal tests have both high *sensitivity*, the extent to which there are no false negatives, and high *specificity*, the extent to which there are no false positives. Sensitivity and specificity are often used in reference to medical tests, such as occult blood tests, mammography, or urine tests for cocaine use, but they are also important characteristics of psychological and behavioral measures, such as the CES-D that measures the level of depression in an individual (Radloff, 1977) or the SF-36 that measures overall health and functioning (Ware, 2000; Ware et al., 1995). The sensitivity and specificity of medical tests as well as of psychological or behavioral measures influence the accuracy of estimating the magnitude of a health problem or condition within a population.

Precursors of the Problem

Another category of data is information about the precursors of the health problem or condition. Precursors can be thought of as the physical or contextual antecedents, as well as the determinants of the health condition. *Antecedents* to the health condition are those elements that must be present in order for the health problem to come into existence. Thus, antecedents can include factors such as genetic predisposition, being in the right place at the right time, prior exposure and vulnerability, or legal or policy conditions. From an asset perspective, antecedents might also include factors such as the political clout of the local representatives or the existence of economic empowerment zones. *Determinants* are those elements that influence whether the health problem will manifest, given the antecedents. Depending on the health problem, determinants might include factors such as exposure to the health hazard, susceptibility, or the virulence of the hazard. From an asset perspective, determinants might include factors such as health knowledge, the existence of healthy food choices in local grocery stores, the existence of environmental pollutants, the existence of road safety features (intersection lights), or the accessibility and availability of local health and social service agencies.

From a public health perspective, a health problem also has contributing factors. *Contributing factors* are those elements that have the potential to either exaggerate or lessen the presence of the health problem. Again, depending on the health problem, contributing factors might be laws and policies or social support. The contributing factors are more likely to directly affect the health problem than the more immediate health indicators that will be addressed by the health program. Complex and interacting relationships exist among antecedents, determinants, and contributing factors. In Exhibit 4.2 the determinants, antecedents, and contributing factors that both hamper and cause health problems are given for four different health problems.

Although the model of determinants, antecedents, and contributing factors is used throughout this text, it is important to acknowledge that a strong epidemiological model does exist and is used widely for infectious diseases and injuries. From an epidemiological perspective, the precursors to a health problem are understood in terms of agent, host, and environment. Haddon (1972), in studying childhood injuries, developed a model for integrating those epidemiological factors with the determinant and contributing factors to a health problem—namely

Exhibit 4.2   Determinant, Antecedent, and Contributing Factors for Four Health Problems (Layetteville Example)

Health Problem	Health Indicator	Determinant Cause	Determinant Hampering Factor	Antecedent Cause	Antecedent Hampering Factor	Contributing Cause	Contributing Hampering Factor
Intentional handgun injuries	Rate of gun-shot wounds	Availability of handguns	Laws regulating handgun sales	Gang presence	Visibility of religious leaders	Unemployment rates	High school completion rates
Birth defects	Rate of neural tube defects	Folic acid, genetics, environmental hazards	Eating habits (nutrition), genetic counseling	Age, culture	Prenatal care, knowledge about folic acid	Paternal factor	Food availability
Adolescent pregnancy	Rate of adolescent pregnancy	Sexual activity	Use of birth control methods	Peer pressure	Knowledge and self-efficacy	Media messages	Family support
Diabetes	Prevalence of type II diabetes	Physiological processes	Specific health behaviors	Heredity	Knowledge about prevention	Inadequate medical supervision	Safe place to exercise, walk

the human, physical, environmental, and sociocultural factors. Exhibit 4.3 is based on Haddon's model, but with the addition of the health care system as another element in analyzing the health problem or condition. Each cell of the table contains either a definition of what might go in that cell or a few examples. For any single health problem that is the focus of a needs assessment, data can be placed into the cells in Exhibit 4.3, thus giving an overview and a preliminary analysis of precursors to the health problem or condition. This format, while

Exhibit 4.3 Haddon's Typology for Analyzing an Event, Modified for Use in Developing Health Promotion and Prevention Programs, with Examples of Possible Factors

Stage	Agent Factors	Human Factors	Physical Environment	Sociocultural Environment	Health System Environment
Pre-event	Latency	Genetic makeup, motivation, knowledge	Proximity, transportation, availability of agent (i.e., alcohol or drugs)	Norms, policy and laws, cultural beliefs about causes, family dynamics	Accessibility, availability, acceptability
Event (Behavior)	Virulence, addictiveness, difficulty of behavior	Susceptibility, vulnerability, hardiness, reaction	Force	Peer pressure	Iatrogenic factors, treatments
Post-event	Resistance to treatment	Motivation, resilience, time for recovery	Proximity, availability of agent (i.e., alcohol or drugs)	Meaning of event, attribution of causality, sick role	Resources and services, treatment options, emergency response

Adapted from Haddon, W., Jr. (1972). A logical framework for categorizing highway safety phenomena and activity. *Journal of Trauma, 12,* 193–207. Cited in Grossman, D.C. (2000). The history of injury control and the epidemiology of child and adolescent injuries. *The Future of Children, 10,*(1) 23–52.

useful for some health problems, particularly for pathogens and injuries, demonstrates the complexity of data that might need to be analyzed in order to understand the health problem or condition.

Population Characteristics

Population characteristics data, the third category of necessary information, relates mainly to the social model of needs assessments. It involves collecting data on characteristics, such as distribution of age categories, income levels, educational levels, and occupations within a community. However, if the who has been narrowly defined in terms of location—say, a prison—the population characteristics can be very specific. Prison inmate characteristics, such as types of crime committed, length of time incarcerated, or race, can become part of the population characteristics data collected for the community (prison) health assessment.

Attitudes and Behaviors

The fourth category of information concerns the attitudes and behaviors of the population being assessed, with particular attention to the attitudes and behaviors of the target audience. Data about attitudes and behaviors help complete or flesh out the description of the antecedents, determinants, and contributing factors in a health problem. Some attitudes and behaviors are antecedents to health problems or conditions. For example, culturally held beliefs about illnesses, illness prevention, and treatments, along with beliefs concerning appropriate health behaviors and the sick role can be viewed as antecedents. Other lifestyle behaviors contribute to the existence of health problems. For example, secondhand smoke contributes to childhood asthma, and regular aerobic exercise contributes to reduced health problems. Still other attitudes and behaviors have a more direct, determinant relationship with health problems. Distrust in medical providers and thus a failure to obtain preventive health services lead directly to severe morbidity conditions in some populations. In other words, attitudes toward health promotion and disease prevention behaviors must be considered as well as attitudes toward health care services and providers in order to have a complete community health assessment.

Collect Data: Approaches

Numerous types and sources of data are used in a community health assessment. Each has the potential to contribute to an understanding of the parameters of the health problem or condition. However, each also has limitations and caveats that need to be considered.

Archival data constitute one type of data, and include medical records and other types of agency records. Archival data can provide information on the demand or need for a source, as well as on the characteristics of program participants. The types and uses of archival data are discussed more fully in Chapter 9. One limitation to archival data is that the data may not include key information that is sought. A potential problem with archival data is its degree of completeness and the extent to which the data were accurately collected initially. These factors will influence the data's overall usefulness and trustworthiness.

Another type of data is public data. Falling into this category are national surveys, vital statistics, and census social indicators. These public data may not be immediately useful but can be used in secondary analyses that enhance the community health assessment. Alcaiti and Glanz (1996) used a wide range of publicly available data in their efforts to develop a cancer control program. Some of the lessons they shared are that the data were useful in making decisions about specific cancers, targeting populations, identifying barriers, and influencing health policy. However, these data sets were not useful in determining which interventions were most effective.

There are also primary data, such as those specifically collected around a need of interest. A wide variety of methods can be used to collect primary data, including interviews, surveys, community forums, focus groups, and interviews with key informants and service providers.

Sullivan, Basta, Tan, and Davidson (1992) interviewed women in a domestic violence shelter. The information gained from the program participants was useful in informing future programs for women who had experienced domestic violence. However, data from participants in a program are rarely used as a sole source of data for a community health assessment. While the program participants can provide valuable insights into the perceived needs of the target audience, that information needs to be considered in light of the fact that the participants are already in the program. This makes them potentially dissimilar to those targeted by the program. Campbell, Sengupta, Santos, and Lorig (1995) used a balanced incomplete block design to collect information from program participants and found the method readily applicable to a needs assessment. Their study highlights that a high level of attention and rigor can be used to collect needs assessment data from program participants.

Providers are another source of data, and can be interviewed for their perspective on the needs of a target audience. For example, Ford, Young, Perez, Orermeyere, and Rohner (1992) surveyed community mental health case managers to assess the needs of their clients. The case managers reported that clients needed medication monitoring, therapy, and day and vocational activities. Although these data are useful in identifying specific service needs of the target population, the information must be viewed as revealing the normative needs only. That is, providers are notorious for having views of what is needed that differ from the views of their clients. An interesting example of this dichotomy is seen in the findings of Donath (2000), who found that people were significantly less likely to consider themselves overweight than their body mass index (BMI), a normative measure used by providers, would indicate. In addition, providers are seeing only those individuals who are accessing the programs, again giving a potentially biased picture of needs. Making program development decisions based only on provider data is likely to result in programs that are not attractive to the intended audience. However, in terms of having organizational needs assessment data, providers are critical. One technique for collecting data from providers is to use focus groups. Siden (1998) used focus groups of providers to assess the need for a telehealth link between a local and tertiary care medical center. The focus group themes yielded insights into the views and opinions of the providers that shaped the design of the program.

Another possible source of data is proprietary data sources—in other words, data that are owned by an organization and can be purchased for use. The American Hospital Association, the American Medical Association, and health insurance companies own databases about their members that can contain information needed for a comprehensive community health assessment. Like archival data, the information that can be gained from proprietary data is limited to what has already been collected.

A case study is yet another potential source of data for a community health assessment. Case studies involve multiple sources and types of data that are descriptive of one or more specifically selected cases, whether the case is a clinic, a program, or an individual. Although they are time intensive, case studies about health agencies, communities, or community action groups may be constructed as a part of a community health assessment. Their advantage is that they provide comprehensive information, although it may not be generalizable to the current situation. Case study methodology is discussed in greater detail in Chapter 12.

Unobtrusive (Webb, Cambell, Schwartz, & Sechrest, 2000) or nonreactive (Webb, Campbell, Schwartz, Sechrest, & Grove, 1981) measures are another source of data. These sources of data are particularly relevant to community characteristics. For example, walking around a neighborhood and observing how many blocks have abandoned buildings or storefront churches are unobtrusive measures. Going through the garbage to count the number of liquor bottles, counting the number of billboard advertisements for unhealthy behaviors, estimating the ratio of bars and pubs to banks, watching the interactions among residents in a local bakery, and collecting local community newspapers are all examples of data collection of the least invasive nature. Each of these examples provides some clues to the character, strengths, and problems in the community unit as a whole. The use of unobtrusive measures is inexpensive and can provide interesting clues about the antecedents and contributing factors to the health problem.

Finally, but not of least importance, the published literature is an excellent source of information, particularly for determining relative and normative needs. It is an inexpensive, reliable source of information that ought not be overlooked in a community needs assessment.

In addition to the various existing and collectable sources of data, it can be important to collect data from sources that are not readily available. This is called "going beyond the street lamp," which derives its name from a little story. One night, a drunk lost his keys. He began to look for them, crawling around on his hands and knees beneath a street lamp. Before long, a stranger stopped and asked the man what he was doing on his hands and knees. He replied that he was looking for his keys. The stranger offered to help and asked where he had lost his keys. The drunk replied, "Over there," pointing to a dark area down the block just outside the bar. So the stranger asked, "Then why are you looking over here?" To which the drunk replied, "Because there is light over here." In other words, the information you need may not be the same as the data to which you already have access. You need to go beyond the street lamp. Some of the sources of data just described are available under the street lamp, and others are not available and will require primary data collection. What determines the extent to which data need to be collected from beyond the street lamp are factors such as time constraints, fiscal resources, level of expertise, and endorsement or expectations of those who will be using the community health assessment.

Collect Data: Methodological Issues

When collecting any type of data, one must address several factors in order to enhance the quality of the data collected. These methodological issues are discussed here in the context of conducting a community health assessment, rather than within the more typical research framework.

First of all, when one is attempting to uncover what is occurring, there is a temptation to ask those experiencing the problem to provide information about the problem. As was mentioned earlier, the trouble with this approach is that those receiving services may be systematically different from those not receiving services. Also, there are likely to be latent needs that are not uncovered, meaning that some needs may not be manifested in an easily recognizable form. Going back to the earlier example of the community that wanted a swimming pool, there was a latent need to have an inequity addressed, as manifested in their perceived need for recreational opportunities.

Another methodological problem is that asking a question has the potential to bias the answer. In other words, when asked about their needs, community members may take the opportunity to express all kinds of frustrations, wants, and needs. In addition, asking about needs, problems, and deficits does not allow for understanding the assets, strengths, potential, resources, and capabilities. Thus, data collection methods are best designed to enable the collection of data that would fall on both sides of the equation.

Community health assessments can take up to a year to accomplish, particularly if the assessment is comprehensive in scope and involves community members in the process. Time constraints are a reality that can heavily influence both the quality and quantity of data collected. Realistic strategies and designs for collecting data must match the timelines; otherwise, only partial data will be collected and will most likely be imbalanced in nature.

As was mentioned earlier, the measures used to collect data must adhere to scientifically rigorous standards. The instruments used must have validity and reliability. *Validity* is the degree to which the instrument measures what is intended to be measured. *Reliability* is the degree to which the instrument will yield the same results with different samples. Epidemiological measures, such as mortality, have high validity; death is rarely misdiagnosed. However, the underlying cause of death as reported on the death certificate is prone to both validity and reliability problems. The validity problems stem from conceptual issues of whether the cause of death ought to be the immediate or underlying cause. The reliability problems involve how the death certificate was completed and coded. Similarly, other epidemiological measures, such as adequacy of prenatal care, have been questioned with regard to validity and reliability. In terms of conducting a community health assessment, the point is that no data are perfect, and the imperfections can lead to inaccurate numbers and hence faulty program planning decisions. Therefore, the user should openly discuss the limits of the data and take reasonable scientific steps to obtain the best data possible.

The issue of determining from whom to collect the community health assessment data will always be important. This is a sampling problem. Sampling is a science, with numerous strategies possible, depending on the degree to which the community health assessment needs to be representative of the entire target population. Epidemiological and social approaches would focus on employing strategies to have individuals included in the sample who look as much as possible like the target audience. However, if primary data are being collected, developing and employing strategies to achieve this can be very costly. Less expensive, but also less scientifically rigorous, sampling strategies are possible. (Sampling strategies are reviewed in Chapter 10.) The underlying decision that needs to be made is how important it is to be able to describe the population with a high degree of accuracy, based on data from less than the entire population.

An overarching concern is the cultural appropriateness of the data collection methods and the cultural competence of the data collectors and interpreters. As was discussed in Chapter 2, culture, language, and ethnicity influence the responses of individuals to survey questions.

One other issue is the need to have community-level indicators—that is, data about the community rather than data about individuals that are aggregated by the community. For example, daily intake of fat is an individual-level indicator, and an average of percentage of daily intake based on all residents in the community is still an individual-level indicator. The percentage of grocery store shelf space allocated to low-fat foods is a community-level indicator. The percentage of workers at a work site who smoke is an individual-level indicator, but the number of anti-smoking posters or announcements in the work site is a work-site-level measure. There are very few ready sources of measures or indicators of aggregates such as work sites or communities. It takes creativity, working with the community members, and careful consideration to develop community-level indicators and then to reliably collect data. But it is worth the effort. For many of the health problems targeted by health promotion or disease prevention programs, what exists in the community will be extremely important as a component of assessing the antecedents, determinants, and contributing factors to the health problems.

Using the community-level data, planners can develop community-level interventions. Community-level interventions may sometimes be necessary when interventions at the individual level need to be reinforced with community-level changes. For example, Fikree, Khan, Kadir, Sagan, and Rahbar (2001) suggested that to increase the use of family planning methods, community-level interventions are needed, such as engaging religious leaders in family planning programs or encouraging outreach efforts by community outreach workers. Only by collecting community-level data as part of the community health assessment can planners identify community-level interventions that are relevant to addressing the health problem.

In summary, there are five "principles" of collecting data for a community health assessment. One, collect data from more than one source. In other words, use multiple methods and multiple sources, and be multicultural. Two, involve members of the community in the design and collection of the community health data: be inclusive and be empowering. Three, give full disclosure and then get informed consent from individuals from whom data are being collected: be forthright, be honest, and be safe. Four, go beyond the street lamp and collect data from unlikely but enlightening sources: be creative, be inventive, and be open. Finally, be as scientifically rigorous as time and other resources allow: be scholarly, be interdisciplinary, and be systematic.

Analyze Numeric Data

Given that most community health assessments involve some population-based data, it is worth reviewing basic epidemiological techniques. More complete and in-depth presentations are available in traditional epidemiology textbooks, such as the one by Mausner and Baum (1974). For a direct application of epidemiology to community health assessment, Dever's (1980) book is a classic. However, the more recent publications by Dever (1997) and by Fos and Fine (2000) also cover basic epidemiological techniques, but from the point of view of health care executives planning for population health. Health program planners would do well to have at least one text like this on the shelf for quick reference. With the widespread availability of computer spreadsheet and database programs, the calculation of most statistics is less a matter of doing the math and more a matter of understanding which numbers to use and how to make sense of the numbers generated by the software. This section on statistical tests is not intended to be comprehensive but to show how and when to use specific statistics in the community health assessment.

Descriptive and Inferential Statistics

Descriptive statistics provide an amazing wealth of information. The simplest descriptive statistic is the frequency or count of occurrences. Based on the frequency, other very informative and simple descriptive statistics can be calculated—namely the average, a measure of central tendency, and the variance or standard deviation, measures of dispersion. Graphical displays of frequency that are commonly used include the bar graph and line graph. A bar graph of frequencies provides a rough picture of the distribution and thus reveals whether there is something approximating a normal curve in the data. The standard deviation is related to the range of values in the data and thus indicates the dispersion of the data. Remember that 68.3% of data are contained within one standard deviation, 95.5% within two standard deviations, and 99.7% within three standard deviations.

Descriptively, the magnitude of a problem is conveyed in measures such as rates and proportions. In epidemiological terms, it is a matter of numerators and denominators. The denominator is generally the total number in the population or the total number in the population that is potentially at risk. The numerator is generally the number of individuals who have the health problem or condition or who are actually found to be at risk. With these basic numbers, a wide variety of commonly defined rates and proportions are used in health (Exhibit 4.4). Increasingly, the rates and proportions for various health problems are available online at the websites for local and state health departments and federal agencies, such as the National Center for Health Statistics, housed within the CDC. Descriptive statistics easily convey the magnitude of a health problem, as well as provide relative need information.

Exhibit 4.4   Table of Numerators and Denominators for Selected Rates Commonly Used in Community Health Assessments

Rate	Numerator	Denominator	Per
Crude death rate	Total number of deaths in a given time period	Total population	1,000
Cause-specific death rate	Number of deaths due to a specific cause in a given time period	Total population	100,000
Birth rate	Number of live births in a given time period	Total population	1,000
Fetal death rate	Number of fetal deaths of 28 weeks' gestation or more that occur in a given time period	Number of fetal deaths of 28 weeks' gestation or more plus number of live births that occur in a given time period	1,000
Neonatal death rate	Number of deaths of infants 28 days old or less that occur in a given time period	Number of live births that occur in a given time period	1,000
Infant mortality rate	Number of infants (from birth to 1 year of age) who died in a year	Number of births in a year	1,000

Inferential statistics are those that allow for estimating the extent to which the data gathered from a sample are like the data that would represent the whole population. They allow us to know the probability that our sample mean is similar to the true population mean. In statistical language the standard error is used to determine whether our sample mean is within one or more standard deviations of the true mean. Most of the statistical tests reviewed in Chapter 11 are inferential in nature. Inferential statistics would be used in community health assessments to determine whether one group was statistically different from another group with respect, say, to income or number of emergency department visits.

The statistical tests that help estimate the likelihood of having or getting a given health problem are the odds ratio (OR) and the relative risk (RR). Relative risk is calculated as the cumulative incidence in the exposed population divided by the cumulative incidence in the unexposed population. It compares two cumulative incidences, thus providing a direct comparison of the probabilities. This makes RR preferable over OR (Handler, Rosenberg, Kennelly, & Monahan, 1998). Relative risk ranges from 1.0 to 0.0; the smaller the RR, the greater the association of the health problem with exposure. The OR is calculated as the odds of having the health problem if exposed divided by the odds of having the problem if not exposed. In contrast to the RR, the OR ranges from 0.0 (no association) to 10 or higher; the larger the OR, the more likely one is to have the health problem. The odds ratio does not use the population in the denominator, making it less accurate than the relative risk. However, when the health problem is rare, the OR begins to approximate the RR. Both the RR and OR are used widely in community health assessment. They both convey information about the comparative influence of determinants, antecedents, and contributing factors (all of which would be listed as "exposure") on health outcomes. Having this information allows one to prioritize which of these factors to address in a health program. Often in conducting a community health assessment, planners obtain the OR and RR from published studies because having data on exposure usually requires epidemiological research.

Population Parameters

The statistic that helps planners understand whether the likelihood that the score (mean value) for some health condition that is based on a sample is like the score of the true population is the confidence interval (CI). The CI indicates the range of values between which the value for the true population is likely to fall. Confidence intervals, like standard deviations, provide a level of assurance that the mean value for the variable falls within a given interval. They thus help planners interpret means. For example, if a mean is within the

CI, then the mean falls within a range that is reflective of the larger population. However, if the mean falls outside the CI, then that mean can be viewed as being important for not being reflective of the population. Thus, CIs help during the community health assessment by focusing attention on areas (means) that are unusual and thus merit attention. They also provide a clue as to relative need, in that areas (means) outside the CI are "abnormal" relative to the population.

Tests of Significance

Tests of significance indicate the degree to which the finding would happen just by chance. There are several different types of tests of significance, and which one is used depends upon the nature of the data and on what is being compared. Regardless of which test is used, the interpretation is the same. For example, if a test of significance is reported as <.05, it indicates that there is less than a 5 percent chance of the finding occurring by random chance.

In analyzing community health assessment data, planners might find it critical to know whether the difference between two communities or two groups is just a random variation or whether it is sufficiently large to raise the question of whether something else is contributing to their difference. A test of significance, such as a t test or a z test, depending on the type of data used, would answer the question. To learn whether the difference in the variance of a score between two communities or groups is within a possible random fluctuation, one might use an F test of significance. The various types of tests of significance are covered in basic statistical textbooks. Unlike the CI, these tests say nothing about the relative importance of the finding.

Associations

The statistics that show the degree to which an association exists between a health condition and something else are the family of chi-square statistics. If the information is collected as a nominal variable—that is, in a yes/no format (this includes dead/alive, exposed/not exposed, with/without a health condition)—a chi-square test can be used to estimate the extent to which, if a factor is present, the health condition will also be present. It is based on the classic 2-by-2 table, with the outcomes (yes/no) as the columns and the factors (exposed/not exposed) as the rows. A chi-square statistic does not indicate the strength of the relationship nor the direction of the relationship. The significance of a chi-square, the t score, is interpreted in the same manner as a p value—that is, the degree to which the chi-square would occur by chance. The chi-square tables are easy to understand visually and thus facilitate communicating needs assessment information. Having a significant chi-square between a health outcome and a determinant, antecedent, or contributing factor further helps prioritize the focus of a health program. Calculations of the chi-square require having data to fill all four cells of the 2-by-2 table. Having such data may be beyond the scope of a community health assessment, in which case using published chi-square information is appropriate.

There is another family of statistical tests that show association: correlational analyses, such as Pearson's correlation coefficient and the beta coefficient of regression analyses. These association statistics require that the data have a mean and variance. In other words, data from sources such as surveys are more appropriate for these statistics. For example, if the community health assessment includes survey data, such as reported blood pressure (health problem) and number of days walked (antecedent), then the degree of relationship between walking and blood pressure can be estimated. As with the chi-square, these measures of association do not provide information regarding which came first; having high blood pressure may lead to not having energy to walk, or not walking may lead to having higher blood pressure.

Synthetic Estimates

In reviewing available data, planners may find that data for a specific group or location are lacking, yet it may be important to have some estimate of the magnitude of a health problem for that group. Synthetic estimation is a technique that converts rates or means of a known group into frequencies (counts) that can then be used to calculate an approximate number (count) for the other group (Dever, 1980). For example, the percentage of whites and blacks with diabetes is known for the state but not for the neighborhood included in the community assessment. To estimate the number of whites with diabetes in the neighborhood, you would multiply the percentage of whites statewide with diabetes by the number of whites in the neighborhood. Next, you would multiply the percentage of blacks in the state with diabetes by the number of blacks in the neighborhood. These two synthetic estimates yield the approximate number of blacks and whites in the neighborhood with diabetes. The calculation steps are repeated for each health problem and each group of individuals for whom synthetic estimates are needed. Clearly, synthetic estimates have deficiencies. One is that there is no way to know how accurate they are. Another is that they do not take into account environmental or social factors that can affect the health problem or condition. In addition, synthetic estimates based on a total population are affected by differences within the population characteristics, such as age and race. Nonetheless, in some instances a synthetic estimate gives a hint at whether or not a health problem or condition might warrant further assessment, as well as the relative need of the groups.

Geographic Information Systems: Mapping

Historically, a subcategory of the epidemiological assessment model is the geographic mapping of health problems or population characteristics. With the advent of mapping software, the usual display on maps of the distribution of health problems or conditions can be done not only at the level of state and county but also for a census tract, zip code, or street address. Mapping at very specific levels of geography provides an extremely refined picture of what is where. The same geographic mapping technology can accommodate social data and asset data, thus enabling a more rapid and potentially more interesting analysis of the intersection of needs or problems and resources. One example of using the visual representation of assets in conjunction with a health problem is the development of a map with hospitals overlaid on rates of chronic health conditions. The map reveals that the highest rates of chronic health conditions are in geographic areas with the lowest density of hospitals. Mapping of health problems, determinants, antecedents, and contributing factors provides very engaging information and thus can be crucial in gaining a consensus or attracting the attention of key stakeholders. Mapping, however, does not provide "hard" information, as in statistical evidence of association, importance, or need. It does lend itself to creative thinking that can lead to additional searches for that "hard" data.

Small Numbers

Small numbers are a big problem, whether one is looking at epidemiological data or social data. If a geographic area has a small population (denominator), then a small variation in the occurrence of a health problem (numerator) leads to a large change in the rate or proportion of that health problem. This instability of the rate affects the conclusions that can logically be drawn from the data. Several statistical techniques exist for addressing the small numbers problem, utilizing counts, rates, or proportions (Dever, 1997). One set of these techniques is based on comparing the small area (population) with a larger area (population) or a standard. Another set of techniques is based on comparing two small areas.

Small numbers can also be a problem if the data collected are of a social or qualitative nature, as might be the case in an asset assessment. If the number of respondents to a community survey or the number of participants in a community focus group is small, then the information they provide has a higher likelihood of not being representative of the range of views and opinions in the community. Once data are collected, there is rarely an opportunity to go back and gather more data. Therefore, careful planning and execution of the data collection must be done to avoid having too few respondents.

State the Need or Problem

Data collected for the community health assessment can be organized in terms of a community profile, a wellness profile, a behavioral profile, or a service profile (Paronen & Oje, 1998). Regardless of which format is chosen, the community health assessment ought to lead to some statement of what was found, phrased in such a way that stakeholders, constituents, community members, and multidisciplinary health professionals can understand the health problem. There is no one right way to make the statement; various formats have been proposed and used. Different formats are given here with the intent of demonstrating the potential usefulness and appeal of each. A diagnosis-type formula was suggested by Muecke (1984) as one technique for synthesizing needs assessment data into a statement that can be understood by various health disciplines. Exhibit 4.5 shows the way in which the elements contained in the community health assessment statement are related to both program

Exhibit 4.5   Relationship of Problem Definition to Program Design and Evaluation

Diagnosis:	Problem →	Program →	Evaluation
Risk of:	Health problem or condition	Program goal	Outcome variables
Among:	At-risk population or group, target audience	Recipients	Sample, control and intervention groups
As demonstrated in:	Health indicators	Program objectives	Impact variables
Related to determinants:	Specific characteristics	Interventions or treatments for the target population	Impact evaluation
Secondary to contributing factors and antecedent factors:	Heredity, lifestyle, environmental factors, socioeconomic characteristics	Interventions or treatments for the population at risk	Intervening, mediating, and other confounding variables in impact evaluation

design and program evaluation. It is important to indicate what health indicators or measures were used to identify the health problems. The health indicators will be important later, both in writing program objectives and in determining evaluation measures. The format of the diagnosis-type statement is as follows:

Risk of [*health problem*] among [*population/community*], as demonstrated in [*health indicators*], as related to [*associated characteristics of the community and its environment*].

Note that the population or community is the who of the community health assessment. Using the example of the Layetteville community health assessment described earlier, the statement would read

Risk of *handgun violence* among *residents of Layetteville*, as demonstrated in the *high rate of gunshot injuries at the local hospitals*, as related to the *gang presence and high unemployment*.

This format can be modified to incorporate findings about antecedent, determinant, and contributing factors in place of the associated characteristics. The resulting format, which has more of a public health tone, is as follows:

[*Health problem*] among [*population/community*], as indicated by [*health indicators or measures*], is related to [*determinant factors*], given [*antecedent and contributing factors*].

Continuing with the Layetteville community example, the public health format statement would read

Intentional handgun injuries among *residents of Layetteville*, as indicated by *police reports and rates of emergency room admissions for ICD-9 coded intentional injures*, are related to *availability and use of handguns*, given *gang presence and high unemployment rates* in Layetteville.

Neither of these two formats includes any mention of community assets or strengths. If we consider that assets and resources have the potential to hamper, diminish, or prevent the health problem, then including assets in the community needs assessment statement is key. We thus need to build further on the public health statement format to include factors that both cause the health problem and hamper the health problem (resources/assets). As a result of the community health assessment, it is likely that numerous health problems or conditions will have been identified as potentially needing to be addressed. For each health problem, a statement can be developed. Exhibit 4.2 is an example of how data collected during the community assessment can be presented in a table format. It contains examples of information for the four health problems identified in the community assessment, both causative and hampering factors. These factors identified through the community assessment can now be used to develop the community needs statement:

> [*Health problem*] among [*population/community*], as indicated in [*health indicators*] is related to [*determinant causative factors*], given [*antecedent and contributing factors*], but as influenced by [*hampering, determinant, antecedent, and contributing factors*].

This format has the advantage of including assets. Again, using the Layetteville example and the information listed in Exhibit 4.2, a complete community needs statement now reads as follows:

> *Intentional handgun injuries*, among *residents of Layetteville*, as indicated in *police reports and rates of emergency room admissions for ICD-9 coded intentional injures* are related to *availability and use of handguns*, given *gang presence and high unemployment rates*, but as influenced by *gun laws, the high visibility of religious leaders' opposition and low high school drop-out rates*.

A similar community health statement can be written for the birth defects health problem:

> *Birth defects*, as indicated by *the rate of neural tube defects* among *residents of Layetteville*, are related to *low folic acid in the diet, genetic and environmental hazards*, given the *mother's age and culture/ethnicity and paternal factors*, but as influenced by *good nutrition, genetic counseling, use of prenatal care, knowledge about folic acid, and availability of food high in folic acid*.

A statement ought to convey information about the health problem in such a way that it stands as a well-articulated base from which to engage in the prioritization process and the subsequent program designing process. The descriptive statements can be used in priority setting, as discussed Chapter 3.

Exhibit 4.6 Diagram of the Need or Problem Statement

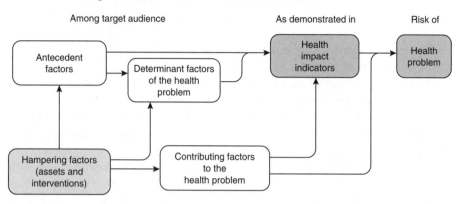

Statements about health problems can be compared with regard to the extent to which the determinants, antecedents, and contributing factors are amenable to change, as well as the level of seriousness or importance of the health problem. It is possible that, although a health problem is initially considered a high priority, data from the community health assessment will lead to a reprioritization of the problem. In short, prioritization and assessment are often iterative processes, rather than a straightforward linear process. This hints at the extent to which planners need to be flexible and act as guides through the planning–assessment process.

A graphic representation of elements of the community health assessment statement is shown in Exhibit 4.6. This generic diagram becomes the basis for developing a logic model and program theory, as discussed in the next chapter. It is critical to note that the program interventions that will be developed can be targeted either at reducing the causative (determinant, antecedent, and contributing) factors *or* enhancing the hampering (determinant, antecedent, and contributing) factors.

ACROSS THE PYRAMID

At the direct services level of the pyramid, heath problems and conditions are viewed as individual problems that are best addressed by individual practitioners. Thus, at this level, assessments are of a focused needs type. A needs assessment is likely to focus on describing the magnitude of a specific medical problem. In addition, such an assessment would describe a subsystem of the community, namely the diagnostic and treatment capabilities of the direct service providers within that community. Individual characteristics that are antecedents, contributing factors, and determinants will need to be identified for the health problem or condition being addressed (Exhibit 4.7).

At the enabling services level of the pyramid, health problems and conditions are viewed as individual problems that are direct results of nonindividual factors and that require community-based or social service interventions. Thus, assessments at this level would focus on describing the social context of individuals with the health problem or condition, as well as the community subsystem in terms of local infrastructure capabilities and human services agencies. Again, antecedents, contributing factors, and determinants related to the health problems of aggregates, whether communities or groups with a common characteristic, can be identified and used in a community health statement. Such a statement ought to flow logically into the development of enabling services.

Exhibit 4.7   Examples of Antecedents, Contributing Factors, and Determinants Across the Pyramid

Factors	Individual and Direct Services	Community and Enabling Services	Population-Based Services	Infrastructure
Antecedents	Health beliefs, attitudes, values	Legal or policy conditions, economic empowerment zones	Genetic predisposition	Mission
Contributing	Lifestyle practices, family, norms	Culture	Income level, education level	Socioeconomic environment
Determinants	Lifestyle practices, health practices, patterns of health services utilization	Road safety features, accessibility and availability of local health and social service agencies	Exposure to hazard	Resources allocated, capacity

At the population services level of the pyramid, health problems are viewed across a population. Thus, assessments at this level are likely to be epidemiological in approach, with attention to describing the magnitude of various health problems or conditions. However, social science approaches to assessment with population data on social indicators provide valuable information about contributing and antecedent factors to the health problems and conditions.

At the infrastructure level of the pyramid, the concerns are with the capabilities of the organization or the health delivery system to address the health problems or conditions at the individual, enabling, and population services levels of the pyramid. In the more ideal sense, the community health assessment is most appropriate for this level because it encompasses understanding both the health problems and conditions within the social context of the target population and the assets that are available to address those health problems and conditions. In addition, the organizational assessment fits at this pyramid level because it focuses on identifying the resources, capabilities, and mission currently available. The findings of the organizational assessment, when considered in conjunction with the findings of the community health assessment, ought to be a solid foundation for garnering resources and planning health programs at the corresponding optimal level of the pyramid.

DISCUSSION QUESTIONS

1. Select one of the perspectives on assessment. In what way does that perspective change, alter, or influence each step in the process of doing a needs assessment?

2. Why is each type of assessment relevant to health program planning?

3. Do a search on Internet sites about community assessments. One suggestion is to begin with state health departments or the Community Tool Kit. What perspective on assessment is reflected in the context of the Interent site? Which of the steps described in the chapter received more or less emphasis by the authors of the Internet site? What implications does that have for the problem statement?

4. Discuss the relevance of each perspective for developing programs at each level of the pyramid. What effect might choosing one perspective have on the level of the subsequent program?

References

Alciati, M. H., & Glanz, K. (1996). Using data to plan public health programs: Experience from state cancer prevention and control programs. *Public Health Reports, 111,* 165–172.

Baker, T. D., & Reinke, W. A. (1988). Epidemiologic base for health planning. In W. A Reinke (Ed.), *Health planning for effective management.* New York: Oxford University Press.

Billings, J. R., & Cowly, S. (1995). Approaches to community needs assessment: A literature review. *Journal of Advanced Nursing, 22,* 721–730.

Blum, H. L. (1981). *Planning for health: Generics for the eighties* (2nd ed.). New York: Human Sciences Press.

Blum, H. L. (1982). Social perspective on risk reduction. In M. M. Farber & A. M. Reinhart (Eds.), *Promoting health through risk reduction.* (pp. 19–36). New York: Macmillan.

Bradshaw, J. (1972). The concept of social need. *New Society, 30,* 640-643.

Campbell, B. F., Sengupta, S., Santos, C., & Lorig, K. R. (1995). Balanced incomplete block design: Description, case study, and implications for practice. *Health Education Quarterly, 22,* 201–210.

Cottrell, L. S. (1976). The competent community. In B. H. Kaplan et al. (Eds.), *Further explorations in social psychiatry.* New York: Basic Books.

Denham, A., Quinn, S. C., & Gamble, D. (1998). Community organizing for health promotion in the rural South: An exploration of community competence. *Family and Community Health, 21,* 1–21.

Dever, G. E. (1980). *Community health assessment.* Germantown, MD: Aspen Systems.

Dever, G. E. (1997). *Improving outcomes in public health practice: Strategy and methods.* Gaithersburg, MD: Aspen Publishers.

Donath, S. M. (2000). Who's overweight? Comparison of the medical definition and community views. *Medical Journal of Australia, 172,* 375–377.

Evaneshko, V. (1999). Mental health needs assessment of Tucson's urban Native American population. *American Indian & Alaska Native Mental Health Research, 8(3),* 41–61.

Fikree, F. F., Khan, A., Kadir, M. M., Sagan, F., & Rahbar, M. H. (2001). What influences contraceptive use among young women in urban squatter settlements in Karachi, Pakistan? *International Family Planning Perspectives, 27,* 130–136.

Ford, J., Young, D., Perez, B. C., Overmeyere, R. L., & Rohner, D. G. (1992). Needs assessment for persons with severe mental illness: What services are needed for successful community living? *Community Mental Health Journal, 28,* 491–503.

Fos, P. J., & Fine, D. J. (2000). *Designing health care for populations: Applied epidemiology in health care administration.* San Francisco: Jossey-Bass.

Goeppinger, J., Lassiter, P. G., & Wilcox, B. (1982). Community health is community competence. *Nursing Outlook, 30,* 464–467.

Green, L.W., & Kreuter, M. W. (1991). *Health promotion planning: An educational and environmental approach.* Mountain View, CA: Mayfield Publishing.

Haddon, W., Jr. (1972). A logical framework for categorizing highway safety phenomena and activity. *Journal of Trauma, 12,* 193–207.

Handler, A., Rosenberg, D., Kennelly, J., & Monahan, C. (1998). *Analytic methods in maternal and child health.* Vienna, VA: National Maternal and Child Health Clearinghouse.

Herman, J. L., Morris, L. L., & Fitz-Gibbon, C. T. (1987). *Evaluator's handbook.* Newbury Park, CA: Sage Publications.

Lochner, K., Kawachi, I., & Kennedy, B. P. (1999). Social capital: A guide to its measurement. *Health and Place, 5,* 259–270.

Mausner, J. S., & Baum, A. K. (1974). *Epidemiology: An introductory text.* Philadelphia: W. B. Saunders.

Muecke, M. (1984). Community health diagnosis in nursing. *Public Health Nursing, 1,* 23–35.

National Association of City and County Health Officers. (2000). Research and development: Assessment Protocol for Excellence in Public Health (APEXPH). *http://www.naccho.org/prjoect47.htm* (accessed 8/12/01).

Paronen, O., & Oje, P. (1998). How to understand a community-community assessment for the promotion of health-related physical activity. *Patient Education and Counseling, 33* (Suppl.), S25–28.

Phillips, J. M., & Belcher, A. E. (1999). Integrating cancer risk assessment into a community health nursing course. *Journal of Cancer Education, 14,* 47–51.

Radloff, L. S. (1977). The CES-D scale: A self-report depression scale for research in the general population. *Applied Psychological Measurement, 1,* 385–400.

Rossi, P. H., Freeman, H. E., & Lipsey, M. W. (1999). *Evaluation: A systematic approach* (6th ed). Thousand Oaks, CA: Sage Publications.

Scriven, M., & Roth, J. (1990). Special feature: Needs assessment. *Evaluation Practice, 11,* 135–144.

Sherman, R. E., Gillespie, S., & Diaz, J. A. (1996). Use of social indicators in assessment of local community alcohol and other drug dependence treatment needs within Chicago. *Substance Abuse and Misuse, 31,* 691–728.

Siden, H. B. (1998). A qualitative approach to community and provider needs assessment in a telehealth project. *Telemedicine Journal, 4,* 225–235.

Sullivan, C. M., Basta, J., Tan, C., & Davidson, W. S., 2nd (1992). After the crisis: A needs assessment of women leaving a domestic violence shelter. *Violence and Victims, 7,* 267–275.

Ware, J. E. (2000). SF-36 health survey update. *Spine, 25,* 3130–3139.

Ware, J. E., Kosinski, M., Bayliss, M. S., McHorney, C. A., Rogers, W. H., & Raczek, A. (1995). Comparison of methods for scoring and statistical analysis of the SF-36 health profile and summary measures: Summary of results from the Medical Outcomes Study. *Medical Care, 33* (Suppl.), AS264–279.

Webb, E. J., Campbell, D. T., Schwartz, R. D., & Sechrest, L. (2000). *Unobtrusive methods* (Rev. ed.). Thousand Oaks, CA: Sage Publications.

Webb, E. J., Campbell, D. T., Schwartz, R. D., Sechrest, L., & Grove, J. B. (1981). *Non-reactive measures in the social sciences* (2nd ed.). Boston: Houghton Mifflin.

Witkin, B. R., & Altschuld, J. W. (1995). *Planning and conducting needs assessments: A practical guide.* Thousand Oaks, CA: Sage Publications.

CHAPTER 5

Program Theory and Interventions Revealed

After developing statements about health problems that have been ranked as a high priority, the next steps involve more intellectual and creative efforts to articulate an explanation of what caused the problem. This is a critical step toward identifying which intervention or group of interventions will be most effective in addressing the health problem. Wild guesses, past experience, and personal preferences might be used, but a more rational approach is to identify existing scientific knowledge and theories that can be used to develop a program theory.

A theory is essentially a description of how something works. It is a set of statements or hypotheses about what will happen and thus contains statements about the relationships among the variables. We use working theories in everyday life, usually in the form of working hypotheses, such as, "If I ask the children to clean their room, they are not likely to do it." We also use theories based in science. For example, based on theories of thermodynamics and heat conduction, we can predict how long a turkey needs to bake.

With regard to planning a health program, a primary consideration is to specify what is to be explained or predicted with a theory. The health problem is what needs to be explained, from a programmatic perspective. To explain how to change or affect the health problem, a theory must contain salient variables, or factors, and must indicate the direction of the interactions among those variables related to the health problem. Identifying the salient antecedent, contributing, and determinant factors of the health problem gives planners the foundation for developing a working theory of how the programmatic interventions will lead to the desired health outcome. A difficult part of this task is to identify where a health programmatic intervention can have an effect on those factors. As more details and more factors are included in the explanation of the health problem and how the programmatic interventions will work, the theory becomes more complex.

The theory development phase of program planning requires thinking rather than doing, and therefore it often receives less attention than is needed to fully develop an effective health program. However, using a systematic approach to developing a program theory and to engaging stakeholders in the development of the theory has big, long-term payoffs that outweigh any delay or costs associated with developing the theory.

PROGRAM THEORY

A sound basis for developing the health program and for guiding the program evaluation is the use of a Program Theory. Rossi, Freeman, and Lipsey (1999) acknowledged that the need for a Program Theory has long been recognized by evaluators. Only recently, however, has the usefulness of a Program Theory for program development and improvement been widely recognized. "Program Theory" is one of the various names given to the comprehensive overview of how the program is to work; other names are logic model, causal model, outcome line, program model, and action theory. These names all refer to a conceptual plan, with some details about what the program is and how it is expected to work. Whether one is developing a new health program or designing an evaluation for an existing health program, understanding and articulating the Program Theory is essential.

There are two main components of Program Theory (Exhibit 5.1). The theory about resources and actions is called the process theory, and the theory about interventions and outcomes is called the effect theory. Although this language may seem cumbersome, the development of a Program Theory and its components leads to a stronger program and a more convincing argument for the program's existence.

Process Theory

The process theory includes three components: the organizational plan, the service utilization plan, and specifications of their outputs. This depiction of process theory developed by Rossi et al. (1999) can be integrated with the language currently used in public health of inputs, which are part of the organizational plan; activities, which are part of the service utilization plan; and outputs, which are by-products of the service utilization plan.

The organizational plan, according to Rossi et al. (1999), encompasses the nature of the resources needed for the program. As such, the organizational plan includes: specifications about personnel and the organization of resources to be used in the program, as well as elements of capacity, such as infrastructure,

Exhibit 5.1   Logic Model of Program Theory

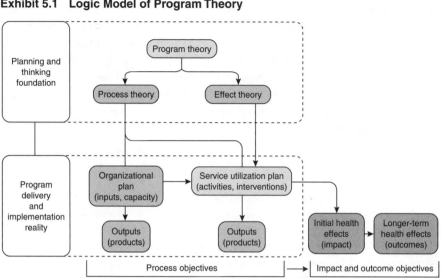

Source: Rossi, P., Freeman, H., & Lipsey, M., *Evaluation: A Systematic Approach, Sixth Edition*, page 101, Copyright 1999 by Sage Publications, Thousand Oaks, CA. Adapted with permission of Sage Publications, Inc.

information technology, fiscal resources, and personnel. The organizational plan is a theory to the extent that it contains explicit "if-then" statements. For example, if program staff are adequately supported with regard to supplies and managerial support, then program staff will deliver the interventions as planned. These "if-then" statements are useful not only for checking the logic behind requesting specific resources, but also for guiding the portion of the evaluation plan that focuses on the processes behind the delivery of the health program.

The service utilization plan, according to Rossi et al. (1999), specifies how to reach the target audience and provide the programmatic services to that audience. This is the "nuts and bolts" of providing the program and of implementing the program plan. The service utilization plan includes the specifics about social marketing of the program, the accessibility and availability of the program, screening procedures, and other logistics of providing the program. Development of the service plan ought to reflect cultural sensitivity and appropriateness of the services and intervention, given the target audience.

Within the context of planning a program, the organizational plan needs to be in place before the program can begin. Both the organizational plan and the service utilization plan need to be developed using the results of the community health assessment, particularly with regard to incorporating existing resources into the plans and addressing structural issues that can affect the delivery of the program. The organizational plan is influenced by the service utilization plan and the effect theory. Likewise, the service utilization plan evolves as the effect theory is revised. Thus, both the organizational plan and the service utilization plan are likely to be continually adjusted throughout this phase of program planning. Although the adjustments and revisions may be frustrating, it is much easier to make the adjustments at this stage of planning, than it is to do so after the program has begun.

Effect Theory

The effect theory is the explanation of how the programmatic interventions will affect the antecedent, determinant, and contributing factors of the health problem and thus of the relationship between the programmatic interventions and the desired immediate and long-term outcomes for program participants. There are four sets of relationships, or "theories," that constitute a comprehensive effect theory (Exhibit 5.2). They are determinant theory, intervention theory, impact theory, and outcome theory. Depending on the health problem, it can be useful to develop each of the four theories. Often these "theories" are implicitly stated and understood by health professionals

---

Exhibit 5.2   Elements of an Effect Theory, Incorporating Need or Problem Statement Components

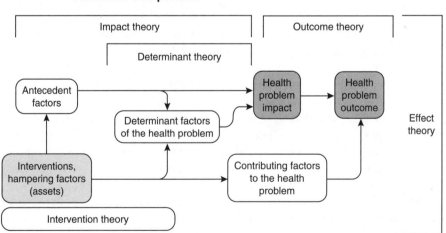

and program staff. By explicitly expressing and discussing each of the theories, planners can refine programmatic interventions, thus increasing the likelihood of program success. The set of four theories, and the associated informally stated hypotheses, constitute the effect theory of the Program Theory. Although Rossi and Freeman (1993) called it the program impact model rather than the effect theory, calling it the effect theory makes it clear that the theory is about both impacts and outcomes. Generating each of the four theories that comprise the effect theory may seem complicated. Program experts agree on the complexity of constructing an effect theory as well as on its central role in program evaluation (Patton, 1997; Rossi & Freeman, 1993; Rossi et al., 1999).

INTERVENTIONS

Interventions are those actions that are done intentionally to have a direct effect on those with the health problem. Interventions are the verbs that tell what is being done to make a change in program recipients. Using this definition allows for the inclusion of a broad range of actions, such as medical treatments, pharmacological treatments, and education, as well as psychological strategies and policy formulation. This broad definition of interventions also allows for the inclusion of strategies not typically considered treatments, such as providing transportation (an enabling service) or community development (an infrastructure-level intervention). Clearly identifying and labeling the interventions as such not only makes developing the intervention and impact theories easier, but also makes developing outcome objectives easier and helps distinguish outcome from process objectives.

Be aware that in some presentations about program planning, such as in the United Way book (1996), interventions are couched in terms of "activities" and thus become indistinguishable from the myriad of activities done as part of the organizational or service utilization plans, which are supportive of the interventions but do not contribute to the interventions. Interventions are the heart of all health programs. A clear understanding and statement of the role of interventions is made in the intervention and determinant theories, which are discussed below.

Finding and Identifying Interventions

Selecting and then articulating the interventions chosen is the cornerstone of health programs. It is important when planning a health program to draw upon existing knowledge in multiple disciplines. A literature review can generate ideas and information with regard to existing theories that have been used to explain what leads to the health problem, as well as explanations of why some interventions have been effective and others have not.

The use of existing theories can expedite the development of the effect theory and lend it credibility. Heany and van Ryn (1996) provided a nice example of this. The health problem was work-site stress. They wanted to develop a health program to reduce work-site stress but were concerned that existing programs had been designed for a target audience of middle class employees within the cultural majority. Heany and van Ryn sought to improve the effectiveness of work-site stress reduction programs for employees of low status or of a cultural minority. The premise was that the potential exists for different subgroups to vary in both their participation in and benefit derived from a program. They began by reviewing the literature on stress and coping. From this literature, they constructed a theoretical model of stress and coping and identified the major variables, along with the direction of the interaction among those variables. They also reviewed the literature on the content of work-site stress reduction programs and the sociological literature on status, class, culture, and stress. From their literature reviews, Heany and van Ryn were able to identify potential program interventions that would alter specific variables in the stress and coping model. This became part of their effect theory for the work-site stress reduction program for low-status minority workers. Unfortunately, for many health problems there are not widely accepted theories that can guide the development of an effect theory or the selection of interventions. Calhoun and Clark-Jones (1998) argued that this was the case for violence. However, health program planners and the planning team have options for how to proceed.

Types of Interventions

One way to begin selecting the intervention is to think in terms of types of interventions. Various classification schemes of interventions have been developed across the health disciplines. The most common typology in public health is primary, secondary, and tertiary prevention. Primary prevention includes those activities that are done to prevent a disease or illness from beginning, such as getting adequate exercise, having good nutrition, immunizations, and wearing seat belts. Secondary prevention involves screening for undiagnosed problems so that the disease can be treated before it manifests. Blood pressure screening at health fairs and the use of occult fecal blood tests and cholesterol tests fall into secondary prevention. Tertiary prevention involves activities to limit the extent of an existing disease and thus include taking blood pressure medications, receiving physical rehabilitation after an injury, and stress management classes for individuals with cardiac problems.

This classification scheme is a good starting point, but very different classification is more applicable to health program planning. The intervention typology (Exhibit 5.3) as originally developed by Grobe and Hughes (1993) had seven categories of interventions. An eighth category was added by Issel (1997) when studying case management of pregnant women. This typology, by providing an encompassing perspective, can aid in identifying the various activities that are actually programmatic interventions. In addition, each of the eight types of interventions exist at the direct services, enabling services, and population levels of the public health pyramid (Exhibit 5.3). The typology also accommodates both secondary and tertiary prevention, as these are activities of health professionals undertaken with the intent of having an effect on the participant. Primary prevention is not included in the typology, because providers cannot do primary prevention for or to the participant. Rather, individuals receive education about primary prevention, are encouraged to engage in primary prevention, and might be monitored for the extent to which they are practicing primary prevention. This is one example of how such a typology of interventions forces program planners to be specific about the strategies and actions that are undertaken to affect the health condition or situation of the target audience.

Specifying Intervention Administration

Many health program interventions differ from medical interventions in that they are thought of in more general terms, like "hand out informational flyers" or "provide emotional support." Nonetheless, health program interventions also need to be thought of in terms of dosage, route of administration, and site of administration. Dosage refers to the amount of intervention required to have an effect, whether in hours of education, days of respite, micrograms of fluoride, or weeks of counseling. For many health problems, research reports can provide information on what doses are needed to be effective. For example, studies are now showing that a minimum of 30 minutes of moderately intense physical activity on most days of the week is optimal for physical well-being (Fletcher et al., 2001). The route of administration can be thought of as the medium used to deliver the intervention, whether it be interpersonal communication, mass media campaign, or educational brochures. Again, research can provide guidance on the optimal route to deliver programmatic interventions. The mode of administration can also be quite important; it involves whether the intervention is provided by a health professional of a particular discipline, a lay health

Exhibit 5.3   Examples of Interventions by Type and Level of the Pyramid

Intervention Type	Direct Service Level	Enabling Services Level	Population Level
Treating	Medical or dental procedures, medications, physical manipulations, tertiary prevention	Respite care, exercise classes or groups	Water treatment and fluoridation, mass immunizations
Assessing	Determination of needs and preferences by asking individuals, secondary prevention	Determination of needs and preferences by needs assessment	Use of epidemiological data to identify trends and rates of illnesses and conditions
Coordinating	Care coordination, client advocacy, referral, linking to services	Case coordination, local provider networks and collaborations	Systems integration, records and data sharing, state child health insurance plans
Monitoring	Reassessment, followup	Local trends and news reports	Trends analysis
Educating	Skills building, information giving	GED programs, job training programs	Media campaigns
Counseling	Psychotherapy, emotional support, marital counseling	Group counseling, family counseling, grief counseling for groups	News alerts and advice
Coaching	Role modeling, empowerment, encouragement	Community development	Policy formation
Giving tangibles	Giving vouchers for food or clothing	Medical supplies loan programs	Income supplements, insurance supplements

worker, or a paraprofessional. For some heath problems, the cultural values attached to a physician may be a key factor in the effectiveness of the intervention, whereas for other health problems and programs, a community member will have more credibility. Once these are specified, the information on intervention administration is incorporated into the service utilization plan.

Interventions and Program Components

One of the challenges in selecting an intervention strategy is to decide on whether a single intervention is warranted or whether a package of interventions would be more effective in addressing the health problem. A program component is an intervention, or set of interventions, with the corresponding organizational plan. Thus, if a health program includes multiple interventions because multiple pathways from antecedent, contributing, and determinant factors have been selected, then the program has multiple program components.

Using program components is appropriate if, to address the health problem, changes must occur across levels, such as family and community. Levels are nested within other levels, and each can be the focus of the program. It is extremely difficult to have a single intervention that can affect all or most determinants, antecedents, and contributing factors at multiple levels. Thus, program components are needed. For example, if individuals as well as the community as a whole in which those individuals live are both targets for the intervention, then interventions tailored to individuals and communities will be needed. If, to address the problem of birth defects, both individual behavior of women and actions of industry are targeted, then different interventions (program components) are needed.

Another reason to have program components is to address micro and macro health problems. Blum (1982) suggested that some health problems or risks require individual behavioral changes, while others require group behavioral change. From a public health perspective, an individual behavioral change needed to protect against a health risk is called active protection, whereas protection that does not require individuals to make a behavioral change but is instituted through policy, laws, or some other means that does not involve the individual is called passive protection. Passive protection often occurs at a macro level, in that it encompasses more than a small group of individuals. However, macro-level changes can also involve active protection, such as the immunization of all infants. Immunization involves individual parental behavior but is intended to have a population effect. In contrast, health programs focused on fluoridation or reducing factory pollutant emissions provide passive protection of a population. The distinctions between micro and macro programs, as well as between active and passive protection, may be important in developing the interventions and the effect theory. If the health program is intended to be community based or community focused, then there quite likely will be program components at the micro level as well as the macro level.

Because each program component will have a slightly different impact, acknowledging the components as such is important in subsequent evaluation plans. The intervention, impact, and outcome theories will vary slightly for each program component and for each of the different units of intervention of the program.

Criteria for "Good" Interventions

The final choice of an intervention or a package of interventions can be evaluated against a set of criterion for useful interventions. One of the most important criterion for a good intervention is that it be *technologically feasible* (Blum, 1982; Rossi & Freeman, 1986). That is, the problem must be changeable with the available knowledge of how to change it. Feasibility also refers to the logistical reality of doing the intervention. In addition, there also needs to be expertise among the program planners for designing the intervention and activities so that those activities actually affect the health problem. As was discussed in Chapter 3 in terms of prioritizing the health problems, the changeability of a health problem is considered to be one aspect of its importance. In terms of interventions, a more technologically feasible intervention ought to result in a more changeable health problem. A component of technological feasibility is that the intervention fits the characteristics of the target population, including their cultural beliefs and ethnic values. Technological feasibility is further enhanced if the intervention has been tailored to the audience, such as age or cultural appropriateness, or if the target audience has been screened for eligibility for the health program.

A second criterion is that *health gains* must result from the intervention. This acknowledges that some interventions may have severe side effects (the "Just Say No" campaign comes to mind) and that some are ineffective (Avegard et al., 2001; Brown, 2001). This criterion also speaks to an advantage of fully articulating the effect theory. It is common to jump to a favorite solution, one that may not necessarily be a good match for addressing the health problem. One technique to avoid jumping to a solution is to articulate the theories that make up the effect theory. In other words, health gains are more likely to occur by going from theory to intervention. In some scenarios, interventions could be useful and effective with regard to one type of outcome but may not lead to the impact or outcome of interest. For example, health education about family planning methods may be effective in reducing the birth rate in a target audience but may not be effective in reducing sexually transmitted diseases. Again, having done the work of developing the effect theory helps planners be certain that the intervention will lead to the desired health gains.

The third criterion of a good intervention is that it be *politically feasible*. Not all interventions are equally acceptable to the target audience, to funding agencies, or to other stakeholders. During the assessment phase, preferences and the willingness of various stakeholders to endorse different types of interventions ought to have been determined. Interventions need to be culturally appropriate and sensitive as a first step toward being politically feasible. There are several strategies that can be used to design culturally sensitive and competent health program interventions for use with ethnically or racially distinct target populations. These strategies include using focus groups and pretesting (Resnicow, Baranowsky, Ahuwalia, & Brathwaite, 1999). A corollary to the political feasibility criterion is that meeting this criterion helps the planner to survive. Proposing interventions that are not politically feasible can result in the planner being used as a scapegoat and being blamed for a "bad" intervention.

The fourth criterion is that the intervention must address *societal priorities*; in other words, the problem must be important in the larger picture. Sufficient agreement first needs to exist with regard to the importance of the health problem. This would have been established during the priority setting and assessment phases. A lack of the desired health or a high prevalence of the problem contribute to its high priority. There are many effective interventions that can be used to address trivial problems that are not a high priority. It is possible that one role played by health program planners and evaluators to raise the issue so that the health problem becomes a priority. To some extent, the societal priority is set by celebrity spokespersons for specific health problems and by the nightly news covering the current health research. These societal pressures may conflict with the local assessment data. The intervention nonetheless must be in line with the societal priorities of health problems in order to receive public credibility and backing. Also, the new behavior or health state must be important to the target audience; otherwise they will not make attempts to change. Although the importance of the health problem to the target audience may have been included as an element in the community needs assessment, it can resurface during program theory development in terms of societal versus individual health priorities.

The fifth criterion is that the intervention must be *manipulable* (Rossi & Freeman, 1993). Manipulability refers to the ability of the program planners and program staff to adjust the intervention to the specific needs of the participants. A major element of manipulability is dosage—that is, how much is received and how often. If the "dosage" of the intervention can be tailored to the target audience, it is likely to meet the manipulability criterion. Effective and efficient interventions are tailored to some extent to the variations among potential participants.

Related to manipulability is the ability to gain synergy by taking into account other programs that are already in place. For example, Guidotti, Ford, and Wheeler (2000) described a project that was specifically designed to be delivered along with existing community initiatives. By building on existing programs and interventions, the new program could mutually reinforce the effects of the other programs. Thus, the intervention was manipulated to be compatible with existing interventions. The approach of intentionally developing a program intervention to maximize the effects of all programs being delivered to a community is increasingly important as communities become saturated with health promotion programs.

Another aspect of manipulability is that the intervention must be designed to overcome influences on the health problem that are not directly addressed by the health program. The strength of the intervention needs to be made sufficient to overcome those factors. In some instances, existing theories can be helpful in manipulating the intervention so that it is sufficiently strong. An example of theory-based nutritional interventions is the Gimme 5 intervention (Baranowski et al., 2000). Guided by social cognitive theory, the researchers designed the intervention to address interrelated environmental, personal, and behavioral factors. The use of social cognitive theory facilitated manipulating the interventions in ways that increased the likelihood that the interventions would be effective with the school-age children in the program. Another example is provided by Brenton (1999), who argued for the use of chaos theory in planning prevention and mental health interventions. In chaos theory, critical moments are followed by transitions and then stable states that are better adapted to the existing environment. Based on this theory, he argued that prevention programs could focus on the critical moments and thus target groups at risk. Using the concept of sensitivity to initial conditions, he argued that programs would have the greatest impact at the beginning of life. This is just one example of how a theory that is not usually used by health professionals can guide thinking and foster creativity in the selection of interventions and the planning of health programs.

The sixth and final criterion is that the *cost* of the intervention must be reasonable rather than prohibitive. The cost of the intervention will depend upon many factors, such as the extent to which the health behavior or problem is resistant to change, the duration of the program, and the number of program components. Estimating the cost of the intervention, generally considered under the service utilization theory, is discussed more fully in subsequent chapters.

IMPACTS AND OUTCOMES IN PUBLIC HEALTH

Just as it is important to carefully consider the interventions that will be used in the health program, so too must program planners carefully consider what impacts are anticipated from the program. Several factors can distract program planners from having a clear vision of the relevant impact. One is that a plethora of possible impacts from programmatic interventions may exist. Another is that there are many ways to think about changes resulting from programs (Patton, 1997). Yet another distraction is extensive stakeholder involvement. Their involvement can lead to becoming sidetracked and thus planners may end up with an extensive list of what "our program could do." For these reasons, having the problem statement, as written at the conclusion of the community needs assessment, helps those involved in the planning process stay focused on the health problem, as well as the health impacts and outcomes that are directly related to the health program.

Further complicating the choice of key health impacts is that change is not always the purpose of health programs; some are intended to stabilize, prevent, or maintain a health state. Because health is multidimensional, Patton (1997) suggested that changes can occur in multiple arenas: life circumstances, health or economic status, behavior, functioning, attitude, knowledge, or skills. This is particularly true if the health problem being addressed has antecedent or contributing factors that are not physiologically based, but relate to one of these other arenas.

Behaviors, such as primary prevention behaviors, are often the focus of health and public health programs. If the desired health impact is a behavior, there are criteria for selecting which behavior ought to be changed. Ideally, the behavior ought to be free from outside influences, such as peer groups or economic factors beyond the control of the program. The behavior also ought to be critical to achieving the desired health outcome. In addition, a knowledge of how to develop the preferred behavior needs to exist; in other words, there needs to be a scientific basis for the behavioral intervention. Naturally, the new behavior must be important to the learner, in the same way that a health state ought to be important to the target audience. Experts need to agree that the new behavior is an important link to the health outcome. A pervasive lack of the behavior would be equivalent to a health problem of large magnitude and would influence choosing the behavior as the focus of a health program.

Another challenge in developing the effect theory is to match the level of intervention with the level of impact and outcome. Health programs can have target audiences that are individuals, families, aggregates, or populations, each of these being a different unit for intervention. Programmatic interventions need to be tailored to reach the target audience—in other words, to match the unit of intervention. For example, if the programmatic intervention is designed to affect family eating patterns, then the health impact sought ought to be family nutritional health, rather than reducing anemia in children or increasing the daily consumption of milk in a neighborhood. The notion of the unit of intervention is pivotal because the unit of intervention becomes the unit of analysis in the evaluation phase (Jackson, Altman, Howard-Pitney, & Farquhar, 1989). Therefore, there also needs to be a corresponding match between the health impacts that are selected and the programmatic intervention.

Generating the Effect Theory

After having considered the type of intervention and the criteria for choosing an intervention, the next step is to more fully articulate the effect theory by enumerating the determinant, intervention, impact, and outcome theories that constitute the effect theory. Articulating these is an iterative process that requires going back and forth between the needs assessment, priorities, and intervention choice. Developing or generating the effect theory is guided by several strategies suggested by Patton (1997).

Inductive and deductive approaches can be used to generate an impact theory. Theory development can proceed through a deductive process that uses reason and existing knowledge, or it can occur through an inductive process that uses experience and intuition. Either approach will lead to a program theory. In practice, a combination of both inductive and deductive approaches is typically used and is optimal. Generating a program theory need not be a daunting task. There are several steps, and they can be done either in sequence or iteratively.

Determinant Theory

The first theory to be developed or understood is the explanation of the process that currently underlies the health problem, the determinant factors leading to the health problem. To use a term borrowed from Rossi and Freeman (1993), this is called the *determinant theory*. It includes statements or hypotheses that describe relationships among the determinant factors causing the health problems. The determinant theory ought to be derived from data collected during the community needs assessment phase of program planning.

Using the handgun example from the previous chapter, the determinant theory is that intentional handgun injuries are due to the availability of guns as influenced by restrictive gun laws. Following up with another example from the previous chapter (Exhibit 5.4), in Layetteville, pregnant women have a high rate of neural tube birth defects [health problem]. The determinant theory in this example is that the high rate of neural tube defects results from poor nutritional intake, particularly folic acid; genetic predisposition; and exposure to environmental hazards [determinants].

Intervention Theory

The *intervention theory* is developed to explain how interventions affect the determinant factors, antecedent factors, and contributing factors. In other words, it contains hypotheses about the relationships among the programmatic interventions and the causative theory. Because clarity about interventions is so

---

Exhibit 5.4   Elements of an Effect Theory: Example for Improving Newborn Health Status

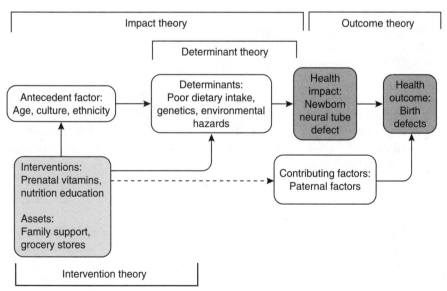

important, what the interventions are and how to identify them is discussed in a separate section later. It is actually within the intervention theory that the program works its magic, so to speak. Developing an intervention theory can help refine the number of interventions that are carried out as part of the health program. Interventions found to have a limited effect on the determinants, antecedents, or contributing factors can be excluded. This will result in a more effective and efficient program.

In the birth defects health problem, the intervention theory is that nutritional education [intervention] changes the behavior of the woman with regard to eating dark green vegetables and taking prenatal vitamins. Prenatal vitamins [intervention] compensate for any nutritional deficit not overcome by changes in dietary intake. Together, receiving nutritional education and taking supplements change eating behaviors and beliefs about preventing birth defects. As this example shows, not all determinants, antecedents, and contributing factors need to be or can be addressed by a single health program. An equally plausible intervention theory would be that community activism [intervention] would change the practices of industry and businesses that have high emissions of teratogenic substances. The decision regarding which intervention theory to use as the basis of a program is influenced by the preferences of stakeholders, the mission of the organization, and the science regarding which determinants are more readily changeable.

Impact Theory

Another step is to develop the *impact theory*, or what Rossi and Freeman (1993) referred to as the action theory. The impact theory is the set of statements describing the relationships connecting interventions and impact, meaning the short-term or immediate consequences of the interventions. Whereas the intervention theory describes factors leading to the health problem, the impact theory describes how the interventions affect the health problem. It is possible for a program to alter or affect some of the contributing or determinant factors yet have no immediate effect on the health problem. Therefore, impact theory helps further articulate the connection between the programmatic intervention and the intended effect on the health problem. Having an impact theory explicitly stated and understood by the program staff directly affects the success of the program.

At this point, the distinction between health indicators and health problems becomes helpful in terms of developing the effect theory. The health indicator becomes the health impact in the effect theory, whereas the health problem becomes the health outcome. It is also important to note that in the evaluation literature the use of the terms "impact" and "outcome" is not standardized. For the sake of clarity, "impact" is used in this text to refer to the immediate consequences of a health problem as seen in health indicators, whereas "outcome" is used for the long-term consequences, as in the more global health problem.

Continuing with the birth defects example, the impact theory is that nutritional education and prenatal vitamins will have an effect on the rate of neural tube defects.

Outcome Theory

The final element of effect theory is the outcome theory, or conceptual theory (Rossi et al., 1999), in which statements about how the impacts lead to outcomes are explicated. Whereas impacts are the immediate, direct effects of the programmatic interventions, outcomes are the broader, more long-term effects of the health program. Usually, a health program has a very limited number of health outcomes that it seeks to affect. Outcome theory helps substantiate the sometimes seemingly wild and wishful claims of program planners about the effects of their program because it specifies the relationship between the immediate impact of the program and the long-term, ultimate changes to the health problem. If one of the program components involves having a community coalition, then its role in contributing to the health impacts and outcomes needs to be articulated (Gabriel, 2000). It is possible to have multiple outcome theories for one long-range outcome, particularly if multiple intervention theories are being used within a single program. Given the complex nature of many health problems and conditions, this is a likely scenario. Continuing with the birth defects example, the outcome theory is that prevention of neural tube defects leads to fewer neural tube defects, which in turn leads to a decrease in the rate of birth defects.

It is not uncommon for funding agencies to specify program outcomes, for example, a decrease in infant mortality or an increase in early detection of preventable disease. These might be stated as program goals that the funded programs are to achieve. In such cases, program planners must essentially work backward to generate the outcome theory, which then affects the impact and intervention theories. Another way in which outcome theories are relevant is that they show the links and explain the relationship between objectives and goals, an important factor that is discussed in the next chapter.

In summary, the effect theory encompasses the determinant, intervention, impact, and outcome theories. These theories are all needed to explain the complexity of a health problem. Exhibit 5.4 brings together all of the components of the effect theory in the birth defects example.

Involving Key Stakeholders

Generating a program theory is not a solitary task; it is a task that requires brainpower, diverse ideas, and sustained energy. Involving key stakeholders not only makes good ideas evident, it also leads stakeholders to become invested in the health program and to address the health problem. This is a critical step toward having a politically feasible intervention.

Potential program participants and providers have their own working explanation, or theory, of how a program affects participants. One type of theory is an espoused theory. Argyris and Schon (1974) were among the first to understand the importance of espoused theories. They found that employees had explanations for why things happened in their organizations. These stated explanations are the espoused theories. People know what they are supposed to do or say, regardless of whether or not they do or say it. It is the stated and repeated explanation that is the espoused theory. For example, staff providing a cardiac rehabilitation program may say that the program works because they are teaching the patients what to eat and how to exercise. This is the espoused theory of how the program improves participants' cardiac conditioning.

Argyris and Schon (1974) also found that espoused theories were not always congruent with the behaviors they observed. What people do in order to achieve their ends is their theory-in-use, sometimes called a theory-in-action. The theory-in-use becomes crucial in program evaluation; it is the interventions that actually make up the health program and affect participants. Returning to the cardiac rehabilitation program example, if the staff in the cardiac rehabilitation program become friends with the patients and provide encouragement in a supportive manner but rarely focus on teaching patients, then their theory-in-use is coaching or social support rather than education.

As seen in the cardiac rehabilitation example, espoused theories and theories-in-use may not be the same. It is the theories-in-use that denote how the program is implemented and that are the source of the effects on participants. Determining whether the theories-in-use differ from the espoused theories of program staff is an important reason for conducting process evaluations. Relying only on the espoused theory as a basis for evaluating a health program can lead to a set of profound difficulties. Findings from the program evaluation may be confusing or misleading if the espoused theory and the theory-in-use are incongruent. Implementation of the program may be inconsistent, with some staff providing the program according to the espoused theory and others providing the program based on their theory-in-use. One way to avoid incongruity between the espoused theory and the theory-in-use is to explicitly include the theory-in-use in the effect theory. Being aware of the differences among espoused theories, theories-in-use, and effect theories (Exhibit 5.5) can help planners to generate an effect theory that incorporates useful elements of the espoused theories and the theories-in-use. If the program has been in existence for some period of time, an alternative is to decide either to incorporate the theory-in-use into the program theory or to explicitly exclude the theory-in-use as an element of the program. Modifying the Program Theory based on the practical experience gained through the theory-in-use may be efficient and prudent if the theory-in-use has had the desired effect on program participants.

Drawing upon the Scientific Literature

Articles published across the health disciplines ought to be reviewed for information that can help generate the theories by providing information on the relationships among the determinants, antecedents, and contributing factors. Abstracts available through online databases are another good source of ideas that can be incorporated into the effect theory. The published literature is also

---

Exhibit 5.5   Comparison of Effect Theory, Espoused Theory, and Theory-in-Use

	Effect Theory	Espoused Theory	Theory-in-Use
What It Is	Explanation of how program interventions affect participants	What staff say about how the program affects participants	What staff do to affect participants
Where It Resides	Manuals and procedures; program descriptions	Minds of program staff; program manuals and descriptions	Actions of program staff; on-the-job training
How It Is Identified	Review of scientific literature, program materials	Listen to staff describe the program, read program materials	Watch what staff do in providing the program
Importance	Guides program and evaluation; basis for claiming outcomes	Becomes what staff, clients, and stakeholders believe and expect of the program	Is the actual cause of program outcomes

helpful in developing the process theory, particularly with regard to the service utilization elements.

Existing theories from multiple disciplines can be used to develop the effect theory. If the health program is intended to have a physiological effect or address a pathology, then theories about biochemistry, pharmacology, or physiology might be useful. If the health program addresses mental health or family problems, then theories about psychopathology, stress, coping, or family functioning might be used to explain the health problem. If the health problem is related to the knowledge and abilities of individuals or communities, then theories about learning, cognition, memory, and attention could be used to explain how knowledge, skills, and abilities are gained. If a health program is intended to foster or maintain lifestyle behaviors and self-care, then theories about motivation, decision making, change, and self-efficacy are among the suitable theories. Many existing theories can help develop intervention theories for health problems and situations. The examples listed in Exhibit 5.6 are grouped by the type of health outcomes anticipated by the program, as a reminder that ultimately the program impact theory needs to be matched with both the health problem and the desired outcomes of the program. There are also existing theories that can be used in developing the process theory; examples of such theories are shown in Exhibit 5.7.

Existing theories relevant to the health problem also can be gleaned from the literature. Svenkerund and Singhal (1998) drew upon two theories in the

---

Exhibit 5.6   Examples of Types of Theories Relevant to Developing Causative Theories Within the Effect Theory, by Four Health Domain Impacts

Physical Health	Psychosocial Health	Knowledge and Abilities	Self-Care and Lifestyle Behaviors
Pathophysiology	Psychopathology	Learning	Peer pressure
Immunology	Social cognition	Communication	Decision making
Endocrinology	Stress and coping	Cognition	Self-efficacy
Pharmacology	Family functioning	Attention	Self-worth
Wound healing	Addiction	Memory	Risk taking
Biochemistry	Violence	Diffusion of innovation	Social stratification
Metabolism		Acculturation	

Exhibit 5.7   Examples of Types of Theories Relevant to Developing the Organizational Plan and Service Utilization Plan Components of the Process Theory

Organizational Plan	Service Utilization Plan
Social network	Social marketing
Communication	Marketing
Leadership	Queuing
Accounting	

planning and delivery of an HIV/AIDS prevention program in Thailand, namely diffusion of innovation theory and social marketing theory. They found that certain concepts and strategies drawn from each theory were effective but that neither theory alone was adequate. This suggests that creativity is needed in applying an existing theory to the development of a health program. It also suggests that theories based on studies of one population may not accurately predict what will occur in another population. This may have been the case in another study. Jenings-Dozier (1999) found that the theory of planned behavior did not predict the actual behavior of African-American and Latina women with regard to the use of pap smear screening. It is therefore important to be aware of possible problems with using the literature. Not all theories are equally applicable to all populations.

Diagramming the Causal Chain of Events

Diagrams that depict the effect theory, the process theory, and the Program Theory can be done with paper or using graphics software. Most software packages include some drawing features that can be used to create diagrams. A picture showing how each intervention changes a characteristic of the participants provides an expedient means of engaging program staff and getting feedback from other professionals in the field. As the scientific literature is reviewed and assimilated, additional relevant variables and their interrelationships can be incorporated into the map of the causal chain of events. Including every possible variable is neither realistic nor desirable; only those variables that relate to the essence of the program and that, according to available scientific literature, are mostly likely to influence the success of your interventions should be included.

There are instances in which a health program is started in response to a mandate or a health policy initiative and thus may not have an explicit program theory. If a program has been in existence or is ongoing, the development of a program theory is still possible and can contribute to program improvements. In such cases, the espoused theory of program staff is a good starting point for the development of a program theory. Observation of program staff would help identify the theory-in-use. Together with the literature, these could be formalized into a program theory. It is quite possible that new areas for program monitoring and evaluation would emerge from such an exercise with program staff. In addition, program staff may come to see the value of their work and become more committed to the program and the participants. Involving program staff in reconciling their espoused theories and theories-in-use can lead to new program approaches and the identification of areas of inefficiencies.

For some health programs, timing is critical, and some intervention components must be accomplished before other intervention components. If there are stages to either the intervention or the impacts, these need to be reflected in the map of the causal chain of events.

Checking Against Assumptions

The overall program theory, and the effect theory in particular, need to be checked against alternative assumptions about theories. Patton (1997) referred to these as validity assumptions. One assumption is that the theory is really about the phenomenon of interest. This means that the program theory is about the health problem or condition that is the focus of the health program. Through the multiple interactions and discussions with stakeholders, this assumption can inadvertently be violated.

Another assumption is of parsimony. Improving the health of individuals, families, and communities is a complex task. Most health programs address only one aspect of a complex puzzle of factors affecting health. Including too much in a program theory can lead to confusion, diffuse interventions, and frustration, not to mention exorbitant expenditures. Parsimony is a crucial characteristic of a good theory, including a program theory. Relying on the priorities set earlier in the planning process by focusing on the most important factors about the target audience helps achieve parsimony.

FUNCTIONS OF PROGRAM THEORY

Having an articulated theory of how the health program will lead to improved health, and, specifically, how the interventions will affect participants, serves several purposes (Bickman, 1987) that range from providing guidance and enabling explanations to forming a basis for communication.

Provides Guidance

A program theory that can be stated in one or two sentences provides a description of what is being implemented. To say that a program is helping asthmatic children is less compelling or descriptive than saying that a program teaches children how to be aware of their bodies and thus avoid situations that may trigger an asthma attack. The latter is a description of how the program works to reduce asthma attacks and provides direct guidance on what to include in the program.

In a world of complex and interactive health problems, identifying the specific health problem and the appropriate target audience for a program can be difficult. Blum's (1982) caution against the failure to analyze problems adequately is avoided by developing the Program Theory, which specifies the problem and target audience. If the program theory is inordinately difficult to develop, it may indicate that the health problem has not been sufficiently narrowed, the target audience is not specific enough, or too many program components have been included. Having a target audience that is too broad can lead to a program theory that is too complex to be of value in designing and implementing the program.

The Program Theory guides what to measure in both the monitoring and outcome evaluations of the program. In terms of the monitoring evaluation, the Program Theory specifies what needs to be measured with regard to the delivery of the intervention. In terms of the outcome evaluation, the effect theory specifies the desired effects and thus what needs to be measured. In instances in which a health program has several possible impacts, the effect theory clarifies which impact is most directly a result of the intervention. Knowing this makes the evaluation of impacts and outcomes more efficient because the evaluation will be designed to find program effects that are arguably the result of the program.

Just as theory is used to guide the development of the health program, so can theory be used to guide the development of the evaluation. For example, Newes-Adeyi, Helitzer, Caulfield, and Bronner (2000) used ecological theory to guide their formative evaluation of the New York State Women, Infant and Children (WIC) Nutritional Program. Their use of ecological theory strengthened the evaluation in terms of its design and ability to explain how the program worked. Their report also serves as a reminder that the same underlying social or psychological theory that guides the effect theory can be applied to the impact evaluation as well.

When a new health program is first provided, its evaluation helps refine the subsequent delivery of the program. A Program Theory helps identify needed inputs as well as what needs to be evaluated and where improvements or changes in the delivery of the interventions are appropriate.

Enables Explanations

Theory helps identify which interventions are likely to have the greatest effect on program participants, and helps clarify how the interventions cause the desired effect in program participants. In this way, the theory enables planners and evaluators to more easily explain how the program should and does work. One task of program planners is to anticipate the unintended. Careful attention to the development of the program theory can help uncover unintended consequences that may result from the program. Having an effect theory helps generate plausible explanations for unintended consequences of the program. Identifying such as an exercise in speculation helps avoid another reason programs do not succeed: failing to examine and compare relevant possible interventions (Blum,1982).

A Program Theory also enables the evaluators to distinguish between process theory failure and effect theory failure (Exhibit 5.8). If the evaluation results show no effect on program participants, then the evaluator must explain what failed. A successful program is one that is provided and that sets into motion the interventions (causal processes) that lead to the desired outcome. However, if a program is not effective, the evaluator needs to identify the roots of the failure. A lack of program success can result from the program not being provided; this is process theory failure. A lack of program success also can result from an ineffective intervention; this is effect theory failure. This distinction between process and effect theory failures, based on the notions of program and

Exhibit 5.8 Two Roots of Program Failure

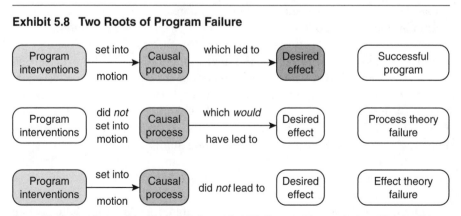

Source: Evaluation Research by Weiss, C.H. Copyright 1972. Reprinted by permission of Pearson Education, Inc., Upper Saddle River, N.J.

theory failure of Weiss (1972) helps evaluators sort out what went wrong or right with the program and explain the evaluation findings to stakeholders.

Forms a Basis for Communication

Health programs compete for resources. A program theory helps convince organizational or legislative policy makers that the program is worthy and deserving of support. The causal chain of events outlined in the program theory serves to frame discussions on a more rational basis, leading to a more rational decision-making process about the health program. The effect theory also helps policy makers understand the extent to which the program interventions are ideologically compatible with their stance and are based on science rather than biases and opinions. In other words, the program theory provides a basis for clear communication of the program intent and content.

Starting and maintaining a program requires that key stakeholders agree on supporting the program. Gaining consensus from stakeholders, whether program staff, administrators, or legislators, is an important step in assuring the success and acceptance of the health program. If stakeholders understand the program theory, it is easier to gain consensus on the usefulness of the program. Having gone through the exercise of developing the determinant, intervention, impact, and outcome theories, the program planners are in the position of being better able to anticipate questions and provide alternative rationales for the health program. Stakeholders can be included in the development of the program theory as a way to gain consensus on the program interventions. In controversial programs, such as sexuality education or family planning for adolescents, consensus on the program theory could be critical to the survival of the program.

Provides a Scientific Contribution

In a sense, every health program is an experiment that tests the program theory. This means that every evaluation has the potential to contribute to our understanding of human nature and health. Evaluations based on the program theory can be used to modify existing theories relevant to the target population and types of interventions used.

ACROSS THE PYRAMID

At the direct services level of the public health pyramid, because the health problems are related to specific individuals, the relevant theories will be about individual behavior and intra-individual responses to treatment or pathology. In other words, the focus is on the micro level. As a result, the interventions are delivered one-on-one, with providers directly delivering the interventions to their clients. Examples of direct services interventions are given in Exhibit 5.3. If the program is to have components, those components would involve different types of interventions that are delivered directly to individuals.

At the enabling services level, because the health problems are related to aggregates of individuals, the relevant theories will be about the interaction of individuals with family or community characteristics. As enabling services are still provided to individuals, the focus continues to be at the micro level. Hence, interventions are delivered one-on-one, as well as to groups with similar characteristics. Different intervention types can be applied at the enabling services level (Exhibit 5.3).

At the population level, because the health problems are related to entire populations, the relevant theories will be about group responses that lead to the health problem, cultural theories that explain behaviors and beliefs related to the health problem, and social theories about interactions among groups. Liddle and Hogue (2000) described an intervention for high-risk adolescents. One key feature of their intervention model was that the theoretical foundation included risk and protection theory, developmental psychopathology theory, and ecological theory. This blend of theories is consistent with the intent of the program. In terms of the pyramid, however, the use of ecological theory reflects the theoretical awareness of the program planners that the population level influences the enabling level (i.e., the family) and the individual level. At the population level, the interventions are designed and intended to have a macro focus. Interventions are more likely to be delivered through the mass media or to involve policy formation. While having program components at the population level can create synergies that enhance the intervention, such program components may be prohibitive in terms of feasibility, manipulability, and cost.

At the infrastructure level, because the problems are related not to individuals but to processes and structures that enable the delivery of health programs, relevant theories might include those about organizational behavior, management and leadership style, personnel motivation, political action, and communication. The interventions can be delivered one-on-one with personnel, as well as with groups of workers or entire organizations. For example, McQuiston (2000) suggested that empowerment theory is useful to enhance the workers' participation in program evaluation. Although he focused on workplace safety programs, the same reasoning can apply to the infrastructure workforce and programs intended to increase the workforce capacity.

DISCUSSION QUESTIONS

1. Select a health program with which you are familiar.

   A. Briefly state the hypotheses that constitute the effect theory of the program.

   B. What are the intervention components and the specific interventions?

   C. Develop a logic model of the program theory used by the program, with attention to the abstract program theory discussed in this chapter.

2. What are the relationships between the possible functions of the effect theory and the selection of optimal interventions?

3. Which of the theories that make up the effect theory are likely to be affected by the cultural, ethnic, or racial differences of target populations? In what ways might you make those theories culturally appropriate or sensitive?

4. Identify possible primary, secondary and tertiary prevention interventions for each level of the pyramid.

References

Argyris, C., & Schon, D. A. (1974). *Theory in practice: Increasing professional effectiveness.* San Francisco: Jossey-Bass.

Aveyard, P., Sherrat, E., Almond, J., Lawrence, T., Lancashire, R., Griffin, C., & Cheng, K.K. (2001). The change-in-stage and updated smoking status results from a cluster-randomized trial of smoking prevention and cessation using the transtheoretical model among British adolescents. *Preventive Medicine, 33*, 313–324.

Baranowski, T., Davis, M., Resnicow, K., Baranowski, J., Doyle, C., Lin, L., Smith, M., & Wang, P. T. (2000). Gimme five fruit, juice, and vegetables for fun and health: Outcome evaluation. *Health Education and Behavior, 27*, 96–111.

Bickman, L. (1987). The functions of program theory. *New Directions for Program Evaluation. 43*, 5–18.

Blum, H. L. (1982). Social perspective on risk reduction. In M.M. Farber & A.M. Reinhart (Eds.), *Promoting health through risk reduction.* (pp. 19–36). New York: Macmillan.

Brenton, J. J. (1999). Complementing development of prevention and mental health promotion programs for Canadian children based on contemporary scientific paradigms. *Canadian Journal of Psychiatry, 44*, 227–234.

Brown, J. H. (2001). Youth, drugs and resilience education. *Journal of Drug Education, 31*, 83–122.

Calhoun, A. D., & Clark-Jones, F. (1998). Theoretical frameworks: Developmental psychopathology, the public health approach to violence and the cycle of violence. *Pediatric Clinics of North America, 45*, 281–291.

Fletcher, G. F., Baladay, G. J., Amsterdam, E. A., Chaitman, B., Eckel, R., Fleg, J., Froelicher, V. F., Leon, A. S., Pina, I. L., Rodney, R., Simons-Morton, D. A., Williams, M. A., & Bazzarro, T. (2001). Exercise standards for testing and training: A statement for healthcare professionals from the American Heart Association. *Circulation, 104*, 1694–1740.

Gabriel, R. M. (2000). Methodological challenges in evaluating community partnerships and coalitions: Still crazy after all these years. *Journal of Community Psychology, 28*, 339–352.

Grobe, S. J., & Hughes, L. C. (1993). The conceptual validity of a taxonomy of nursing interventions. *Journal of Advanced Nursing, 18*, 1942–1961.

Guidotti, T. L., Ford, L., & Wheeler, M. (2000). The Fort McMurray Demonstration Project in social marketing: Theory, design, and evaluation. *American Journal of Preventive Medicine, 18*, 163–169.

Heaney, C. A., & van Ryn, M. (1996). The implications of status, class, and cultural diversity for health education practice: The case of worksite stress reduction programs. *Health Education Research, 11*, 57–70.

Issel, L. M. (1997). Measuring comprehensive case management interventions: Development of a tool. *Nursing Case Management, 2*, 3–12.

Jackson, C., Altman, D. G., Howard-Pitney, B. & Farquhar, J. W. (1989). Evaluating community-level health promotion and disease prevention interventions. In M. T. Braverman (Ed)., *Evaluating health promotion programs.* San Francisco: Jossey-Bass.

Jenings-Dozier, K. (1999). Predicting intentions to obtain a pap smear among African-American and Latina women: Testing the theory of planned behavior. *Nursing Research, 48*, 198–205.

Liddle, H. A., & Hogue, A. (2000). A family-based, developmental-ecological preventive intervention for high-risk adolescents. *Journal of Marital and Family Therapy, 26*, 265–279.

McQuinston, T. H. (2000). Empowerment evaluation of worker safety and health education programs. *American Journal of Industrial Medicine, 38*, 584–597.

Newes-Adeyi, G., Helitzer, D. L., Caulfield, L. E., & Bronner, Y. (2000). Theory and practice: Applying the ecological model of formative research for a WIC training program in New York State. *Health Education Research, 15*, 283–291.

Patton, M. Q. (1997). *Utilization-focused evaluation* (3rd ed.). Thousand Oaks, CA: Sage Publications.

Resnicow, K., Baranowsky, T., Ahuwalia, J. S., & Brathwaite, R. (1999). Cultural sensitivity in public health: Defined and demystified. *Ethnicity and Disease, 9*, 10–21.

Rossi, P., & Freeman, H. (1993). *Evaluation: A systematic approach* (5th ed.). Newbury Park, CA: Sage Publications.

Rossi, P., Freeman, H., & Lipsey, M. (1999). *Evaluation: A systematic approach* (6th ed.). Thousand Oaks, CA: Sage Publications.

Svenkerund, P. J., & Singhal, A. (1998). Enhancing the effectiveness of HIV/AIDS prevention programs targeted to unique population groups in Thailand: Lessons learned from applying concepts of diffusion of innovation and social marketing. *Journal of Health Communication, 3*, 193–216.

United Way of America (1996). *Measuring program outcomes: A practical approach.* Alexandria, VA.

Weiss, C. (1972). *Evaluation.* San Francisco: Jossey-Bass.

CHAPTER 6

Program Objectives and Setting Targets

Written with Deborah Rosenberg, Ph.D.
Research Assistant Professor
Division of Epidemiology and Biostatistics
University of Illinois at Chicago, School of Public Health

In this chapter, the focus is on setting the parameters by which the program is judged as successful—in other words, developing goals and objectives for the program. Setting goals and objectives may sound like a mundane exercise in administrivia. However, the activity of developing goals and objectives is informative in terms of forcing further clarity and specificity about implementing the program and later evaluating its effects. After a logic model has been developed, this is the next step in program planning.

PARAMETERS OF THE PROGRAM

One of the first decisions facing program planners is to define for whom the program is designed. Although general agreement may exist about who is the focus of the program based on the needs assessment and the logic model, further specificity is required. The *target population* is the entire population in need of the program, whereas the *target audience* is the segment of the population for whom the program is specifically intended. The term "recipient" is used to refer to those who actually receive or participate in the program. For programs at the population level of the pyramid, the target population is also the target audience and, hopefully, also the recipient. However, at the direct services and enabling services levels, the program cannot accommodate all those in need and may be designed for a subpopulation. For such programs, "target audience" is a better term. The distinction between the target population or audience and the recipients is critical in terms of both budgetary issues and program implementation and evaluation issues. The program can have an impact only on the recipients, and therefore the evaluation will focus primarily on this group, but it is also necessary to quantify the broader target audience in order to estimate underinclusion and overinclusion in the program and describe how these may have an impact on the evaluation.

Inclusion: Underinclusion and Overinclusion

Ideally, only those in the target audience would receive the program. However, these ideals can be difficult to achieve, resulting in overinclusion or underinclusion. Overinclusion and underinclusion in the program are two closely related concepts. *Overinclusion* occurs when there are participants in the program who are not part of the target audience. It can be minimized by having procedures to correctly exclude individuals who are not members of the target audience. For example, in a dental sealant program, children who are younger than 2 years of age, as well as children who are between the ages of 5 and 14 who already had sealant treatment, would be excluded in order to avoid overinclusion (National Institute of Dental and Craniofacial Research, 2001). *Underinclusion* occurs when those who are members of the target audience do not receive the program. Underinclusion can be minimized by having procedures to correctly include members of the target audience for whom the program is designed. Underinclusion in the dental sealant program would be seen as having fewer children of the appropriate age receive the dental sealant than the number of children of that age who need the sealant and who are within the catchment area of the dental clinic. Underinclusion can occur if the program is not well publicized, if there is some characteristic of the program that is unappealing to the target audience, or if a barrier exists to accessing the program. Steps taken to implement the program, as discussed in subsequent chapters, ought to be tailored to avoid underinclusion and overinclusion.

Neither overinclusion nor underinclusion is desirable. In terms of program expenditures, overinclusion can result in a shortage of funds and underinclusion can result in unspent funds that may need to be returned to the funding agency. Underinclusion and overinclusion are also undesirable from the perspective of program evaluation. Overinclusion of those who do not need the program can decrease the measurable effect of the program on participant outcomes. That is, the extent of change experienced by those individuals who do not need the program is likely to be less than that experienced by those who do need the program. This will translate into a decrease in the average amount or degree of change found when all participants in the program are considered. In addition, overinclusion may artificially inflate the normative need for the program. If current enrollment or requests for participation in the program are used for future planning of the program, overinclusion will falsely increase the apparent number in the target audience. Overinclusion also can lead to a decreased availability of funds to include true target individuals in the program. This is particularly plausible if members of the true target audience are more likely not to be the first ones to enroll in the program.

Underinclusion can also affect evaluation results, particularly for programs designed for and delivered at the population level. Having too few of the target audience in the program could make it difficult to find significant small program effects, could increase the amount of program services received by individual participants and thereby falsely increase the program effects, and will definitely increase the cost per participant. At any level of the pyramid, underinclusion can lead to biased evaluation results if those in the target audience who do and do not participate in the program differ from one another in ways that are related to the program's effectiveness.

Several steps can be taken to help minimize overinclusion or underinclusion. The first step comes in developing the process theory, in terms of specifying how those in need of the program get into the program; this is part of the service utilization plan. Another step is to have a solid, thoughtful marketing plan, another element in the service utilization plan.

Once the target population or audience has been clearly specified, screening tests that are both highly sensitive and specific can be used to minimize both overincusion and underinclusion (Exhibit 6.1). Test sensitivity refers to the probability that the screening test will be positive when there is actually

Exhibit 6.1   Relationship of Test Sensitivity and Specificity to Overinclusion and Underinclusion

	Specificity	
Sensitivity	**High**	**Low**
High	Ideal inclusion and coverage; minimal overinclusion and underinclusion	Overinclusion
Low	Underinclusion	Both overinclusion and underinclusion occur

Note: Specificity identifies ineligibles, or those not in need; sensitivity identifies true eligibles, or those in need.

an illness, need, or existing risk factor. Using a highly sensitive screening test to identify individuals who are eligible for the program increases the likelihood that more individuals will be in the program who actually need it, thus reducing underinclusion. Test specificity refers to the probability that the test will be negative when there is no illness, need, or risk factor. Using a highly specific screening test to identify individuals who are not eligible for the program results in fewer individuals in the program who do not need it. This reduces overinclusion. In practice, it is never possible to have a screening test that is both 100% sensitive and 100% specific. Typically, there is a trade-off between sensitivity and specificity, with the screening test being either more sensitive or more specific. Nonetheless, a screening mechanism is often the best way to minimize overinclusion and underinclusion.

Scope: Full and Partial Coverage

The distinction between target population, target audience, and recipient is also critical in determining whether the program has partial or full coverage (Rossi & Freeman, 1993). The distinction between partial and full programs has implications for public health and health policy. *Partial coverage* programs are those designed to serve some portion of the target population, and participation in the program is based on a set of criteria that focuses recruitment strategies and takes account of limited resources. During the planning stage, the decision to have a program that provides only partial coverage generally stems from having limited capacity to serve all those in the target population. Partial coverage programs are likely to be at the direct care or enabling services levels of the pyramid. Examples of partial coverage programs include educational classes for individuals at high risk for a health problem and providing medi-car services to homebound elderly.

Full coverage programs are delivered, or are intended to be delivered, to the entire target population. By definition, full coverage programs are more likely to be at the population services level of the pyramid. Examples of full coverage programs include childhood immunization programs and water fluoridation. Some programs are less easily identified as full or partial coverage because, although the program is designed with the population level in mind, the target "population" is restricted to those meeting the criteria for participation, such as income level for state child health insurance programs, federal WIC programs, or Medicare. Since these programs are intended to serve the entire target population, they are actually full coverage programs, despite the use of what are typically referred to as eligibility criteria. One way to distinguish between partial and full programs is to consider whether the program is primarily designed to make changes at the individual level or at the population level (Exhibit 6.2).

Exhibit 6.2   Examples of Programs with an Individual and Population Focus, by Partial and Full Coverage

	Individual or Aggregate Focus (Direct and Enabling Services Levels)	Population Focus (Population-Based Level)
Partial Coverage	Class-based educational offerings, needle exchange programs, medi-car services	WIC program, state child health insurance plans (SCHIP)
Full Coverage	Speed limits, seat belt laws	Medicare, fluoridation of the water supply

Making the distinction between full and partial coverage programs during the planning phase may not be so easy. It is plausible that stakeholder issues may arise and advocacy positions may be taken regarding whether a program ought to provide full or partial coverage. Some vocal activist groups may want the health program to serve an entire population at risk or in need, regardless of budgetary or logistical issues. Their position needs to be taken into account and reconciled with issues of feasibility in order for the program to be successful in gaining their support or endorsement. Also, if the health program is to be a partial coverage program, eligibility criteria and procedures for prioritizing and enrolling potential recipients must be established. This, of course, can lead to considerable debates over the particulars of the cut-off criteria chosen for program eligibility. The other reason to consider whether the health program will provide full or partial coverage is that the scope of the program affects the design of the evaluation and potentially the cost of conducting an impact assessment of the program.

In addition, the scope of the program needs to be considered with respect to underinclusion or overinclusion. Overinclusion will be much more difficult to detect in a full coverage program than in a partial coverage program because the presumption in a full coverage program is that an entire target population is the intended program recipient. Given that a full coverage program by its nature is likely to have a large number of recipients, it will be difficult to identify the few recipients who are not members of the target population. In a partial coverage program, overinclusion is more likely to occur than underinclusion. The interaction of the scope of a program with the appropriateness of inclusion may have implications that need to be considered when developing the program marketing plan and the program budget as well as when prioritizing among program designs. In addition, an awareness of the interaction may help explain later findings of evaluations of either the process or program effect.

PROGRAM GOALS AND OBJECTIVES

"Goals" and "objectives" are terms that are widely used in program planning and evaluation. *Goals*, in a strict sense, are broad, encompassing statements about the outcomes to be achieved, whereas *objectives* are specific statements about impacts to be achieved and are stated in measurable terms. Goals are always statements about the health outcomes or status of the target audience, generally with a longer time horizon, such as five years. Typically, goals do not incorporate a quantifiable measure but instead refer in broad terms to the most important anticipated effect of the program. A program will have at least one goal, and a well-focused program with several components may have more than one. However, the number of goals is generally quite low. Funding bodies do not use the words "objective" and "goal" in any apparently consistent manner, and for this reason, program planners and evaluators must understand the difference. Making the distinction between objectives and goals is key to subsequently making conceptual distinctions between short-term impacts and long-term outcomes of the program.

An easy format that helps in remembering the parts of a good objective is this: "By when, who will achieve what, by how much." For example, one objective may be, "By 2002, the Bowe County Healthy Start Program will reduce the rate of low birth weight infants among program participants by 2% compared to women not participating." The "by how much" portion of the objective, or the target value, is the quantifiable measure that distinguishes an objective from a goal. The target value is the essence of the objective and, without it, no objective exists. The statement, "The percentage of low birth weight infants among women enrolled in the Bowe County Healthy Start Program during 2002 will be reduced" is a goal, not an objective. A goal may have several objectives that delineate more precisely what achieving the goal entails. Thus, adding a target value would yield the following objective for reaching that goal: "The percentage of low birth weight infants among women enrolled in the Bowe County Healthy Start Program during 2002 will be 8%." The 8% quantifies the reduction and is measurable. The time frame used in the objectives needs to be short term and well within the lifespan of the program. Generally, objectives have no more than a one- to two-year time horizon, although the national Healthy People objectives set targets for a decade.

Goals and their corresponding objectives flow from the logic model and the Program Theory. Involving the stakeholders and program staff in the development of the program objectives and goals can be useful in gaining their support, good ideas, and consensus on what will constitute the program. However, the process of gaining consensus, particularly on objectives, can be a bit of a struggle if stakeholders have vested interests in achieving particular health impacts for their constituents. In addition, there are often tight timelines for preparing a program proposal, making timely involvement of stakeholders a considerable challenge. The efforts devoted to arriving at a set of clearly articulated goals and objectives pay off in terms of having a foundation from which to develop the evaluation and having standards against which to assess the success of the program.

Foci of Objectives

Development of objectives begins with conceptual clarity regarding whether the objective is related to the program's process theory or effect theory. Understanding the distinction between process and effect objectives is covered in this section. The next step discussed is identifying and selecting appropriate indicators for the objectives. The section concludes with a review of the characteristics that distinguish well-constructed goals and objectives.

Process Objectives

The process theory component of the Program Theory, specifically the organizational plan and the service utilization plan, provides a framework for stating process objectives. Because the process theory describes how the program is designed and delivered, the process objectives focus on what is done by program staff to implement and sustain the health program. Following the format for writing objectives, process objectives would then state, "By when, which staff will do what, to what extent" (Exhibit 6.3). Process objectives focus on the activities of the program staff, not benefits to the participants. The organizational plan and service utilization plan provide insights into what ought to be included in each process objective, particularly for the "do what" portion. The "to what extent" portion will be determined based on past experience with the capabilities of the staff and on the amount of work to be done within the time frame. In the fields of public health and mental health, objectives are identified for the capacity of the infrastructure, in terms of personnel qualifications (Perrin & Koshel, 1997). Capacity objectives are best considered as objectives about the organizational plan. Thus a process objective might be, "By month 6, 100% of program staff will have participated in training on health education modules being used in the Bowe County Healthy Start Program."

Exhibit 6.3   Aspects of Process Objectives as Related to Components of the Process Theory

	Organizational Plan	Service Utilization Plan	Outputs
Format of Objective	By when, how many staff with what type of qualifications	By when, how many interactions with participants of what type	By when, how many products distributed by whom and to whom
Example	1.1 By [date], # of staff in the program will have received # hours of training about the program	2.1 By [date], participating women will receive # of prenatal care visits	3.1 By [date], staff will distribute # brochures to women receiving prenatal care at the clinic

Effect Objectives: Impact and Outcome

Effect theory objectives are about the program participants and the benefits they will experience as a result of receiving the program interventions. Following the formula for writing objectives, effect objectives would then state, "By when, how many of which program participants will experience what type of health benefit or state and to what extent."

The effect theory, notably the intervention, impact, and outcome theories, provides the basis for stating intervention, impact, and outcome objectives (Exhibit 6.4). In most program literature, these three are all referred to as outcome objectives. The purpose of distinguishing among the three types is so that during the planning process, connections between the planned interventions and health changes are made explicit. Being explicit at this phase of the planning will facilitate subsequent development of the evaluation, particularly with regard to what changes, benefits, or health outcomes to measure. Because funding agencies generally require objectives about effects, intervention objectives can be included with impact and outcome objectives.

The format for writing good objectives can be used to write objectives in terms of increasing or reducing the level of a certain outcome compared to some benchmark level. The earlier example of "By 2002, the Bowe County Healthy Start Program will reduce the rate of low birth weight infants among program participants by 2% compared to women not participating," uses nonparticipants as the comparison or benchmark. Another approach to writing an

Exhibit 6.4   Using elements of Effect Theory as the basis for writing Program Effect Objectives

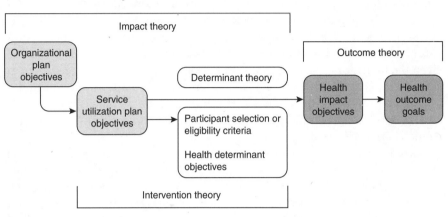

outcome objective is to have the "by how much" reflect a preferred level of achievement or a target value the program seeks to achieve. An objective written in this way might be, "During 2002, women enrolled in the Bowe County Healthy Start Program will have a rate of low birth weight infants of 8%." Regardless of how the "by how much" is stated, the objectives need to reference a time frame, the program participants to be affected, a health outcome related to the program interventions, and a quantifiable target value for that health outcome. Clearly stated objectives that include these components become a major guide to designing the evaluation of program effect.

Objectives and Indicators

One aspect of developing objectives is to consider indicators. Like so many other terms in program planning and evaluation, the word "indicator" has many uses and interpretations. It can refer to the "what" portion of the objective, to the variables used to measure that "what," or to performance benchmarks used to determine the failure or success of a program. There is no easy way to distinguish among these uses or to prescriptively state that one is better than the others. It is, however, important to be aware that the results of the evaluation regarding "by how much" can be influenced not only by the program's true effect, but also by the sensitivity of the measure (indicator) selected. For example, if an impact objective concerns improvement in cognitive functioning of children with special health care needs, indicators of cognitive functioning might be a score on a standardized scale like the Bayles Assessment Scale or the Denver Developmental Assessment Test, or a parental report of cognitive functioning. Because the standardized scales are more sensitive and specific than the parental report, they can detect a smaller true change. By choosing, or at least considering, indicators when developing objectives, planners and evaluators can set reasonable target numbers for how much change is projected, given the indicator chosen. It is also important to be aware that for full coverage programs at the population level, it may be more appropriate to think of indicators in terms of benchmarks. For example, the national standard for a healthy birth weight could be used, as in the objectives for infants born to women in the WIC program.

Most health programs address one or more domains of health or well-being. Typically, these domains are physical, mental, cognitive, behavioral, knowledge, social, and financial. For each of these domains of health, specific variables (indicators) are used to measure the program effect on that domain. Exhibit 6.5 provides some commonly used variables for each health or well-being domain. Each health program would need to select indicators that reflect the specific health

Exhibit 6.5   Domains of Impact on Health Program Recipients and Examples of Corresponding Indicators

Impact Domain	Examples of Indicators (Variables) to Measure Objectives
Physical health	Cardiovascular fitness, weight, lab values, medical diagnoses
Mental health	Motivation, values, attitudes, emotional bonding, diagnostic category
Cognitive processes	Decision making, judgments, problem-solving ability, cognitive processes
Behavior	Lifestyle behavior, health promotion behavior, aggression, parenting behaviors
Knowledge	Skill, ability, performance, education of others
Social health	Marital status, social network, recreation activities, friendship and kinship networks
Resources	Income, insurance source, utilization pattern, housing situation, employment status, education level

domain targeted by the program. Reliance on the effect theory, and knowing which antecedents, contributing factors, and determinants of the health problem are targeted, also help select optimal indicators of program effect.

Various criteria can be used for selecting indicators. The first criteria to consider are the indicators that are required or mandated by the funding agency. For example, the Maternal and Child Health Bureau (MCHB) of the Health Resources Services Administration (HRSA) requires all grantees of Title V funds to use their set of 18 performance measures and 6 outcome measures, plus 8 core health status indicators that are related to the purpose of the Title V funds. MCHB Title V indicators include measures such as the rate of children hospitalized for asthma, the percentage of women with a live birth who have had an adequate number of prenatal visits according to the Adequacy of Prenatal Care Utilization index (Kotelchuck, 1997), and the percentage of live births of less than 2,500 grams (Maternal and Child Health Bureau, n.d.). Although some of the MCHB indicators could be considered related to process, grantees must use these indicators as outcomes. This is not an uncommon situation to which program planners must pay attention.

There are several other criteria for selecting indicators. One is that the data for the indicator (variable) must be feasible to collect and easy to analyze. Indicators (variables) also ought to be scientifically defendable, hence the use of standardized or existing questionnaires and tools. Indicators (variables) also ought to be relevant to users, such as the program managers and program stakeholders. And finally, the indicators (measures) need to be relatively easy to analyze. It is pointless to rely upon an indicator (measure) that is so difficult to analyze that it is not used in program management or improvement.

The other way to think about indicators is by returning to the community health assessment and the statements developed about health problems. In those statements (Chapter 4), the health status indicator can be directly applied to the impact objectives. For example, the health indicators (Exhibit 4.2) of the rate of gunshot wounds, adolescent pregnancy, and neural tube defects are also appropriate as indicators (variables) in the objectives. Exhibit 6.6 provides examples of intervention, impact, and outcome objectives for the goal of reducing birth defects.

Good Goals and Objectives

Obviously, good goals and objectives are ones that are meaningful and useful (Patton, 1997). Of course, the objectives need to be distinctly related to either process or effect. Both process and effect objectives need to be tailored to the specific health program being planned. Thus, program planners are encouraged to adapt rather than plagiarize objectives from similar programs.

Exhibit 6.6   Aspects of Effect Objectives as Related to Components of the Effect Theory

	Intervention Objective from Intervention Theory	Impact Objective from Impact Theory	Outcome Objective from Outcome Theory
Format of Objective	By when, what proportion of recipients will have how much effect from program interventions on which determinant factors that lead to health problem	By when, what proportion of recipients will have how much effect from program interventions on immediate health problem	By when, what proportion of recipients will have long-term or global health changes consistent with the program goals
Example	1.1 By [date], [target #] women in the program will have a decrease of [target %] in exposure to environmental hazards that are teratogenic 1.2 By [date], [target #] women in the program will increase dietary folic acid intake so that ADA standards for pregnant women are met	2.1 By [date] , [target #] women in the program will have normal newborns (no neural tube defects)	3.1 By [date], [target # or %] newborns will not have preventable birth defects

Each objective ought to convey only one idea, so that each statement can be related to only one measure. Ideally, the objectives will be understandable to any stakeholder who might read them. Another important consideration is the ability to imagine that without the program, whatever is stated in the objective would not occur. This is a way to double-check that the program is directly responsible for the elements addressed in the objective. Similarly, the program goals and objectives need to be reviewed for alignment with the needs, problems, and assets identified through the community health assessment.

The use of creative activities, stories, and clear communication can make the writing of goals a positive experience. Although this chapter presents the development of the goals and objectives as being derived from the logic model and the Program Theory, in actuality, discussions that can develop about objectives may lead the program planners and the program stakeholders to revise the logic model or the Program Theory. Similarly, the process of selecting indicators for objectives may cause the objectives to be revised. These iterations ought to be viewed as a positive sign that ways to strengthen and streamline the health program are being identified and are occurring during the planning phase rather than after the program has been implemented.

Good goals and objectives have one other characteristic: they are congruent with and contribute to the strategic plan, whether that be the national (i.e., *Healthy People 2010*), state, or local health plans, or the health care organization's strategic plan. The extent to which the program goals and objectives are compatible with the strategic or long-term plan of the organization can affect the priority given to the program and hence the fiscal support and organizational approval of the program. For health programs being developed by local health agencies or local community-based organizations, this larger context of health programs can be crucial in building synergies within the program as well as between programs with complementary foci.

USING DATA TO SET TARGET VALUES

All types of objectives, whether related to process theory or effect theory, have the "by how much" portion for each "what." A critical step in developing a meaningful objective is choosing a numeric value as the target for the "by how much" portion of the objective.

For process objectives, the procedure for establishing target values for the "by how much" portion relies upon using data from the organizational and marketing assessments. There are not likely to be national standards or objectives to use as a guide. However, there are professional standards that can be used, particularly for organizational plan objectives. For example, there are legal and professional standards for minimum qualifications for personnel. These standards can be used as a starting point for establishing targets—say, for the percentage of program staff with a given certification.

For effect objectives, the target-setting process relies on the effect theory. The assumption is that as long as the objectives are consistent with the Program Theory and the level of programmatic effort, targets can be achieved. What is achievable, of course, depends on a host of factors within as well as outside of the program. Having reasonable target values will directly influence the extent to which a program is perceived to be successful, particularly with regard to impacts and outcomes, and therefore the measurement of success must be scientifically credible. During the development of the objectives and their corresponding targets, planners and evaluators will want to agree on a strategy that accounts for both the Program Theory and extraneous factors, and they will also want to have stakeholders involved during this crucial initial stage.

Developing a rational target-setting strategy, instead of using mere guesstimation, is more likely to lead to targets that are meaningful from a programmatic perspective and that are achievable to the extent that they are an outgrowth of the Program Theory and are based on empirical data. It is certainly possible to choose reachable target values without having a clear analytic strategy, but doing so emphasizes achievability over the Program Theory. To use an extreme example, a target value of 0.0% change among program recipients could be chosen, and achieving this target would for all intents and purposes be guaranteed, but the integrity of the target-setting process, not to mention that of the program evaluation, would be undermined. In contrast, the target-setting approaches outlined here begin with establishing guidelines based on a decision framework and then choosing one or more relatively simple statistical procedures to yield target values consistent with the decisions. These approaches are best suited for setting target values for effect objectives. The framework described in the next section was developed by Rosenberg (1999) as an outgrowth of an effort by the MCHB to provide states with enhanced skills for program planning and evaluation.

Decisional Framework for Setting Target Values

The first and most basic element in developing a target-setting strategy is deciding how program success will be defined. This is a decision that is best made prior to selecting target values. Success can be defined as meeting or exceeding a target, or as making meaningful progress toward the target but not necessarily meeting it. If success is defined as meeting a target, then targets will probably be chosen more cautiously than if success is defined less strictly. If program planners and staff wish to claim success even when a target value is not achieved, then "making meaningful progress" must be quantified, in addition to setting the target value itself. Either definition of program success is acceptable, but the definition that will be used in the later program evaluation needs to be agreed upon and, more importantly, made explicit to all relevant parties during the planning stage.

The way in which program success is defined will influence whether targets will be chosen primarily according to past or baseline indicator values or whether more emphasis will be placed on the values of longer-term objectives for the program. This difference in perspective can have a dramatic effect on a final target value. Referencing targets to past or baseline values is typically a more cautious approach, because the target values will tend to be set to a level that represents a very modest improvement in the health outcome being measured—in other words, a minimum expectation for program effectiveness. In contrast, referencing targets to longer-term objectives is a bolder approach, often resulting in target values that will be somewhat more difficult to reach but that will challenge program planners to continually examine the program implementation and to advocate for changes if necessary. Both approaches are appropriate, and a decision needs to be made as to which focus is more important to the particular program under consideration.

Once program success is defined and the relative importance of past, present, or future indicator values has been generally agreed upon, planners can begin developing a specific methodology for incorporating indicator values into the target. Sometimes only current data values will be used in setting a target; sometimes a combination of current values and trend data will be considered; and sometimes current values, trend data, and a local or national standard will be considered. For example, if data exist over time and there is also an already established objective or national standard specifying a long-term outcome, it may be important to set a target based both on the trend in the data and on how close to or far from the existing standard the outcome currently is. Exhibit 6.7 shows a matrix representing combinations of patterns over time and relationships to a long-term objective. A different target value might be selected depending on which cell is relevant to the outcome of interest. For example, if a program is being implemented for a target population that is experiencing worsening conditions over time and that has a current indicator value far from the long-term objective, the target value might be set more cautiously than if the program were being implemented for a target population that was experiencing gradual improvement and that had a current indicator already fairly close to the long-term objective.

Another component of making decisions about target setting is choosing what types and sources of data will be used. As will be discussed in subsequent chapters, a wide variety of sources of data are often available and appropriate

Exhibit 6.7   Matrix of Decision Options Based on Current Indicator Value, Population Trend of the Health Indicator, and Value of Long-Term Objective or Standard

Population Trend of Indicator	Current Value of the Health Indicator in the Target Audience		
	Better than Long-Term Objective or Standard	Meets Long-Term Objective or Standard	Worse Than Long-Term Objective or Standard
Improving	Set target to *maintain* current level; better than the long-term objective and limits to further improvement	Set target to *surpass* the long-term objective; continuing the improving trend	Set target to a *better* level; accelerate improving trend to approach the long-term objective
No change	Set target to slightly *better level*; better than the long-term objective, but want to see improving trend	Set target to *surpass* the long-term objective; begin improvement in trend	Set target to a *moderately better* level; begin improvement in trend
Deteriorating	Set target to *maintain* current level; stop the worsening trend	Set target to *maintain* current value; stop the worsening trend	Set target to *maintain* current level or adjust it slightly downward; stop or slow the worsening trend

for assessing health programs and measuring objectives. Ideally, multiple data sources should be used in setting target values because each source contributes slightly different information to the target-setting process. For example, one source of data might be police reports on the use of guns, and another source might be medical diagnoses of gunshot wounds in emergency departments. The statistics reported by each of these sources might be similar or might be different. Having access to both would be useful in setting a reasonable target for the rate of intentional gun violence in Layetteville.

The number of data sources available and the consistency of the data across these sources influences the target-setting process. Exhibit 6.8 shows

Exhibit 6.8   Framework for Target Setting: Interaction of Data Source Availability and Consistency of Information

	One or Only a Few Sources	Many Sources
Consistent Information Across Sources	Need to consider whether the available data is of high quality. Need to consider whether it is relevant to the program and objective target being considered.	Can use any of the data sources.
Inconsistent Information Across Sources	If the one data source is markedly different from the literature, need to either change the objective or verify the data.	Need to decide which data source to use, given the strengths and weaknesses of each data source. Need to consider which data source is most relevant to the program and the objective being considered.

the intersection of these two dimensions. For example, if many data sources are available and their data are in reasonable agreement, then arriving at a target value is relatively straightforward because it will be a reflection of the consistent values. Similar target values would be reached regardless of which data sources were used. If, however, many data sources are available but the information is inconsistent or conflicting, then decisions are needed about which data source should be given precedence or what combination of data sources will be used. These decisions should be based on the strengths and weaknesses of each data source, including sample size, data completeness, and other aspects of data quality. The goal is to integrate the data and the information in a way that permits arriving at one target value.

The choice of data source also needs to be congruent with or correspond to the target population or audience. For example, if a target value is being developed for effect objectives for a full coverage, population-level program with a goal of improving birth outcomes, an appropriate data source would be vital records data. In contrast, for Bowe County Healthy Start, which is a partial coverage program for a smaller target audience with the same goal of improving birth outcomes, appropriate data sources are medical records and surveys of the women who are program recipients, as well as the county vital records data. The data sources for setting the target may or may not be the same as the sources of the evaluation data or the data for the community needs assessment. The choice of data source for each of these program planning and evaluation activities must always correspond to the purpose for which the data will be used.

Another factor to consider in the decision-making process is the extent to which disparities exist across or within the target populations. During the community health assessment, some sense of the disparities ought to be evident. If the disparities exist by income or race/ethnicity or geographic location, the data may need to be stratified by those factors. When available data are not stratified, indicator values are simply averages that may mask very different outcomes for different population groups. Left unstratified, for example, the rate of low birth weight infants in a community might appear relatively close to the *Healthy People 2010* objective of 5%, but when births are stratified by neighborhood, it may become clear that the rate of low birth weight infants in one area is far from the national target value and much different from the rate in another area. Target values may or may not be chosen based on stratified data, but program evaluators should certainly incorporate stratified values into their interpretation of why targets are or are not met. With respect to the Program Theory, the antecedent or contributing factors may include factors that can be stratified. Continuing with the low birth weight example, the neighborhood can represent a contributing factor or set of contributing factors to birth outcomes and thus may be a variable that can be stratified.

It is not always possible to stratify data in the way that evaluators may want. The sources of data that have information on the indicator of interest may not include data for the variables to be stratified. For example, the emergency department data is not likely to have information on the education level of the patient, and the police report data is not likely to have information on the severity of the injury. Stratification may also result in having only a few individuals within some strata, which poses statistical and interpretation problems. One approach to addressing the problem of small numbers is to minimize the number of strata by combining data across multiple years, multiple geographic areas, or even across sociodemographic characteristics, if appropriate. For example, while it might be desirable to stratify by age, broad rather than narrow age strata might be defined to ensure adequate numbers in each group. This problem of small numbers is particularly poignant for programs in rural areas or for target audiences with rare health needs or problems.

One technique for explicitly organizing and documenting the process of setting targets is to use logic statements. These can be written as the decision-making process is unfolding as a way to keep the decisions explicit and focused. Logic statements are written in "if, then; otherwise, if, then" format. For example, thinking about how to integrate different data sources, a logic statement for gun violence might be as follows:

If the emergency department data and the police department data do not agree,

> **then** the [one or other of the data sources] will be given precedence in setting the target value.

To integrate different types of data about gun violence, a logic statement might be something like the following:

If trend data for gun violence show steady improvement, but the current value is still far from a long-term objective,

> **then** the target value will be set to reflect an increase in the rate of improvement;

otherwise, if the trend in gun violence shows steady improvement and the current rate is already close to a long-term objective,

> **then** the target value will be set to reflect a continuation of the existing rate of improvement;

otherwise, if no trend data are available,

> **then** the target value will be set to reflect an improvement in the current value of X percent.

Sets of such statements can be drafted for each factor about which decisions are being made, such as data sources, data consistency, data types, existing or perceived disparities, and resource availability. The statements ought to incorporate information obtained during the community health assessment, along with input from stakeholders.

It is important to recognize that although some target-setting decisions can be applied to all of the program objectives, other decisions may vary depending on the objective. Objectives for different health outcomes, the "what" component, will have differing pools of data sources and may exhibit differing trends over time, differing patterns of disparities, and differing importance within a larger context. In addition, objectives for population-based and full coverage programs require a target-setting strategy that is different from that developed for a direct-services-level program that addresses a specific health domain within individuals. It must also be recognized that target setting is an iterative process, taking place over the life of a program. Rarely are target values set beyond one year, making it necessary to revisit the targets on an annual basis for health programs that are institutionalized or that are planned for a longer period of time.

Options for Calculating Target Values

There are many options for calculating target values, and each may be appropriate in some circumstances but not in others. The fact that target values for any one health problem can be calculated in so many ways underscores the importance of having established a consensus on the underlying logic reflected in the "if, then" statements that lead to a particular value. Ten options for calculating target values are described here. The calculations can easily be done using a calculator or a spreadsheet, as shown in Exhibits 6.9, 6.10, and 6.11, based on a program whose goal is to reduce adolescent pregnancy across the state. For this program, impact objectives are needed regarding the extent to which that goal is being met.

The Ten Options

In planning some health programs, the information available on which to base the calculations for the target values may be very limited. This would be the case for innovative programs, programs addressing rare health problems, or programs that are highly tailored to the location in which they are delivered. In such cases, there may only be one piece of information from the community health assessment that can be used, namely a numeric value for the current level of the health problem. There are four options for calculating a target value that can be used in the impact objective under these conditions (Exhibit 6.9).

Option 1 assumes that no change will occur because of the program. This is equivalent to accepting the current level or value. As a default position, it provides a starting point, particularly if the health program is in its first year and there is minimal empirical information on how much change is realistic or possible. It may also be appropriate for health programs that are mature and are seeking to maintain the current value because it is already at an acceptable, healthy level. The formula is as follows:

Target value = current value

Exhibit 6.9 Calculations of Options 1 Through 4 Using a Spreadsheet

	A	B	C	D	E	F	G	H	I	J	K	L
1			Long term									
2	Current Value	% Change	Target Value	Number of Years	Population at Risk		Option	Description	Formula	Target Value	Absolute Change	Percent Change
3	37.6				16,556		1	Default	(none)	37.6	0	0.0%
4												
5	37.6				16,556		2	Use statistically significant change (approx.)	A5–(SQRT(2*(A5*(1000–A3))/E5)*2)	33.5	4.1	−10.9%
6												
7	37.6	−0.02			16,566		3	Use current trend as change desired	(B7 * A7) + A7	36.8	0.8	−2.0%
8												
9	37.6	−0.04	30	5	16,556		4	Use meeting long-term objective				
10												
11								then, Yr 1	(B9 * A9) + A9	36.1	1.5	−4.0%
12								then, Yr 2	(B9 * J11) + J11	34.6	1.5	−4.0%
13								then, Yr 3	(B9 * J12) + J12	33.2	1.4	−4.0%
14								then, Yr 4	(B9 * J13) + J13	31.9	1.3	−4.0%
15								then, Yr 5	(B9 * J14) + J14	30.6	1.3	−4.0%
16								Total improvement			7.0	18.6%

In other words, the target value for the birth rate per 1000 female adolescents ages 15 through 17 is stated in the objective as 37.6 per 1000. This target value is used in the program objective as the "how much" value.

Option 2 identifies a value that, when compared to the current value, results in a statistically significant improvement. This option would be appropriate if the data source is credible, the program has a rigorous intervention, or policy makers need to be convinced that it is a worthwhile program. Because change happens by chance, not just because of the health program, it is important to be able to argue that the amount of change is greater than would occur by chance alone. An approximate z test can be used to derive the amount of change needed to be statistically significant. Typically, the significance level is set at $<.05$, meaning that the probability of reaching that target by chance alone is less than 5 in 100, or 5%. The .05 significance level translates into a z score of 1.96, which is used in the formula to estimate the target value. The formula is quite complex but has been simplified somewhat here so that it can be done using a spreadsheet:

$$\text{Target value} = \text{current value} - \left(\sqrt{\frac{2 \times \text{current value} \times (\text{multiplier} - \text{current value})}{\text{population at risk}}} \times 1.96 \right)$$

This formula assumes that the current value is an integer—that is, it is a percentage or a number per 1000, 10,000, or whatever the usual units are for reporting the indicator. The "multiplier," then, is the unit value. In the adolescent birth rate example, the current value is 37.6 and the multiplier is 1000. In addition, the formula is written so that the target value will be less than the current value. If improvement in an indicator translates into a target value that is larger than the current value, then the minus ($-$) sign in the formula will change to a plus ($+$) sign.

It is important to understand that a test for statistical significance is very sensitive to sample size. For a full coverage program using population data, the sample size is typically big, and so a modest improvement in the current value can lead to a significant result. If the sample size is small, though, as is likely in a partial coverage program using data for only the program recipients, it is likely that an unrealistic target would be needed to achieve statistical significance. In the adolescent pregnancy example, the statistical test is based on more than 16,000 adolescents, and thus a reasonable target value of 33.5 would result in a significant result. In contrast, suppose that this method were to be used in a program serving only 500 adolescents. In this case, a target value of 14.0 would be required to result in statistically significant improvement—clearly an impossible target to meet. Statistical testing, then, should really be used as an aid to understanding what a reasonable target value might be, and not to determine the target value per se.

Option 3 is to select a desired percentage decrease in the health problem or, conversely, a desired percentage increase in the healthy counterpart. This option is the most straightforward approach and can be understood intuitively by stakeholders. It can be used with health programs that are situated at any level in the pyramid and in any health domain. The percentage change chosen can be based on information gained from published literature, or it may merely be a hopeful guesstimate. The formula is as follows:

Target value = (% change desired × current value) + or − current value

If trend data exist for the health outcome, then the percentage decrease (or increase) can be refined based on past and recent experience. The percentage change can be chosen either to reflect a continuation of the observed trend or to reflect a change in the trend, either an acceleration of improvement or a slowing of deterioration, depending on the health outcome of interest. In the example of the adolescent birth rate, trend data indicate an average 2% annual decrease. Using this percentage in the formula for option 3, the target value for the birth rate per 1000 female adolescents is 36.8 (Exhibit 6.9). If a 4% decrease is applied, assuming that the program can accelerate improvement, the target value for the birth rate per 1000 female adolescents would be 36.1. The target value chosen is used in the program objective as the "how much" value. As this exercise reveals, although a 4% decrease in adolescent births may require considerable programmatic resources to achieve, the reduction in the rate may be barely noticeable. It may be useful to repeat the calculation with slightly different percentage changes and consider what in the organizational plan and service utilization plan would need to be modified to achieve those other percentage changes.

Option 4 is used when programs are ongoing, multiyear, or have long-term effects. For such programs, the "by when" portion of the objective may be several years into the future. It is thus necessary to have annual target values that cumulatively reach that long-term target value. Essentially, the total amount of change is dispersed across the time period for the program. Because of this, the target values for each year will be affected by the anticipated length of the program and the starting or current value. Option 4 can be used for programs at any level of the pyramid, but it is appropriate only for objectives related to a long-term goal. To use option 4, the first decision is to select an existing benchmark or standard, such as a *Healthy People 2010* objective that identifies the desired target value for the health problem that is to be achieved over the long term.

Calculating annual target values first involves estimating an approximate amount of annual change needed to get close to the long-term target. The annual percentage change is estimated and then used in calculations like those in option 3 to find the target value for each subsequent year. The set of formulas that are done in sequence are as follows:

> Annual % change = ((long-term objective − current value)/ current value)/ number of years
>
> Next year target value = (annual % desired change × current value) +/− current value
>
> Subsequent year target value = (annual % desired change × past year value) +/− past year value

As seen in Exhibit 6.9, an annual 4% decrease results in an adolescent birth rate of 30.6 at the end of five years, for an overall decrease of 7 births per 1000. This represents an 18.6% decrease in the birth rate among adolescents. Notice that in this example, a rate of 30 births per 1000 was the long-term objective and, using the method described here, this final target value was not exactly met. This is because the rate of improvement was maintained at 4% each year. To exactly reach the long-term objective, the rate of improvement would have to increase slightly each year. The question for discussion among the planning team, however, is whether a 4% decrease every year for five years is possible for the program, and whether the 18.6% decrease over the five years is acceptable to funding agencies and other stakeholders. It will also be important to consider whether the change can be identified using the methods currently planned for use in the impact or outcome evaluation.

Options 5 through 10 are relevant for population-based and multisite programs when the data can be stratified, either by geographic area or by some characteristic such as age, race/ethnicity, or income. The adolescent pregnancy example is a population-based program, using data from 10 counties as well as data on whether the adolescents are below or above the poverty level. When stratification is used for target setting, there is often an assumption that some sites may already have reached a very desirable level and thus are not expected to improve dramatically due to the program. The corollary is that some sites are drastically far from any target that might be set, which means they must make radical improvements to reach any reasonably set target. The extent to which a site may already be at an ideal level warrants attention from the planning team and ought to be reflected in the logic statements and the subsequent decisions about selecting target values.

Option 5 sets the target value as the mean of the rates across the sites, and option 6 sets the target value as the median of the rates across the sites. Options 5 and 6 are likely to give very similar target values, especially if the rates of the health outcome across the sites are normally distributed. However, if there is not a normal distribution, they may not yield similar values. In the adolescent birth rate example (Exhibit 6.10), the county rates range from 11.3 per 1000 females 15 to 17 years of age to 62.4 per 1000 females 15 to 17 years of age, with the mean of all 10 county rates being 33.8 and the median being 31.0. A disadvantage of these two options is that they do not take into account the differing sizes of the target population in each group, such as in each county or in each clinic. If the sites have very different rates and sizes of the target population, and if they are not normally distributed, then options 5 and 6 may not be optimal.

Options 7 and 8 take into account the population sizes of the counties targeted by the program. The overall rate of 37.6 for all counties combined (using the value used in options 1 through 4 as the current value) is the mean for the whole population, but because it combines the data for all of the counties, it obscures the county-by-county information. Options 7 and 8, on the other hand, also calculate overall current values, but rather than using all 10 counties, each option uses only a portion of the population with the "best" outcomes. Options 7 and 8 are based on the idea that the rate achieved by a certain portion of the target audience should be reachable by the whole target audience, and so the target value ought to be set based on that already existing rate. Options 7 and 8 use what is called "the pared means method" (Kiefe et al., 1998). This approach

Exhibit 6.10   Calculations of Options 5 Through 8 Using a Spreadsheet

	A	B	C	D	E	F	G	H	I	J	K	L
1	County	Size of Population at Risk	Number of Teen Births	Teen Birth Rate per 1000		Option	Description	Formula	Current Value	Target Value	Absolute Change	Percent Change
2	O	793	9	11.3					37.6			
3	P	2785	66	23.7			*Not considering*					
4	Q	859	22	25.6		5	Mean rate	Average (D2:D11)	37.6	**33.8**	3.8	−10.2%
5	R	2205	64	29.0		6	Median of the rates	Midpoint between County S and T:D6+((D7-D6)/2	37.6	**31.0**	6.6	−17.4%
6	S	1338	40	29.9								
7	T	994	32	32.2								
8	*Subtotal/Rate for Approx. 50% of Population*	*8974*	*233*	*26.0*			*Considering sample size:*					
9	U	708	24	33.9		7	Rate for "best" 50% of population	50% = B14 x 0.50 = 8,278. Sum sizes until reach 8278, O,P,Q,R,S,T				
10	V	2664	106	39.8				(C8/B8)*1000	37.6	**26.0**	11.6	−30.9%
11	W	302	15	49.7								
12	*Subtotal/Rate for Approx. 75% of Population*	*12648*	*378*	*29.9*		8	Rate for 75% of population (Counties P to	75% = B14 x 0.75 = 12,417. Sum sizes until reach 12, 417, P,Q,R,S,T,U,V,W				
13	X	3908	244	62.4				(C12/B12)*1000	37.6	**29.9**	7.7	−20.5%
14	*Total/Overall Rate*	*16556*	*622*	*37.6*								

reinforces that the target value for a program should aim to move the entire target population to a value already achieved by a portion of the target population. In other words, for options 7 and 8 the target value for the objective would be to have the adolescent birth rate in the 10-county region improve to match the birth rate already achieved by the counties encompassing 50% or 75% of adolescents.

The difference between options 7 and 8 is the proportion of the target population that is used to calculate the target value; option 7 is based on 50% of the target population, whereas option 8 is based on 75% of the target population. The pared means method can actually be used with any proportion of the target population. The higher the proportion, the easier it will be to reach the target; the lower the proportion, the more difficult it will be. Choosing 50% means that half of the target population has already achieved the target but the other half will have to improve; choosing 75% is more conservative, since improvement will have to occur only in 25% of the population. Continuing with the example, to calculate the target value according to option 7, take as many counties as necessary to incorporate 50% of all of the adolescents in the 10-county region who have the lowest (best) birth rates. Then calculate the overall birth rate for this subset of counties. In the example, 6 of the 10 counties need to be used in the calculation in order to include 50% of female adolescents. The calculation is as follows:

Target value = number with the health outcome in the top 50% / number in the target population in the top 50%

Using these data gives a target value of 26.0 births per 1000, which is a 30.9% decrease from the overall, current rate of 37.6. In comparison, if the counties that have 75% of the adolescents are used in the calculation (option 8), then the target value is 29.9, or a 20.5% change.

Options 9 and 10 are examples of approaches to using stratified data (Exhibit 6.11). If data are available on the health status or rates of groups within the target population, then it is possible to use those rates to calculate target values for those groups. Option 9 is simply an extension of the pared means method used in options 7 and 8; it uses the "best" rate of the two groups as the overall target. In contrast, option 10 starts with two separate targets, based on the two strata, by choosing different percentage decreases or increases for each. The different percentages chosen may reflect a more intense programmatic effort aimed at the group with the most urgent need for improvement. Thus, distinct, stratum-specific targets are calculated, but these can then be combined into a target value for the whole population by

---

Exhibit 6.11   Calculations of Options 9 and 10 Using a Spreadsheet

	A	B	C	D	E	F	G	H	I	J	K	L
1	Strata	Size of Population at Risk	Number of Teen Births	Teen Birth Rate per 1000		Option	Description	Formula	Current Value	Target Value	Absolute Change	Percent Change
2	Poverty											
3	Yes	2533	148	58.4		9	Rate for best strata	(none)	37.6	33.8	3.8	–10.1%
4	No	14023	474	33.8								
5	Total	16,556	622			10	Overall rate based on strata specific rates	Step 1. Use Option 2 formula per strata				
6								10% decrease for Poverty = (–0.1 * 16) + 16	58.4	52.6	5.8	–10.0%
7								2% decrease for No Poverty = (–0.02 * 17) + 17	33.8	33.1	0.7	–2.0%
8												
9								Step 2. Calculate final target, weighting by % of population in each group				
10								(J6*(B3/B5))+(J7*(B4/B5))	37.6	36.1	1.5	–4.0%

Exhibit 6.12 **Range of Target Values Derived from Options 1 Through 10, Based on the Data from Exhibits 6.9 Through 6.11**

Option	Description	Resulting Target Value
1	Default, no change, overall rate	37.6
2	Result of statistical testing	33.5
3	Percentage change in health problem: based on trend data	36.8
4	Use existing benchmark or standard to project target values for several years: first-year target	36.1
5	Mean of rates across geography/sites	33.8
6	Median of rates across geography/sites	31.0
7	Overall rate for best 50%	26.0
8	Overall rate for best 75%	29.9
9	Rate for "best" stratum (i.e., adolescents not living in poverty)	33.8
10	Overall rate based on stratum-specific rates	36.0

calculating an average weighted by the size of the population in each group. The formula for this is as follows:

$$\text{Target value}_{\text{Group 1}} = (\% \text{ change desired} \times \text{current value}) +/- \text{ current value}$$

$$\text{Target value}_{\text{Group 2}} = (\% \text{ change desired} \times \text{current value}) +/- \text{ current value}$$

$$\text{Overall target} = (\% \text{ of population in Group 1} \times \text{target value}_{\text{Group 1}}) + (\% \text{ of population in Group 2} \times \text{target value}_{\text{Group 2}})$$

In summary, a variety of techniques can be used to calculate the target value to be used in the effect objectives. Each calculation technique results in a different value (Exhibit 6.12). In the example used, the potential target value for the rate of births to adolescents ranges from a low of 26.0 births per 1000

Exhibit 6.13   Summary of When to Use Each Target-Setting Option

Option	Description of Option	Type of Program for Which It Is Ideal	Advantages of Option	Disadvantages of Option
1	Default, no change	Mature, stable program New program with no historical data for comparison Maintaining ideal	Does not require historical data	Does not require improvement
2	Change based on results of statistical test	Population based or program with large numbers of recipients	Supports argument that improvement was more than by chance	Sensitive to sample size; may result in unreasonable target
3	Percentage change in health problem based on current trend, literature, or hopeful guess	Stable program Stable target population	Very straightforward and easy to understand; can easily take into account trend data if available	Requires some statistical knowledge
4	Use existing benchmark or standard to project target values for several years	Program must show improvement Long-term commitment to program delivery and stability	Comparable programs can be compared	Requires existence of long-term objective or standard; requires long-term program
5	Mean rate across geographic areas	Population based	Easily understood	Requires having data for each area
6	Median of rates across geographic areas	Population based	Easily understood	Requires having data for each area
7	Overall rate for best 50% across geographic areas	Population based or multisite	Takes into consideration the best and the worst values in the target population; moves entire target population to an achievable value	Requires having data for each area; may be more difficult to understand; overlooks sample size

Exhibit 6.13   Summary of When to Use Each Target-Setting Option *(continued)*

8	Overall rate for best 75% across geographic areas	Population based or multisite	Takes into consideration the best and the worst values in the target population; moves entire target population to an achievable value	Requires having data for each area; may be more difficult to understand
9	Rate for best stratum using sociodemographic groupings	Population based or diverse target audience with evidence of disparities	Takes into consideration the best and the worst values in the target population; moves entire target population to an achievable value	Requires having data for each group; may be more difficult to understand
10	Overall rate based on differential targets for each stratum	Population based or diverse target audience with evidence of disparities	Program must show improvement; more intense program intervention aimed at group with the most need for improvement	Requires having data for each group; may be more difficult to understand

using option 7 to a high of 37.6, which is the current value, using option 1. This range of possible and reasonable target values underscores the importance of having a decisional framework for target setting, including developing explicit logic statements in order to realistically define what constitutes the success or effectiveness of a health program. Which target value is ultimately chosen depends upon the Program Theory, the availability of resources, and the strength of the intervention. Although options 2 and 5 through 10 are best suited to population-based programs, they can be adapted to very large programs at the direct services and enabling services levels of the pyramid. To use these options, there must be sufficient data per site and enough sites to have reasonable numbers in the groups. Options 3 and 4 are straightforward and can be used for any program. Exhibit 6.13 summarizes under what conditions each option would be best, and the advantages and disadvantages of each option.

ACROSS THE PYRAMID

At the direct services level of the public health pyramid, process objectives are likely to focus on the ways in which providers interact with program participants and how the program will support the providers in their involvement with the program. Effect objectives for programs at the direct services level will focus on individual client behavior or heath status change. Setting targets for direct services programs may involve translating national objectives into local program objectives. Although national targets may or may not be appropriate for local programs, the national targets need to be considered at least as an accepted benchmark or goal.

At the enabling services level, in addition to the foci at the direct services level, process objectives are likely to include a focus on the involvement of community resources in the program, as well as on interagency collaboration and cooperation. Effect objectives for the enabling services level are likely to address changes in the behavior or health status of families and other aggregates, such as a school or residents of a tenement. Setting targets for enabling services can be more challenging because national or state data regarding the problem being addressed are not as likely to exist. For enabling services, past experience, experiences of similar programs, and data from the community needs assessment may be the only data available for using a rational approach to setting the target numbers.

At the population services level, process objectives will need to include an emphasis on the coordination of efforts necessary to implement the health program, and on the garnering of adequate and appropriate resources to provide a population-based health program. The effect objectives can have either an impact or outcome focus, and the "who" portion will be the community or population. Setting targets for population-based services, particularly those provided to state and metropolitan populations, will draw heavily upon national data.

At the infrastructure level, process objectives will dominate. The infrastructure, by its nature, is about developing and sustaining an organization and about obtaining and managing the resources needed to implement a health program. Nonetheless, effect objectives can be written regarding the infrastructure, most probably about the effectiveness and efficiency of services. For example, Allison, Kiefe, and Weissman (1999) proposed using a pared mean benchmark method to arrive at a target value for the best performing physicians in terms of patient outcomes. There can also be effect objectives that more directly apply to the infrastructure itself. For example, there could be effect objectives regarding impacts from and educational training for staff, or outcomes from employee screening programs.

DISCUSSION QUESTIONS

1. In what ways might you write or develop objectives to minimize underinclusion or overinclusion?

2. The organizational plan and the service utilization plan can have many elements and processes. What would you use as criteria for developing a set of objectives about the process theory? Would you set targets for process objectives?

3. For effect objectives at each level of the pyramid, what sources of data might be commonly used for establishing targets?

4. Imagine that you have been asked to explain to your colleagues in 10 minutes how to set targets for program objectives. Develop an outline for the steps involved.

References

Allison, J., Kiefe, C. I., & Weissman, N. W. (1999). Can data-driven benchmarks be used to set the goals of Healthy People 2010? *American Journal of Public Health, 89*(1), 61–65.

Kiefe, C. I., Weissman, N. W., Allison, J., Farmer, R., Weaver, M., & Williams, O. D. (1998). Identifying achievable benchmarks of care: Concepts and methodology. *International Journal for Quality in Health Care, 10(5)*, 443–447.

Kotelchuck, M. (1997). Adequacy of prenatal care utilization. *Epidemiology, 8*, 602–604.

National Institute of Dental and Craniofacial Research. (2001). Seal out dental decay. *http://www.nidr.nig.gov/health/pubs/sealants/text.htm* (accessed 12/11/01).

Maternal and Child Health Bureau of the Health Resources and Services Administration. (n.d.) Core health status indicators detail sheets. *http://mchb.hrsa.gov/html.blockgrant.html* (accessed 12/11/01).

Patton, M. Q. (1997). *Utilization-focused evaluation* (3rd ed.). (pp. 147–175). Thousand Oaks, CA: Sage Publications.

Perrin, E.B., & Koshel, J. J. (1997). *Assessment of performance measures for public health, substance abuse, and mental health*. Washington, DC: National Research Council.

Rosenberg, D. (1999). Performance and outcome measurement: Methods for setting annual targets. *http://www.uic.edu/sph/cade/citymatch99/targets/slideshow/sld001.htm* (accessed 8/28/03).

Rossi, P.H., & Freeman, H. E. (1993). *Evaluation: A systematic approach* (5th ed.). Newbury Park, CA: Sage Publications.

Section 3

Implementing Health Programs

CHAPTER 7

Logistics of Program Implementation

Implementing the health program, the next step, requires acquiring and overseeing adequate resources to provide the program in a manner that is consistent with the Program Theory and the purpose of the program. It requires the most and longest sustained effort of all the phases of a health program (Exhibit 7.1). This chapter introduces the logistics associated with managing a health program, with particular attention to budgeting and general managerial issues. These logistics fall within the organizational plan and the service utilization plan portions of the process theory (Exhibit 7.2). Health programs are projects that can be viewed as miniature organizations. In the management literature, the organizational plan and the service utilization plan would be considered elements of the tactical plan. A common frame of reference for thinking about health programs is inputs, throughputs, outputs, and outcomes (Kettner, Moroney, & Martin, 1999; Turnock, 2001). In the process theory, there are various inputs into both the organizational plan and the service utilization plan. These two plans also have specific outputs. Distinguishing between the inputs and the outputs of these plans aids program managers in acquiring the appropriate resources and in being able to communicate both programmatic needs and successes.

Accountability and responsibility are cornerstones of program implementation. Being accountable means answering for the success or failure of the program. Being responsible means ensuring that things get done. Program managers are both accountable for the program and responsible for seeing that the program is carried out. They are accountable for the program in six areas (Rossi, Freeman, & Lipsey, 1999). Each area requires attention, planning, and oversight. Three types of accountability relate to the organizational plan. Fiscal accountability refers to the need for sound accounting, careful documentation of expenses, and tracking of revenues, whereas legal accountability encompasses

Exhibit 7.1   Amount of Effort Across the Life of a Health Program

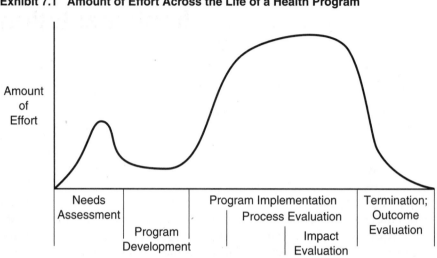

staff acting in accordance with local, state, and federal laws and within their professional licensure limits. Efficiency accountability means that the program is delivered with efficient use of the resources. Two types of accountability relate to the service utilization plan. Coverage accountability relates to the program reaching the intended recipients, and service delivery accountability refers to the actual provision of the program components and interventions. Finally, there is one type of accountability related to the effect theory: impact accountability, which is concerned with the program having an impact on the recipients. Through careful attention to the organizational plan and the service utilization plan, a program manager can achieve each type of accountability.

INPUTS TO THE ORGANIZATIONAL PLAN

The organizational plan encompasses the program inputs and resources, as well as the way in which those resources are organized. The type and amount of resources required for a heath program vary with the interventions to be used. Nonetheless, the expertise of the personnel, the characteristics of the target audience, and the degree of attention paid to acquiring and managing recourses all affect the potential to have a successful program. The organizational plan objectives serve as a guide as to which activities are the most critical for implementing a health program. However, many aspects of the organizational plan will not be in the organizational plan objectives yet will need to be addressed. The following is an overview of key inputs and the rationale for considering them to be key.

Exhibit 7.2   Diagram of the Process Theory Elements, Showing the Components of the Organizational Plan and Service Utilization Plan

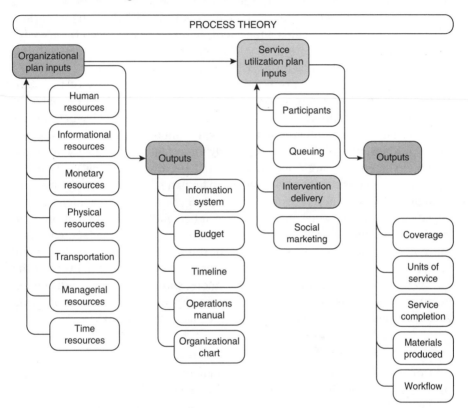

Human Resources

Human resources encompass the quantity and quality of personnel, in terms of their expertise, experience, and capabilities. Human resources come at a cost, and personnel costs are almost always the largest portion of any programmatic budget. The dollar cost of personnel includes not only wages (an amount paid hourly) or salaries (an amount paid monthly) but also fringe benefits as a percentage of the wage or salary. Estimating the dollar cost of personnel is a rather straightforward arithmetic problem, as explained in the later section on budgeting.

Training staff and volunteers for their role in implementing the program is an aspect of human resource management. Training costs include both staff time for this activity and the trainer's time. There are also costs of materials used during training, such as handouts, equipment, and audiovisuals. Training costs can be substantial, but training is necessary for assuring the standardized delivery of the program interventions. Without this standardization, the program could easily be quite different from the intended program, depending upon the personal preferences of the individuals providing the intervention. In other words, training helps align theory-in-use and espoused theory with effect theory. This has serious implications for achieving the desired outcomes and thus for the long-term sustainability of the program.

Training is also necessary for the morale and self-efficacy of the staff. Receiving training helps program staff feel valued, trusted, and capable of providing the interventions. These feelings contribute a sense of having a higher ability to carry out the intervention as designed—in other words, a greater task self-efficacy. Staff self-efficacy is especially important in the delivery of a complex intervention to a target and recipient audience that is resistant or difficult.

A separate consideration with regard to human resources is workforce cultural diversity. As health programs are increasingly targeted to audiences with specific cultural and racial characteristics, it becomes important that program staff are not only culturally competent with regard to the target audience but, more ideally, are themselves members of the target audience. While having program personnel who are culturally diverse may help in the delivery of the intervention, it can lead to other issues among staff. Program managers must be attentive to signs of interracial or cross-cultural tensions among program personnel and address the issues as soon as they are identified.

Volunteers as Human Resources

Community involvement in the development and implementation of health programs can occur by establishing advisory committees and boards, councils or consortia. Through such groups, community members have a structured means to participate. To maximize the benefits of having these groups, they are best considered or approached as being volunteers and a human resource.

Volunteers are also increasingly used to deliver the health program interventions, as was done in Kansas City to deliver a school-based immunization program (Wilson, 2001), in Virginia to detect and prevent geriatric alcoholism (Coogle, Osgood, & Parham, 2001), and in Wellington, New Zealand, to provide hospice care (Roessler, Carter, Campbell, & Macleod, 1999). The use of volunteers in health programs makes them a key human resource requiring particular attention, especially if they create a synergy between themselves and the program recipient (Hintgen, Radichel, Clark, Sather, & Johnson, 2000). In other words, volunteers gain from the experience and participants may benefit in terms of personal attention. In addition, there is evidence that the use of volunteers who are peers of the program recipients (in other words, who are themselves members of the target audience) may lead to a greater achievement of desired health impacts than would the use of professionals (Schafer, Vogel, Viegas, & Hausafus, 1998).

Volunteers are motivated by factors that are different from those that motivate paid employees. Altruism is a major motivation to be a volunteer (Bowen, Kuniyuki, Shattuck, Nixon, & Sponzo, 2000; Roessler et al., 1999). Other reasons include personal gains in terms of pre-employment experience and references, being accepted by the program staff, being valued as an important team member (Roessler et al., 1999), and having personal concerns related to the health condition (Bowen et al., 2000). Older adults are likely to perceive the opportunity to engage in new endeavors as the most beneficial reason to volunteer, although a sense of life satisfaction, being productive, and having social interaction are also important reasons to volunteer (Marrow-Howell, Kinnevy, & Mann, 1999).

Despite sincere and honorable motives, volunteers often come without adequate training or experience with the target audience. This makes training volunteers particularly critical to the success of the health program. Volunteers need not only the skills to effectively implement the intervention, but also emotional support in dealing with challenging clients and knowledge about the clients and the health condition.

Volunteers can be recruited through a variety of techniques. In a study of volunteers of one cancer prevention program, Bowen and associates (2000) found that half of the volunteers were recruited through media, such as television, radio, or newspapers, and from work-related sources. Although these methods are similar to those used to recruit employees, the messages will be different. The messages for recruiting volunteers will focus on motivating factors, such as those just mentioned.

One issue germane to community health programs and the use of volunteers is reflected in a study by Trettin and Musham (2000), who found a difference between program developers and community volunteers in their perceptions of the role of volunteers. This finding hints at an undercurrent in the relationship between program planners and the community—namely, the perception of volunteers that they are being exploited under the guise of being volunteers. In some communities, this undercurrent will be more evident and influential in determining the success of a health program.

Physical Resources

Physical resources or inputs include material resources, facilities, and equipment (Kettner et al., 1999). Material resources are those tangible items that are needed to provide the intervention as well as to provide program support. Intervention equipment might range from blood pressure cuffs to imaging machines. Space, usually called facilities, is another material resource needed for both the intervention and the program support. The costs associated with having or renting classrooms, auditoriums, community meeting rooms, waiting rooms, examination rooms, and offices need to be taken into account. Supplies are another material cost encompassing miscellaneous office supplies (i.e., paper, stationery, pens, clips, and computer disks), specific resources for program staff (i.e., journal subscriptions, resource or reference manuals), and any items needed related to the intervention (i.e., tote bags, clipboards, stopwatches, bandages, syringes). Physical resources may be needed for the evaluation as well, generally office supplies and storage space for data collected. Maintaining an adequate supply, without hoarding, is the function of inventory control; having too many unused supplies drains monetary resources that may be needed for other expenses.

A large category of physical resources is office equipment: computers, printers, cables, fax machines, and photocopiers. If these items exceed an amount set by the organization, the purchase of the item will be considered a capital expense and will require special approval and possibly special ordering procedures. Also, some funding agencies look unfavorably on the purchase of standard office equipment if it exceeds a certain amount. For these reasons, many program managers minimize purchases that are considered capital expenditures.

Transportation

Transportation is a separate type of resource and expense. Transportation must be thought of from the perspective of both program staff and program participants. For staff, the issue is one of reimbursement for any travel related to providing the program. For example, if the health program includes an outreach component, staff need to carefully document their mileage or keep track of expenditures for public transportation. From the perspective of program participants, the issue is accessibility of the program site given the usual mode of transportation used by potential program participants. Thus, in a rural program the transportation issue might be one of travel time required to get to the program site, whereas in an urban program the issue might be proximity to a major mass transit stop.

Informational Resources

Computer hardware and software are costs that will be included in a budget, usually as a physical resource. But information is a key intangible resource. The knowledge and expertise of the staff must be viewed as a resource to be managed. Increasingly, information possessed by individuals is considered an asset for the organization (Kennedy, 1998; Thompson, Warhurst, & Callaghan, 2001). Information is a resource that can be present in the form of professional networks, street smarts that affect program implementation, and professional knowledge and experience. Staff bring professional knowledge to the program and gain additional knowledge through the training sessions. In terms of health programs, this means that the knowledge held by employees involved in the program is valuable to the implementation of the program. As staff become more qualified for other positions based on their knowledge and experience, it can become difficult to retain those personnel. Therefore, the retention of such employees is an issue and becomes an additional reason to make efforts to keep the program personnel satisfied with their job and the organization. Loss of staff is not just an issue of replacing personnel but is more appropriately thought of as replacing knowledge and expertise, hence the importance of maximizing staff retention and minimizing unplanned staff turnover.

Time

Time generally translates into personnel costs, but it must also be thought of as a separate resource. Time is relevant to the overall timeline of a program design and implementation. The sequencing of events, especially in the start-up phase of a program, is very time dependent. A delay in accomplishing one step easily affects the overall timeline. If meeting a start date is essential, then additional personnel resources may be required during the startup phase, thus having an effect on the budget. Time affects the budget in less obvious ways through depreciation, inflation, and interest. These are discussed later in the section on budgets.

Managerial Resources

The qualities and characteristics of the managerial personnel are also key resources. When one is selecting the project manager, Posner (1995) suggested considering the skills required of a person in the position—namely organizational abilities, communication skills, team-building skills, and leadership qualities for coping with complex and ambiguous tasks and environments, and technical skills related to the health program intervention.

Organizational abilities refer not only to the logistics of juggling multiple tasks and persons but also to not losing track of important dates and information. The ideal program manager will also be able to organize the project in terms of structuring the relationships among project personnel, as is usually reflected in organizational charts that denote flow of communication, delegation, and responsibilities. A somewhat different but equally crucial aspect of organizational abilities is the understanding of how the health program fits within the parent organization and how to position the program for success within the parent organization.

Communication skills are not just the ability to communicate verbally with peers but also the ability to guide discussions, communicate nonverbal messages that are consistent with the verbal messages, and, perhaps most importantly, to listen and appreciate various points of view. In addition, written communication skills are essential for a health program manager to function in the larger context of grant writing, report generation, and e-mail communication. The other facet of communication skill is understanding who needs to know what and when. This communication skill is closely linked to the creation and manipulation of information in order to have an effective and efficient health program.

Negotiation is a major component of the communication skills required of program managers. Negotiation is the process by which two or more parties reach a decision when they have different preferences with regard to the available options (Bazerman, 1994). Much research about negotiation forms the basis of what is known about how people think and respond to information. Three pieces of information are needed in a negotiation: each party's best alternative to the negotiated agreement, an analysis of the interests of each party, and the relative importance of each party's interests. With this information, the negotiator enters a process in which the various parties use certain strategies to arrive at an agreement by breaking out of the existing definitions of differences. These strategies include many actions that are common in good communication, such as building trust, asking questions, strategically disclosing information, and making many offers simultaneously (Bazerman, 1994). Program managers will negotiate not only with funding agencies but also with program staff and community stakeholders. Thus, a rudimentary understanding of negotiation techniques is important.

Team building is another essential managerial skill, especially for health programs that are participatory, community based, or multidisciplinary in nature. The ability to mobilize a group, foster group cohesion, and facilitate teamwork are elements of team building. Information about team building and teamwork can be found in both the lay managerial literature available at most bookstores and the professional management journals. Managers must consciously attend to the quality of interactions within a team and to the quantity of teamwork. Problems can quickly arise and must be expeditiously addressed. Otherwise, the team can become dysfunctional and drain resources rather than be a resource. One aspect of team building is the use of stories. As program staff begin to develop as a team, stories will be told about clients, about managers, about events. These stories, which are ubiquitous in organizations, serve the function of building team norms and establishing communication among the team members.

Leadership is the ability to inspire and motivate others into action that is purposeful and organized. Program managers are rarely thought of as leaders, yet they must motivate staff, be role models of productivity, and generate enthusiasm for the health program. These are qualities often attributed to good leadership (Kouzes & Posner, 2000). Therefore, program managers need to be knowledgeable about the motivational process in regard to both staff and program participants. Motivation of program staff results in everyone doing what they were hired to do in a timely, efficient, and high-quality manner.

The technical skills required of program managers involve skills related to the health program intervention. In most health programs, the manager must have basic scientific or practical knowledge about the health problem and the type of interventions that are provided. There are situations in which the program staff, the program participants, or the funding agencies will not view the health program favorably if the program manager does not have some professional credibility. Technical skills are also necessary in order to adequately supervise the program staff and assure the integrity of the program intervention.

Monetary Resources

The category of monetary resources is generally listed on the income side of a balance sheet or budget, as it refers to funding and to income generated through fees and billing. Monetary donations are another resource that needs to be tracked and included in accounting records. However, if participants are given any cash for participation, then monetary resources also fall on the expense side of a budget.

OUTPUTS OF THE ORGANIZATIONAL PLAN

Not all of the inputs into the organizational plan will be directly linked to specific organizational plan outputs; some will be linked to service utilization plan outputs. The following are examples of outputs that could be measured or at least used to document effective use of the organizational plan inputs.

Timeline

A timeline is a graphic representation of the dates, time span, and sequence of events involved in planning, initiating, sustaining, and evaluating the health program. Timelines vary from the simple to the intricate. At a minimum the timeline ought to reflect the activities necessary, be related to the expenses detailed in the budget, and be easily understood by those who will use it (Exhibit 7.3). A timeline can be created using the table function in a word processing program, a spreadsheet, or specific project management software. It is a communication tool that conveys responsibilities and deadlines. It also helps keep activities coordinated and sequenced, communicates accountability for assigned tasks, and helps estimate personnel and material costs.

Operations Manual

The operations manual contains the policies, procedures, guidelines, and protocols related to the health program. It also includes job descriptions and workplace polices and procedures. One element of many health program operations manuals is a section on safety. For both staff and participants, safety is an issue—not only in their car as they are coming to or from the program site, but also on the street surrounding the program site. Particularly if program staff are outreach workers, their safety must be considered, and safety strategies need to be part of their job training and procedures related to their work.

Organizational Chart

Most organizations have a graphic representation of the relationships among work units, departments, and individuals. As a result of having personnel designated to the health program and having program accountability, health programs will have their own organizational chart. One aspect of the health program organizational chart that may be different from the charts of other work units is the inclusion of any community-based consortium or council that is used as an advisory committee to the health program. The inclusion of any such groups is important, as it reflects, in a legitimate and visible fashion, the involvement of the community in the health program. Also, the health program ought to be specifically identified within the appropriate organizational chart. For health programs that are population based, such as state child health insurance, the program needs to be reflected somewhere in the organizational chart of the state agency, as well as with the community organizations involved in promoting or providing the program.

Information System

The information system has outputs that are part of the organizational plan. Upgraded hardware and software are outputs, as are reconfigured and

Exhibit 7.3   Example of an Abbreviated Timeline for a Short-Term Health Program (Created with the Table Function in Microsoft Word)

Activity	Month	1	2	3	4	5	6	7	8	9	10	11	12
Convene program planning group		X											
Conduct community needs and asset assessment		X	X										
Translate assessment information into objectives			X	X									
Formulate Program Theory, articulate process theory				X	X								
Initiate process to obtain human subjects protection					X	X							
Advertise for program personnel						X							
Hire and train program personnel						X							
Advertise the health program (social marketing)							X						
Deliver the health program								X	X	X	X		
Conduct a process evaluation								X	X	X	X		
Conduct an impact evaluation											X		
Analyze the evaluation data											X		
Produce report							X					X	
Disseminate report													X

programmed computers that accommodate data generated by the health program. New report capacities are also information system outputs.

Planning via Budgets

Budgets are mechanisms for planning and tools for communicating and refining priorities. They are projections of dollar amounts that enable the program planner to assess the fiscal feasibility of doing a project. Developing a budget for a program highlights the programmatic changes that may be needed to be fiscally responsible and efficient. For example, changes might be needed in the size of the program to achieve a more efficient participant-to-staff ratio.

Each organization will have its own particular format for developing budgets and, possibly, special software. The financial officer in the organization will set forth the rules and accounting specifics used across programs and departments within the organization. This chapter discusses more general budget principles that apply across formats and organizations. The intent is to introduce basic program budget concepts so that heath program planners can communicate with financial personnel, funding agencies, and administrators in order to present the program in a positive light.

Budgeting Terminology

The broadest categories within budgets are expenditures and revenues. Expenditures are classified in various ways: as fixed or variable and direct or indirect.

Fixed costs are those that do not vary with the number of clients served. Examples are rent, salaries of administrative personnel, and insurance costs. In contrast, costs that do vary with the number of clients served are *variable costs*. Examples of variable costs are copying for program handouts, program advertising, and refreshments for participants. Depending upon how the health program is designed and implemented, and how the organization does its accounting, costs will be counted as fixed or variable. For example, if program staff are paid regardless of how many clients show up, then personnel is a fixed cost. But if the program uses staff on a part-time, as-needed basis, then personnel costs are variable. Budgets prepared based on the distinction between variable and fixed costs are more likely to be useful for program management via fiscal monitoring and for conducting economic and accounting analyses of the program.

Another way to think about costs are as direct or indirect. In the purest sense, *direct costs* are those that are used directly in the delivery of the program. Generally, staff providing the intervention is a direct cost, as are materials or supplies used with clients. Similarly, in the purest sense, *indirect costs* are those not associated with the delivery of the program, but more generally with supporting the program. Thus, utilities, telephone, and staff travel to present the program at scientific conferences are examples of indirect costs. In general, however, indirect costs of overhead expenses (e.g., rent, utility, facilities management, shared clerical support staff, and office equipment) are estimated at a standard rate, and that rate is set either by the program funding agency or the organization's financial officer. Indirect costs as a percentage of direct costs can vary from 8% as limited by funding agencies up to 51%. Thus, it is important to obtain the correct rate at which indirect costs are applied to the expenditure side of the budget.

Revenues are a bit simpler. Funds for health programs come mostly from grants from funding agencies, fees collected from program participants, and charitable fund raising. State or federal agencies might also match local dollars allocated to the health program. A critical distinction is made between the costs of providing a service and the charge for that service. The cost of the service is the simple sum of all the resources required to provide the service. However, clients are charged more than the cost; charges typically include the cost plus a profit margin and administrative costs. When budgeting, the program planners must consider both the cost of the service and the amount charged for the service, given that ultimately the charges influence participation in and acceptance of the program.

One frequent source of revenue is invisible, in-kind donations. These are services provided to the program free of charge but for which the program would have to pay if they were not donated. A common example of an in-kind donation is printing. Volunteer time is another in-kind donation for staff time. In some not-for-profit agencies, the in-kind donations can be substantial. It is important to track these for two reasons. One, the use of in-kind donations is looked upon favorably by funding agencies as an indication of community support for the program. Also, if the in-kind donations are not received, a contingency plan for paying for those services must exist and be implemented.

Most grant proposal budgets focus on the major categories of direct costs, as is seen in the commonly used federal grant budget page of the PHS 398 form (Exhibit 7.4). However, some federal funding agencies have begun to ask for budgets that are more directly linked to the program objectives, while others ask for budget by pyramid levels. Such budgets enable the funding agencies and program managers to determine the merit of the budget in terms of what is planned and the anticipated outcomes. While creating such a budget can be challenging and can require some degree of speculation, assigning costs per program objective can be a powerful motivational and managerial tool.

Break-Even Analysis

After the program budget is complete and nearly final, it is possible to do a break-even analysis. A break-even analysis is the mathematical determination of the point at which the expenses related to providing the program are equal to or less than the revenues generated for or from the program. A break-even

Exhibit 7.4   Example of program budget using the PHS 398 form

DD   Principal Investigator/Program Director   (Last, first, middle):   Jones, Sally

DETAILED BUDGET FOR INITIAL BUDGET PERIOD DIRECT COSTS ONLY					FROM 06/01/02	THROUGH 5/31/03	

PERSONNEL (Applicant organization only) NAME	ROLE ON PROJECT	TYPE APPT. (months)	% EFFORT ON PROJ.	INST. BASE SALARY	DOLLAR AMOUNT REQUESTED (omit cents) SALARY REQUESTED	FRINGE BENEFITS	TOTALS
Sally Jones	Principal Investigator	9	25%	51,542	$12,886	$3,300	$16,185
Sally Jones	PI - Summer	2	25%	51,542	$2,863	$733	$3,597
Richard Smith	Co-Inv.	12	20%	67,751	$13,550	$3,470	$17,020
Pat Garcia	Co-Inv.	9	20%	74,050	$14,810	$3,793	$18,603
To Be Named	Proj Manager	12	50%	32,000	$16,000	$4,098	$20,098
To Be Named	Proj Staff	12	50%	22,000	$11,000	$844.80	$11,845
To Be Named	Proj Staff	12	50%	22,000	$11,000	$844.80	$11,845
To Be Named	Community Liason	12	50%	25,000	$12,500	$3,201.00	$15,701
To Be Named	Admin Assist	12	50%	26,000	$13,000	$998.40	$13,998
	SUBTOTALS				$107,609	$21,283	$128,892

CONSULTANT COSTS
Stress reduction consultant ($10,000); Evaluation consultant ($6,000) — **$16,000**

EQUIPMENT (Itemize) — **$0**

SUPPLIES (Itemize by category)
Software($300),Office Supplies($1,500),Copying-stress reduction materials($500),Copying-survey duplication($5,000) — **$5,100**

TRAVEL
Staff to community-based intervention sites -600mi@.32=192.00
PI to professional meeting related to project ($1200) — **$1,392**

PATIENT CARE COSTS — INPATIENT / OUTPATIENT

ALTERATIONS AND RENOVATIONS (Itemize by category)

OTHER EXPENSES (Itemize by category)
Insurance ($13,110)   Participant Incentives($20,000)
Telecommunications($200)   Postage/Fed Ex($200)
Laboratory(cortisol)($10,000) — **$43,510**

SUBTOTAL DIRECT COSTS FOR INITIAL BUDGET PERIOD	$ **$194,894**

CONSORTIUM/CONTRACTUAL COSTS	DIRECT COSTS FACILITIES AND ADMINISTRATION COSTS	$0

TOTAL DIRECT COSTS FOR INITIAL BUDGET PERIOD (Item 7a, Face Page)	$ **$194,894**

PHS 398 (Rev. 4/98)   (Form Page 4) Page   DD

analysis uses the price of the service—in other words, the charge—the vari-able costs of program, and the fixed costs of the program. The rather straight-forward formula (Finkler, 1994) for a break-even analysis is as follows:

$$\text{Quantity of services} = \frac{\text{fixed costs}}{\text{price per client} - \text{variable costs per client}}$$

When the total fixed costs associated with the program are divided by the difference between the amount charged per participant and the variable costs per participant, the result gives the number of services that need to be provid-ed in order to break even. Exhibit 7.5 is a narrative example of a break-even quest, and Exhibit 7.6 is the analysis done using a spreadsheet program, Microsoft Excel.

Even programs provided by not-for-profit agencies would be wise to con-duct a break-even analysis. This rudimentary process provides useful insights into the amount of funding needed. Too often public agencies and public pro-grams neglect their fiscal accountability and efficiency accountability by not conducting a break-even analysis. If clients are not paying for services, as is often the case in public heath programs or mass media campaigns, the price an individual might be willing to pay for the service or other such information can be used in place of the charge or price. For example, if residents of a com-munity are willing to pay only 10 cents for information on how to prevent sexually transmitted diseases, then the "safe sex" mass media campaign will need to reach a very high number of persons to theoretically break even.

Thinking in terms of break-even analyses may seem unethical or contrary to the public heath ethic. However, the use of break-even analyses is a fiscally responsible way to make decisions among programs or programmatic options.

Exhibit 7.5 Example of a Break-Even Analysis, Bright Light Example

> Your community agency, Lighthouse, has decided to implement a new program, Bright Light II. In the past, Lighthouse billed Medicaid and insurance companies $75 for a similar service (Bright Light I), and it plans to charge the same for Bright Light II. Operational expenses for Bright Light I for the past year totaled $4,300, but Bright Light II will share those fixed costs with Bright Light I. Because Bright Light II is an educational program and Lighthouse tries to have a consistent ratio of teachers to clients, the number of teachers varies with the number of clients. For every 10 clients, Lighthouse employs 1 teacher, at a salary of $500. Lighthouse can provide classes to only 100 clients per year. Using this information, how many clients must be served, billed, and pay for Bright Lights II to break even? What recommendation would you make to Lighthouse?

Exhibit 7.6   Break-Even Analysis on an Excel Spreadsheet

	A	B	C	D	E	F
1	**Fixed Costs (annual)**		$4,300			
2	Rent	$2,000				
3	Clerical support	$1,200				
4	Cleaning service	$500				
5	Financial service	$600				
6						
7	**Revenue**					
8	Charge per class	$75				
9						
10	**Variable Costs**		$5,000			
11	Teachers	$500				
12	Number students	10				
13						
14						
15	Quantity to break even =		(c3/2)/(b9–(5000/100))			
16	Break-even number of students =	86				
17	The choices are: 9 teachers with 9.5 students, or 8 teachers with 10.5 students					
18						
19				9 teachers		8 teachers
20		**Formula**		*Option A*		*Option B*
21	Fixed costs	c3/2		$2,150		$2,150
22	Variable costs	9 or 8 * $500		$4,500		$4,000
23	Expense subtotal			$6,650		$6,150
24						
25	Revenue	86 * $75		6450		6450
26						
27	Balance	Revenue – expenses		–$200		$300
28						
29	Number to break even d29/$7			2.666667		

It also provides a quantifiable rationale for proceeding with or modifying a health program. Importantly, a break-even analysis may reveal that additional funding is required to provide the program as intended; it is far better to identify this potential problem before the program is initiated.

Budget for Evaluation

The budget must also include expenses related to the program evaluation. Whether the program staff will be involved in the evaluation activities or a consultant will be hired, funds must be allocated to the evaluation before the program begins. Retrospectively acquiring funds to conduct an evaluation can be difficult. In general, program grant proposals and budgets that do not include evaluation funds receive lower priority scores. Evaluation expenses generally fall into the same categories as program expenses, although material expenses are generally limited to supplies and copying costs. Incentives given to individuals to participate in the evaluation can be a substantial portion of the evaluation budget. However, as with program costs, personnel will be the largest expense. At a minimum, a meaningful evaluation cannot be done for less than 10% of the direct program costs.

Budget Justification

Budget justification is a requirement for virtually all grant proposals, although the degree of detail expected varies by funding agency. A safe rule of thumb is to provide a very detailed budget justification; more detailed budget justifications demonstrate a more thorough program implementation and evaluation plan. Most budget justifications involve some narrative explanation of why the dollar amounts are requested, but they must also include fairly detailed arithmetic formulas that show specific costs. For example, budget narratives typically show the cents per mile paid to staff for travel, the estimated number of miles staff are expected to travel, and the number of staff traveling those miles. Even if a health program is being sponsored by a parent organization, a budget justification is presented to departmental administrators or advising boards when requesting their support.

INPUTS TO THE SERVICE UTILIZATION PLAN

The service utilization plan can be thought of as the point-of-service aspect of the program. Before delivering the program, however, people need to know about and want the program; this is the purpose of social marketing. Determining through the process of screening based on eligibility criteria who will receive or participate in the program is another aspect of the service utilization plan. Other elements of the service utilization plan include how queuing is addressed and the actual delivery of the program intervention.

Social Marketing

Kotler (1989) was one of the first authors to advocate for social marketing as a method to reach a wide audience with health or social messages. Walsh, Rudd, Moeykens, and Moloney (1993) defined social marketing as the design, implementation, and control of a program calculated to influence the acceptability of social ideas. More recently, Maibach, Rothschild, and Novelli (2001) stressed that the purpose of social marketing is to influence voluntary behavior of the target audience.

Social marketing adapts the four P's of classical marketing: promotion, place, price, and product. Product refers to the service, tangibles, or ideas that are delivered with the intent of being beneficial to the target audience. Social marketing focuses on the beneficial aspects and on understanding from the perspective of the recipient how those benefits are valued and perceived. Price in social marketing is a cost of any type that poses a barrier to accessing or using the product. Price considerations focus not only on the charge for the service, but also on the secondary costs, such as transportation or loss of peer group status. Place refers to where the product is available, whether it is in a clinic, on a billboard, or found in a convenient location within a store. Making the product accessible, convenient, and visible are qualities of place that merit attention. Promotion encompasses the more visible publicity type of activities, including paid media, public service media, and word of mouth by opinion leaders.

These principles from social marketing have been used successfully in a variety of health educational programs to get the health program to the target audience (Maibach et al., 2001). In this way, the development and implementation of the social marketing strategy is an input into the service utilization plan, as it enables the health program to reach the target audience.

Eligibility Screening

Having a procedure to actually screen for program eligibility is another input to the service utilization plan. The screening procedure is necessary to assure that the program is provided to members of the target audience, thus minimizing underinclusion or overinclusion. Despite the inclination to want to provide the program to anyone interested, screening enhances the efficiency and effectiveness of the program. Efficiency is enhanced by having only program participants to whom the intervention is tailored, thus making it less likely that the program intervention will need to be individually tailored. Effectiveness is enhanced because only those who need the program, and thus who are more likely to experience the benefits of the program, are included in the impact and outcome evaluations.

Queuing

Waiting to be seen for services, being on hold, and having to wait until services are available are all aspects of being put in the queue. Waiting lines and wait times are the result of the degree of match between the capacity to provide the service and the demand for the service. The service utilization plan ought to include a plan for handling waiting lists. For example, if an immunization clinic is being held, the service utilization plan ought to include the anticipated number of individuals seeking immunizations balanced against the rate at which individuals can be processed for the immunization, the length of time to give the immunization, and the number of program staff to implement the immunization clinic. An imbalance will result in either people waiting for long periods or staff not having work. Because the particulars of studying queues can be complex, large health programs, particularly those that are ongoing, may find it valuable to hire an operations specialist to study the issue of queuing so that the health program will be provided in the most timely and efficient manner possible.

Intervention Delivery

The fact that this discussion of intervention delivery occurs halfway through this text is no accident. The actual delivery of the intervention, while it takes the most effort (Exhibit 7.1), is relatively easy if the planning has been done well and the process theory has been thoroughly thought out.

Delivery of the intervention ought to follow the protocols and procedures developed specifically for the health program. This ensures that the intervention is delivered in a standardized and consistent manner. The level of detail included in the protocols and procedures will vary across programs. For example, if the health program intervention is secondary prevention of breast cancer with mammography screening, then the intervention protocol will include considerable details about performing the actual mammogram, taking a history before performing the mammogram, and notifying and referring those screened. In contrast, if the health program is a citywide mass media awareness campaign about the value of breastfeeding, then the intervention protocol will need to allow for flexibility in accessing and communicating with media contacts while providing guidance regarding whom to approach, what topics to address and avoid, and which products (public service announcements, video clips, flyers) to distribute to which media sources.

One aspect of the intervention that makes common sense, but is often neglected, is pilot testing the program. Prior to full program implementation, it is best to pretest the program, with attention to the different program components. Pretesting can take a variety of forms, such as having focus groups review materials and make comments, providing the program free to a small group, or having experts comment on the program design and materials.

Marketing materials and media messages in particular ought to be pretested. The characteristics to be assessed include the attractiveness, comprehension, acceptability, and persuasion of the program materials. Also, any materials that will be read by program participants need to be tested for readability. Currently, computer word processors include features that will determine the reading difficulty and the grade level at which the material is written. The rule of thumb is that the lower the reading level the better; no one wants to struggle with technical language, complex sentences, or large words. For example, this paragraph contains 200 words and is written at a 12th grade level. Generally, an 8th grade reading level is recommended for program materials. Exhibit 7.7 shows this paragraph rewritten at an 8th grade level.

Pretesting the interventions ought to include pretesting the evaluation instruments that will be used during the program and after the program has been completed. As more funding agencies require health programs to document their success, the evaluation becomes more integral to the actual intervention and overall program delivery.

OUTPUTS OF THE SERVICE UTILIZATION PLAN

The outputs of the service utilization plan are the number of units of service provided and the quantity of service completions. "Units of service" is a term used to refer to the agency- or program-specific quantification of what

---

Exhibit 7.7   Paragraph Re-written at 8th Grade Reading Level

It makes common sense to try out a program before it begins, but this is often not done. Before starting a program, try out the handouts and the program parts. There are many ways to see if the people in the program will understand the handouts and program. One way is to have a focus group that looks over the materials and makes comments. Another way is to give the program free to a small group of people and see if there are any problems. Also, experts can help by making comments on the program and the handouts. Advertisements and media messages need to be tried out before they are used. Look at how attractive they are, how easy it is for people to understand them, whether people will accept the message, and how good the message is at convincing people. Also, handouts need to be checked for how easy they are to read. Today, computer word processors can check them and show the grade level it is written at. The rule of thumb is that lower grade levels are better because no one wants to work at reading technical words, long sentences, or large words. For example, this paragraph has 213 words and is written a little below the 8th grade level.

was provided, such as hours per client, number of inpatient visits, number of educational sessions, and number of hours of client contact. Because these quantifications can vary widely, it is important for each health program to specify what it considers a unit of service. Assuring that a mechanism is in place to track the number of units of service is a critical managerial responsibility. Another output of the service utilization plan is the number of services that have been completed. For health programs this might be the number of immunization clinics held, the number of completed referrals for medical followup, or the number of health educational courses provided.

The service utilization plan has one other output: the materials developed and produced in order to provide the health program, such as public service announcements, educational videos, annual reports, or curricula. A final key output is the workflow—that is, the extent to which program staff have work over a given time period or that work is done in a coordinated manner.

As the health program is implemented, keeping a record of these outputs is a major component of the subsequent process evaluation activities focused on program implementation, as is discussed in the next chapter.

ACROSS THE PYRAMID

At the direct services level of the public health pyramid, implementing a health program will be very similar to implementing other health services. However, particular attention ought to be focused on tailoring the human resources to the programmatic intervention. The social marketing plan will also be targeted to individuals and individual behaviors.

At the enabling services level, again, a match between providers and the health program intervention is necessary. If the program intervention is an enabling service, the providers (the human resources) are more likely to have a social services background or expertise. Programs at the enabling services level are also more likely to use volunteers. This has implications for the managerial resources needed. The social marketing plan will also need to be tailored to the aggregate targeted by the program. Because many enabling services either require a referral or are accessed via a referral, the social marketing of the program may focus as much on the providers making the referral as on the target audience of clients.

At the population services level, as with the other levels, a match must exist between the abilities and skills of the providers and the health program intervention. Social marketing to a population will have a broad base of appeal and will certainly use mass media.

The infrastructure level of the pyramid is what this chapter is primarily about. Having a highly specified, comprehensive organizational plan and service utilization plan is foundational to implementing an effective health program. Also, having the necessary and appropriate resources for the health program is an indicator of the quality of the infrastructure. The most creative of ideas and the most scientifically sound programs will fail without an adequate infrastructure. Too often, attention is focused on the health program interventions and clients, without the prerequisite attention and effort to developing and maintaining the programmatic infrastructure. Therefore, the organizational plan must include resources for the infrastructure as well as for the activities in the service utilization plan. In addition, if the health program is intended to increase the capacity of the infrastructure, such as to improve workforce capacity, an organizational plan and service utilization plan for such a program are still warranted as steps to assure the success of the program.

DISCUSSION QUESTIONS

1. In what ways might each type of accountability be affected by or related to social marketing?

2. How do the outputs of the organizational plan and the service utilization plan relate to the process theory objectives?

3. For a health program at the direct services level, the enabling services level, and the population-based level, speculate on how fixed and variable costs might change. Discuss the implications these changes have for the results of a break-even analysis.

4. Imagine that you are on a committee to establish an information management system for a new health program. What factors would you argue should be included and what would be your rationale?

References

Bazerman, M. H. (1994). *Judgment in managerial decision making* (3rd ed.). New York: John Wiley & Sons.

Bowen, D. J., Kuniyuki, A., Shattuck, A., Nixon, D. W., & Sponzo, R. W. (2000). Results of a volunteer program to conduct dietary intervention research for women. *Annals of Behavioral Medicine, 22,* 94–100.

Coogle, C. L., Osgood, N. J., & Parham, I. A. (2001). Follow-up to the statewide model detection and prevention program for geriatric alcoholism and alcohol abuse. *Community Mental Health Journal, 37,* 381–391.

Finkler, S. A. (1994). *Essentials of cost accounting for health care organizations.* Gaithersberg, MD: Aspen Publishers.

Hintgen, T. L., Radichel, T. J., Clark, M. B., Sather, T. W., & Johnson, K. L. (2000). Volunteers, communication, and relationships: Synergistic possibilities. *Topics in Stroke Rehabilitation, 7*(2), 1–9.

Kennedy, F. (1998). Intellectual capital in valuing intangible assets. *Team Performance Management, 1214,* 121–137.

Kettner, P. M., Moroney, R. M., & Martin, L. L. (1999). *Designing and managing programs: An effectiveness based approach* (2nd ed.). Thousand Oaks, CA: Sage Publications.

Kotler, P. (1989). *Social marketing.* New York: Free Press.

Kouzes, J. M., & Posner, B. Z. (2000). *Five practices of exemplary leadership: When leaders are at their best.* San Francisco: Jossey-Bass.

Maibach, E. W., Rothschild, M. L., & Novelli, W. D. (2001). Social marketing. In K. Glanz, B. Rimer, & F. L. Marcus (Eds). *Health behavior and health education* (3rd ed.). San Francisco: Jossey-Bass.

Marrow-Howell, N., Kinnevy, S., & Mann, M. (1999). The perceived benefits of participating in volunteer and educational activities. *Journal of Gerontological Social Work, 32,* 65–80.

Posner, B. Z. (1995). What it takes to be a good project manager. In J. R. Meredith & S. J. Mantel (Eds.), *Project management: A managerial approach* (3rd ed.). New York: John Wiley & Sons.

Roessler, A., Carter, H., Campbell, L., & Macleod, R. (1999). Diversity among hospice volunteers: A challenge for the development of a responsive volunteer program. *American Journal of Hospice and Palliative Care, 16,* 656–664.

Rossi, P. H., Freeman, H. E., & Lipsey, M.W. (1999). *Evaluation: A systematic approach.* (6th ed.). Thousand Oaks, CA: Sage Publications.

Schafer, E., Vogel, M. K., Viegas, S., & Hausafus, C. (1998). Volunteer peer counselors increase breast feeding duration among rural low-income women. *Birth, 25,* 101–106.

Thompson, P., Warhurst, C., & Callaghan, G. (2001). Ignorant theory and knowledgeable workers: Interrogating the connection between knowledge, skills, and services. *Journal of Management Studies, 38,* 923–942.

Trettin, L., & Musham, C. (2000). Using focus groups to design a community health program: What roles should volunteers play? *Journal of Health Care for the Poor and Underserved, 11,* 444–455.

Turnock, B. J. (2001). *Public health: What it is and how it works.* (2nd ed.) Gaithersburg, MD: Aspen Publications.

Walsh, D. C., Rudd, R. E., Moeykens, B. A., & Moloney, T. W. (1993). Social marketing for public health. *Health Affairs, Summer, 12,* 104–119.

Wilson, T. (2001). A bi-state, metropolitan, school-based immunization campaign: Lessons from the Kansas City experience. *Journal of Pediatric Health Care, 15,* 173–178.

CHAPTER 8

Process Evaluation: Measuring Inputs and Outputs

Once the health program has started, stakeholders, funding agencies, and program staff want to know if the program is or was implemented successfully and as planned. Answering this question is done through a process evaluation. Process evaluation, monitoring evaluation, implementation evaluation, and formative evaluation are terms that refer to very similar processes and involve similar sets of activities. The term "process evaluation" is used as a generic term that encompasses each of these slightly different approaches to understanding the extent to which the program is being delivered as intended. A process evaluation also measures the inputs into the program, and, according to Rossi, Freeman, and Lipsey (1999), is the systematic examination of programmatic coverage and delivery. Patton (1997, p. 196) defined process evaluation as "finding out if the program has all its parts, if the parts are functional, operating as they are supposed to be operating."

This chapter covers techniques and issues related to conducting process evaluations. The topics are addressed in relation to the components of the program theory, with attention to creating data that can be used to assess the achievement of the process objectives established during the planning phase. Understanding the extent to which the process objectives have been achieved, and at what cost, is a major reason for conducting a process evaluation. In other words, process evaluations help identify gaps between program accomplishments and process objective targets. As with the development of the program interventions and plan, input from volunteers and stakeholders regarding key factors to include in the process evaluation, as well as their contributions to gathering and interpreting the process evaluation data, enrich the health program implementation. Their enthusiasm, insights, and diverse points of view can bring the process evaluation to life and provide a wealth of possible solutions to problems the process evaluation identifies.

PROCESS EVALUATION

All evaluation questions that focus on elements of the organizational and service utilization plans are referred to in this text as process evaluation—in other words, evaluation of the process theory and its components. Ideally, process evaluation occurs during or throughout the program implementation, rather than as a post hoc idea and activity. Of course, this is feasible only if the process evaluation is planned during the program planning stage and is incorporated into the implementation of the program. Attending to the design of the process evaluation during planning allows the choice of what to include in the process evaluation to be more precisely guided by the process objectives that are being developed. It is possible to have process objectives that relate to each element of the process theory (Exhibit 8.1). However, this is not only impractical but also unnecessary. Each program will have a tailored set of process objectives that form the basis of the process evaluation, and will address various purposes.

Exhibit 8.1   Minimum Elements of the Process Theory Included in a Process Evaluation

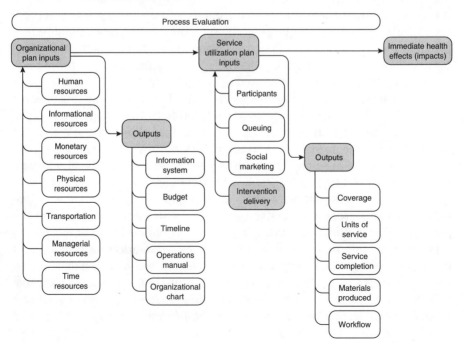

Purposes of a Process Evaluation

Green and Lewis (1986) enumerated different foci that process evaluations can have. Their categories fit into the broader elements of the program's process theory: the organizational plan and the service utilization plan. Organizational factors surrounding the program, the program staff, and the response of individuals in the organization who are involved with the program are one set of foci. These are elements of the organizational plan. Attention to participants and their subjective response to the delivery of the program, and quantification of participation correspond to elements of the service utilization plan. The other major focus Green and Lewis identified is on the implementation of the program interventions, a component of the service utilization plan. As will be discussed later, the actual intervention deserves special consideration.

Understanding how the program is delivered, as revealed through a process evaluation, has at least four purposes. One purpose is to have data about the delivery of the program so that the results of impact and outcome evaluations can be interpreted within the context of the program delivery. That is, if there is no effect on the health problem, it will be important to verify that the program was, in fact, delivered, and to quantify the degree of intensity and faithfulness to the program design. Process evaluations are intended to demonstrate that program specifications are met, and as such are useful for assuring that the work being done by program staff is consistent with the program's process objectives and plan. Process evaluations help identify whether the implementation of the program contributed to the program's failure, as distinct from having an ineffective effect theory (Exhibit 8.2).

The second purpose of process evaluations relates to the dissemination or replication of the health program. The process evaluation provides operational information to the new sites so that the program can be successfully replicated. A third purpose of process evaluations is to meet requirements of funding agencies, specifically regarding demonstrating the extent of program implementation. Required reporting often entails a predetermined set of data that will need to be collected and used in the report to the funding agency. Thus, not all aspects of a process evaluation are under the control of the program administration or evaluators.

Finally, process evaluations, like quality improvement methodologies, can provide data upon which to make midcourse corrections in the delivery of the program. The interactive and iterative nature of planning and implementing a health program requires some degree of flexibility, particularly for programs that are repeated, so that the process evaluation information can be used to modify aspects of the organizational plan or the service utilization plan that are ineffective in accomplishing the process objectives. This flexibility and

Exhibit 8.2   Roots of Program Failure

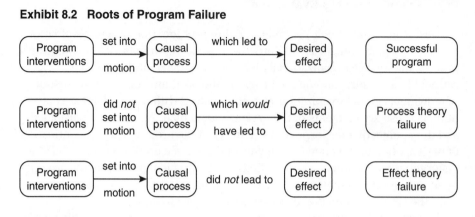

Source: Evaluation Research by Weiss, C. H. Copyright. Reprinted by permission of Pearson Education, Inc., Upper Saddle River, N.J.

change amounts to a corrective managerial practice. Through such actions, issues of accountability and quality are addressed. Overall, the process evaluation functions as an early warning system and provides a basis for making changes to the process theory.

The Three E's

In evaluating programs, one concern is often with whether the program was effective, efficient, or efficacious. These three terms are often used with minimal attention to the important differences among the concepts. However, the differences have implications for the role of the process evaluation, and they reveal underlying reasons for the different evaluation activities needed to quantify each.

Of the three terms, "efficacy" is probably the one most likely to be misused, usually being used instead of "effectiveness." Efficacy is the maximum potential effect under ideal conditions. Because ideal conditions are difficult to create, the efficacy of an intervention is determined through rigorous studies, usually clinical trials, especially randomized clinical trials. Randomized clinical trials, by controlling many of the potential influences, provide a context in which the highest possible effect of a treatment or intervention can be directly attributed to that treatment or intervention. Because of the costs and ethical considerations involved in clinical trials, efficacy evaluations of health programs are seldom done unless they are done as evaluation research. The role of a process evaluation in program efficacy studies is to establish that the health program intervention is carried out precisely according to the intervention protocol.

Effectiveness is the realistic potential for achieving the desired outcome when a treatment or intervention is used in real life. The degree of effectiveness of an intervention thus reflects what can be expected given the normally messy situations that occur when health programs are delivered. Data from impact assessments and impact evaluations, as well as from evaluation research, provide practical experience in the anticipated level of intervention effectiveness. The degree of effectiveness is reflected in several different statistics, depending upon the evaluation design and methods. Any statistic that denotes the degree of difference related to having received the programmatic intervention, whether a difference score, a correlation coefficient, or an odds ratio, is providing information on the degree of effectiveness. In this way, existing studies of the effectiveness of interventions provide a benchmark against which to gauge the success of subsequent or similar programs, and thus such studies have value beyond their specific findings. The role of a process evaluation in effectiveness studies is not only to assure that the program is being provided according to protocol, but also to document situations, events, and circumstances that influenced the delivery of the intervention.

Efficiency is, generically, the relationship between the amount of output and the amount of input, with higher outputs for less inputs being more efficient. With regard to health programs, efficiency is generally thought of in terms of the amount of effect from the program intervention, as the ultimate output, compared to the amount of inputs that went into providing the intervention. In more colloquial terms, efficiency is the "amount of bang for the buck." Process evaluations are essential to estimating the efficiency of a program. Efficiency can be estimated through an accounting-type process evaluation. This type of evaluation involves measuring the amount of inputs as well as the program outputs related to the service utilization plan and the organizational plan. The result is a measure of program efficiency with regard to achieving the process objectives. If program effectiveness is also measured, then the evaluation can also quantify the program efficiency in terms of achieving the impact and outcome objectives.

DATA COLLECTION METHODS

Along with the question of what to measure is the question of how to collect data. There are at least seven categories of methods of data collection that are appropriate for process evaluations. These methods are summarized in Exhibit 8.3 as activity logs, organizational records, client records, observations,

Exhibit 8.3   Methods of Collecting Process Evaluation Data

Method	When to Use	Examples of Measures	Pros	Cons
Activity log	Have list of actions that are discrete and a common under-standing exists for what those are; need quantitative data	Number of ses-sions, number of recipients/ participants; number of times repeated the intervention	Can tailor list and log to the program and the activities to be monitored, easy to use, easy to analyze data, familiar to most people	May become too long; may not get completed on a regular basis
Organizational record	Have existing records that capture the information needed and can legally access those records; need quantitative data	Length of time on waiting list; number of com-puters bought or upgraded; number of hours worked; number of advertising events	Inexpensive, as can use the data directly	May need a data abstraction form; may not be exactly what is needed; may be complex data linking and data analysis
Client record	Have existing records that capture informa-tion needed and can legally access those records; need quantitative data	Program attendance	Inexpensive, as can use the data directly	May need a data abstraction form; may not be exactly what is needed; may be complex data linking and data analysis
Observation	Need to have data on interpersonal interactions or sequences of events	Use of materials produced; quality of inter-action between clients and staff	Data may reveal unexpected results; naturalistic; can quantify observations	Time intensive; need observa-tion checklist; complex data analysis

Exhibit 8.3   Methods of Collecting Process Evaluation Data *(continued)*

Method	When to Use	Examples of Measures	Pros	Cons
Questionnaire	Need to quickly collect data from reliable respondents and have a reliable and valid questionnaire; need quantitative data	Degree of satisfaction with program and with physical environment of the program	Straightforward to distribute and collect pen-and-paper version of questions; easy data analysis (if well constructed), efficient	Requires respondent to have good reading skills and motivation to complete; useless data if not well written
Interview	Have time and need qualitative data or have respondents for whom questionnaire is not appropriate	Commitment of staff to program and intervention	Able to get detailed descriptions during one-on-one interview; possibly new insights	Time intensive; need private place for the interview; need interview question and format, more complex data analysis
Case study	Need to understand the full set of interactions around the program and the context in which it is functioning	Degree to which managerial personnel make changes to assure fidelity of intervention	Gives very thorough picture of program and provides new insights	Extremely complex because uses multiple methods over period of time; time intensive; very complex data analysis

questionnaires, interviews, and case studies. Chapter 9 provides information on developing questionnaires and client records (as secondary data), and Chapter 12 describes techniques for interviewing, observation, and conducting case studies, because these data collection methods are also commonly used to evaluate the effect of the program. The use of activity logs and organizational records tends to be more specific to process evaluation. Regardless of the data collection method chosen, high standards for the quality of the data collected, the reliability of the tools, and the accuracy of data entry must be met. This need for reliability extends to establishing inter-rater reliability in the use of checklists (Sinacore, Connell, Olthoff, Friedman, & Gecht, 1999), and similarly in activity logs. This list of data collection methods does not preclude disciplined creativity in developing and using data collection methods or tools that are uniquely tailored to the needs of the program.

The choice of a method of data collection needs to be congruent with the indicators in the process objectives and the best method for arriving at a conclusion as to whether the process objective target was ever reached. Thus, there are situations in which one method will be a better choice than the others. A few examples of measures that would result from the data collection method are listed in Exhibit 8.3. It is important to note that each method has advantages and disadvantages. These need to be carefully considered when choosing a data collection method.

MONITORING INPUTS TO THE ORGANIZATIONAL PLAN

During the program development stage, specific organizational resources were identified as being key to implementing the health program. An evaluation of the organizational plan determines the extent to which those resources were or are available and used to support the implementation of the program. Both inputs into the organizational plan and outputs of the organizational plan are included in the process evaluation. Although each type of input could be the subject of a process evaluation, evaluating all of them would not be prudent or feasible. Each program will have its own set of concerns and interests with regard to evaluating the organizational plan inputs, as reflected in organizational plan process objectives. Thus, the choice of which organizational plan inputs are evaluated will be influenced by the earlier work of the program planners and the current concerns of program staff.

A comprehensive process evaluation, which is rarely done, would monitor at least a measure of each type of organizational plan input (Exhibit 8.4). A variety of measures can be used to measure each element of organizational plan input and output (Exhibit 8.5), although the specific measure will depend on the program and the objectives. At a minimum, the process evaluation needs to assess the human resources devoted to the program, and thus it is used in the next section as an example of considerations that would be involved in monitoring human resources input. Another example of monitoring organizational plan inputs is focused on physical resources. These discussions are not intended to be definitive, but rather illustrative of how to approach the development of the process evaluation plan.

Exhibit 8.4   **Qualities of the Elements of Organizational Plan Inputs and Outputs That Can Be Measured**

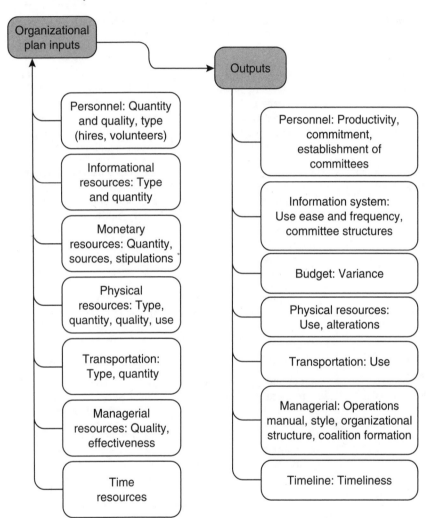

Human Resources

Both the quantity and the quality of the human resources available to the health program ought to be assessed, as they often constitute the largest cost component of a program. Not only is the quantity of personnel relevant, but also their level of commitment to the program, their competencies in terms of

Exhibit 8.5   Example of Measures of Inputs and Outputs of the Organizational Plan

Elements	Examples of Measures of Input	Examples of Measures of Output
Human resources	Number of FTEs, number of new hires, number of volunteers, percentage of licensed personnel, percentage of personnel with certification, educational level of staff, hours of training and orientation	Number of hours worked, staff to recipient ratio, hours per client contact per staff, degree of job satisfaction of staff and volunteers, degree of commitment of staff to program and intervention
Informational resources	Number of computers bought or upgraded, number of program recruitment efforts, availability of communication hardware and software, ease of process data entry and retrieval, ease of impact data entry and retrieval	Degree to which computer and telecommunication systems facilitate delivery of the intervention, availability and accessibility of personnel data, budget, operating, meeting or other reports
Monetary resources	Amount of grant monies and donations, amount of indirect cost deducted from the program, number of proposals submitted for program funding	Dollars or percent variance from budgeted per line item
Physical resources	Number and type of equipment, square footage of office space	Extent changes are made to physical resources needed for intervention delivery
Transportation	Parking fees, total mileage per month, number of bus passes used, program vehicle expenses	Mileage per staff, number of clients receiving transportation assistance, transportation cost per staff or per program participant
Managerial resources	Place in organizational chart, years of experience, educational level, degree of ability to clearly and persuasively communicate	Extent to which is viewed by staff as controlling or delegating, degree to which managerial personnel make changes to assure fidelity of intervention
Time resources	Timeline developed, presence of deadline dates	Number of days delayed, percent of deadlines met, number of repeated requests

knowledge and skills, and their attitudinal performance. The degree of commitment to the program is important to assess, given that program staff who lose commitment to the health program are less likely to fully implement the program as designed. A change in commitment levels may reflect unanticipated challenges to the delivery of the program. For example, the program staff may develop lower levels of commitment because of obvious failures of the intervention, or "side effects" of the program. Thus, monitoring the program staff's commitment to the program and to the interventions is one venue for gaining insights into program implementation.

The extent to which program personnel are competent to deliver the program also provides information on the extent of program implementation. If licensed health professionals are required to deliver the intervention, and there are insufficient fiscal resources to hire such individuals, then the program is not likely to be implemented as planned. Thus, the extent to which the credentials of program staff match the competencies needed for program implementation provides more evidence of the extent to which the designed interventions are delivered. This is not to imply that unlicensed personnel are not qualified. There are many types of interventions and health programs that rely heavily and appropriately on a wide range of qualifications for program staff. The issue is the extent to which the program staff's qualifications actually match what is required to fully implement the program in order to gain the maximum effect for program participants. As the health program evolves, so might the qualifications needed by program staff. This needs to be taken into consideration, and thus the process evaluation may lead to a revision of the process theory.

The empowerment and participation of stakeholders does not stop with the planning process, but continues in the process evaluation. The inclusion of volunteers and stakeholders as human resources in the organizational plan is intended to be a continual reminder that these individuals and groups need to be actively engaged in the various stages of the health program. Ideas from program staff about ways to improve the program can be part of the process evaluation. Their ideas are key for several reasons. One is that their ideas may help increase the effectiveness and efficiency of the program without compromising the integrity of the intervention as conceptualized. Their ideas may also provide some clues as to areas that were not implemented as intended. For example, they are very likely to pick up on and articulate the difference between what they were asked to do and what they are able to do with the given resources.

A major area of increasing importance to federal funding agencies is the monitoring of community coalitions associated with health programs. For example, the Centers for Disease Control and Prevention has an initiative to reduce racial and ethnic disparities across five health conditions. Each grantee is required to report on the status of the indicated community coalition. Similarly, the Maternal and Child Health Bureau has a program to reduce infant mortality. Grantees must have a community consortium and report on the functioning of that consortium. The use of community coalitions also had a strong history in substance abuse prevention programs (Paine-Andrews et al., 1996) and AIDS prevention (Cox, Rouff, Svendsen, Markowitz, & Abrams, 1998). The rationale for using community coalitions or consortia is based on the belief that such groups of individuals from the target population not only foster the development of culturally appropriate health programs but influence the context of the program in ways that enhance the service utilization plan. Therefore, the evaluation of these groups is primarily in terms of the process theory, rather than the effect theory.

Process monitoring data about coalitions can reveal difficulties in mobilizing the community as a whole and the preferential interests of various groups (Higginbotham, Heading, McElduff, Dobson, & Heller, 1999). Process evaluations provide indicators of the extent to which coalitions continue to be true to their constituents (Armburster, Gale, Brady, & Thompson, 1999). Process evaluation data help assess whether coalition activities have contributed any program effect. For example, Hays, Hays, DeVille, and Mulhall (2000) found that the structural characteristics of a coalition, particularly membership diversity and sectorial representation, were differentially related to community impacts of the health program. Such process information can be important for future coalition development, as well as program development.

Physical Resources

For some programs, the extent to which facilities are adequate in terms of the types of rooms needed to provide the health program, or the accessibility of equipment needs to be assessed, given the critical role of these resources in the success of the program. If the necessary physical resources are not available or used, it may indicate that the program has not been fully implemented. For example, if a health promotion program includes both an educational component requiring only a classroom and a cooking demonstration component requiring a kitchen, then the use of both needs to be evaluated. If no kitchen facilities have been used for the program, then only the educational component of the program has been implemented. When it is time to evaluate the impact of the program, knowing that facility limitations have affected the program and that only one component of the program has been implemented provides an explanation for a weak program effect on the stated outcomes. The simplest measure of physical facilities would be a simple dichotomous variable of yes/no as to whether the facilities or equipment specified in the process objective were used. Once it is decided that a yes/no type variable is acceptable, data must be collected and recorded in a manner that will enable the evaluator to arrive at an answer.

QUANTIFYING OUTPUTS OF THE ORGANIZATIONAL PLAN

Just as only key organizational plan inputs are evaluated, only key organizational outputs can realistically be evaluated. Those with process objectives are the minimum to be included. For some programs it may be important to understand the organizational structure, such as where in the organizational hierarchy the health program director is located. The program director's position in the organizational chart can indicate the relative importance of the health program and hence the ability of the program manager to garner resources for the program. In the next sections, two organizational plan outputs, information system and budget, are used as examples of different approaches to the measurement of organizational plan outputs.

Information Systems

Before computers, program staff maintained their own catalogs of cases, tick sheets of telephone calls, tickler files of dates for follow-up contacts, and such. These were difficult to aggregate across the staff. Computerized systems enable program managers to collect the same data in the same format from all program staff, thus enabling easier aggregation across staff members. The ability to process this type of data and generate needed reports is an output of the information systems. Given the increasingly central role played by information systems in acquiring program funds and documenting program implementation and effects, mechanisms ought to exist for monitoring the extent to which the computer hardware and software are capable and programmed to generate the needed reports. This may range from a quarterly report from the information systems department to a simple tally of the number of computers with specific software. Tracking the number of problems, requests, and complaints would be another approach to measuring the information system outputs.

Attending to the information systems is particularly critical as more of the process and impact evaluation data are captured through computerized databases. Ideally, the process evaluation is developed sufficiently in advance of beginning the program with which the data elements needed for the process evaluation can be computerized. This requires that a database be created based on knowing what data elements will be needed. If program staff are expected to contribute process evaluation data through the computerized system, staff training on how to use the computerized system will be necessary. The importance of correctly entering data in a timely manner must be explained in terms of their role in assuring that the data are reliable and thus useful for all concerned. Testing the system, including the personnel involved in using or maintaining the information system, involves checking that relevant data are collected and stored, that the data can be manipulated to provide information and answers to programmatic questions, and that those inputting the data are doing so reliably. Of course, the same information system or a comparable one will likely be used for evaluating the effect of the program. Part of the process evaluation may include an assessment of the system's capacity to handle the impact and outcome evaluation data.

Monetary Resources: Budget Variance

On an ongoing and regular basis, usually monthly, the program manager ought to determine the extent to which current expenditures exceed (or not) the projected program expenditures. The difference between the budgeted and actual expenditures or income is called the budget variance. The variance is calculated for each category or line item as a simple subtraction of expenditures from the budgeted amount, which can be easily done with the use of spreadsheets. Because of delays associated with billing and organizational fiscal reports and the various dates selected by the organization at the beginning of a fiscal year, the actual expenses and income will always be based only on what is available at any given time. As reports are received, the expenditures must be updated. The variance ought to be no more than 10 to 20 percent of the projected budget. Program managers, by monitoring the budget variance, can make needed adjustments throughout the fiscal year, so that the year-end variance is within an acceptable range. Severe negative variances can be due to overexpenditures or inadequate income, whereas severe positive variances can be due to underexpenditures or greatly increased income. Either way, the presence of a significant variance is an alert that the program is not being delivered as planned and needs attention.

MONITORING INPUTS TO THE SERVICE UTILIZATION PLAN

Process evaluation typically is equated with elements that are included in an evaluation of the service utilization plan, namely data on the participants and program delivery (Exhibit 8.6). As was mentioned with regard to evaluat-

Exhibit 8.6   Qualities of the Types of Service Utilization Plan That Can Be Measured

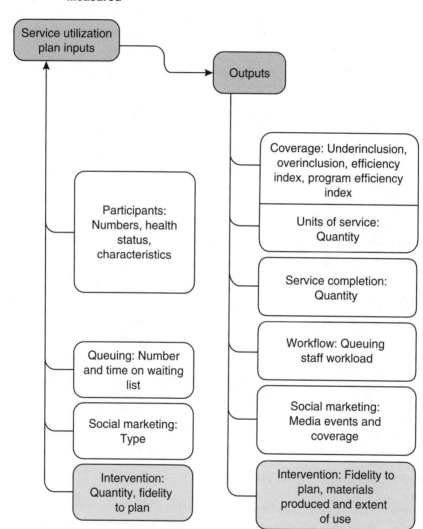

ing the organizational plan, the process objectives are a guide as to what, of all possible inputs and outputs, is crucial to evaluate. Exhibit 8.7 provides some examples of measures that are useful for service utilization plan monitoring.

Exhibit 8.7   Examples of Measures of Inputs and Outputs of the Service Utilization Plan

Elements	Example of Measures of Input	Examples of Measures of Output
Participants	Number of recipients/ participants, number of persons denied program or not qualified for program, number of requests for program	Percentage undercoverage, percentage overcoverage, efficiency index, program efficiency index, degree of satisfaction with program
Queuing	Number on waiting list, presence of system to move individuals from waiting list to program or alternative programs	Length of time on waiting list, evenness of work among staff and across time (workflow)
Social marketing	Type of social marketing, quality of marketing, extent of social marketing analysis	Number of advertising events, number of requests for program based on social marketing efforts
Intervention	Number of meetings to standardize program, extent of revisions based on previous cycle of intervention delivery, extent of revisions based on new research evidence	Fidelity to intervention plan, number of sessions, hours of program delivery, number of participants completing intervention (service completion), number of requests for additional program delivery, use of materials produced

Participants and Recipients

There are several types of data about program participants that are reasonable to include in a process evaluation. One type is simple, straightforward demographic characteristics. This is necessary for determining the extent to which the target audience has been reached. These data provide insights into whether the social marketing approaches used to reach the target audience were effective. Demographic data can be readily collected during program sign-in or intake procedures, especially for direct and enabling services. Demographic data on recipients of population-focused programs may be more difficult to obtain directly, given that many population-based or focused health programs do not require that recipients be physically present at a given location. For example, it would be very difficult to determine the number of recipients of health messages delivered via billboards or a health policy.

Participant satisfaction with the program is an element of process evaluation and not a health impact or outcome of the program. This perspective is in contrast to the general vernacular of classifying satisfaction as an outcome. The rationale for thinking of satisfaction as a process output stems from the definition of satisfaction: the degree to which participants receive what they expect to receive and the extent to which their expectations are met with regard to how they are treated (Parasuraman, Zeithaml, & Berry, 1985). What is subsequently received, what is expected, and how one is treated are all aspects of the service utilization plan, rather than parts of the effect theory of how participants are changed by the program. In addition, the satisfaction of clients and patients with the information they receive is subsequently related to impacts, such as adherence to medication regimens (Horne, Hankis, & Jenkins, 2001). Satisfaction with services has received considerable attention in the health services (Seibert et al., 1999), with various standardized tools having been developed for use in various settings. There are tools for use across a variety of settings, such as primary health care settings (Drain, 2001; Steine, Finset, & Laerum, 2001), prenatal care services (Raube, Handler, & Rosenberg, 1998), physical therapy (Roush & Sonstroem, 1999), and mental health services (Pellegrin, Stuart, Maree, Fruech, & Ballenger, 2001).

The reality is that most funding agencies are interested in knowing the satisfaction level of participants. Most participants, clients, or patients report being satisfied to very satisfied with the services they receive. This is because it is difficult to measure satisfaction in a way that does not lead to a "ceiling effect." A ceiling effect occurs when the measurement tool is constructed so that respondents do not have an opportunity to distinguish among levels at the high end of the scale. In other words, if the satisfaction scale is a five-point Likert scale, the difference between 4 as somewhat satisfied and 5 as very satisfied will lead to 5 being chosen more often than 4. One remedy for this is to use a scale of 1 to 10, which then allows respondents to distinguish among 7, 8, 9, and 10 as levels of satisfaction. The other difficulty in developing a measure of satisfaction stems from the conceptual definition of satisfaction, which entails a match between expectations and experience. Developing a scale that focuses on the difference is surely to be longer and more challenging to analyze as a difference score. For these reasons, the use of an existing satisfaction measure is highly recommended. The last difficulty in measuring satisfaction concerns the scope of what is important in terms of satisfaction.

For example, inpatient satisfaction questionnaires generally include items about parking and food service alongside items about the courtesy of staff (Gesell, 2001; Mostyn, Race, Seibert, & Johnson, 2000; Seibert et al., 1999). Ideally, only items that are related to elements in the organizational and service utilization plans should be included in the satisfaction questionnaire.

INTERVENTION DELIVERY

How well the intervention was delivered and whether the intervention was provided as designed and planned are essential elements of a process evaluation. There are three ways in which the intervention can fail, and each is related to its delivery. The process evaluation needs to be designed so that the presence of any one of these failures can be detected. Adequate and timely monitoring evaluations can then help prevent the failure due to inadequate program implementation.

Nonprogram

One way in which an intervention can fail is the lack of a program (nonprogram, no treatment), meaning that the program was not provided. If the intervention requires a sophisticated delivery system, it may not be delivered. For example, a program that involves coordinating services among a variety of health professionals employed by different agencies can easily result in no program. An alternative way for no treatment to occur is if the delivery of the intervention in some way negates the intervention. Having program staff who are not supportive, encouraging, or empathetic would negate intended program interventions that require such qualities in staff. Similarly, physical resources, say a building with limited and difficult access, would negate interventions for those with disabilities.

Nonrobust Intervention

The second way that interventions can fail is if an intervention other than the designed and planned intervention was provided, or the intervention was drastically diluted in some way. For example, if an educational program was designed to cover five topics and only one topic was covered despite holding the classes for the designated number of hours, the program was dramatically diluted, possibly to the point of having no effect on participants. The process objectives that specify the program content and quantity can be used to assess whether the strength (dosage) of the intervention was as intended. It is also possible that the intervention or impact theory was flawed and thus, although delivered as planned, the intervention was inadequate as conceptualized.

Unstandardized Intervention

The third way interventions can fail is if the intervention was provided in an unstandardized manner, thus becoming an unstandardized treatment. To assure that the intervention is responsible for the outcomes, a standardized intervention is necessary. If the program personnel or practitioner uses discretion and alters the intervention, there is no assurance that the intervention as planned is responsible for the impacts and outcomes. One approach to minimize this potential source of program failure is to incorporate the program theory in the training of program personnel, so that they appreciate the need to follow the guidelines for delivery of the program. Of course, policies, procedures, and standardized materials need to be in place and used as tools to help standardize the program, hence inclusion of the operations manual as an organizational plan output.

Unstandardized intervention can also have a more insidious and hidden cause. Both program participants and program staff have their own working explanations or theories of how a program affects participants. One type of theory is an espoused theory, which is the stated or espoused explanation for how things happen (Argyris, 1992). The effect theory, as it is known and understood by program staff, becomes the espoused theory. People know what they are supposed to say, expected to espouse, regardless of whether they believe it or their actions match their espoused theory. For example, staff providing a cardiac rehabilitation program may think that the program is effective because they are teaching the patients what to eat and how to exercise. This is the espoused theory of how the program intervention affects health. Argyris also found that the espoused theory was not always congruent with behaviors. The actions taken to achieve the ends are their theory-in-use; they are the actual interventions that are delivered and that affect participants. Therefore, identifying the theory-in-use is crucial, as it provides insights into what intervention was provided, especially if it was not the programmatically espoused theory. All three theories—effect, espoused, and theory-in-use—need to be assessed during the process evaluation (Exhibit 8.8). Returning to the cardiac rehabilitation program, if the staff become friends with the patients and provide encouragement in a supportive manner but rarely focus on the educational content, then their theory-in-use is coaching or social support, not education. Naturally, some programs will be more prone to inconsistency than other programs; the

Exhibit 8.8   Comparison of Effect Theory, Espouse Theory, and Theory-in-Use

	Effect Theory	Espoused Theory	Theory-in-Use
What It Is	Explanation of how program interventions lead to the desired health impact and outcome	What staff say regarding how the program interventions affect participants	What staff do to affect participants
Where It Resides	Manual and procedures, the Program Theory	Minds of the staff, program manuals and descriptions	Actions of program staff, on-the-job training by peers
How It Is Identified	Review of scientific literature, program materials	Listening to staff describe the program, reading the program materials	Watching what staff do in providing the program
Importance	Guides the interventions and evaluations; basis for claiming the impacts and outcomes	Becomes what staff, participants, and stakeholders believe and expect of the program	Is the actual cause of the program effects and impacts

espoused theory and theory-in-use among staff in immunization clinics are likely to be quite congruent, whereas incongruence is likely among staff of health programs that entail complex interpersonal interactions and that address socially sensitive health problems.

Relying only on the espoused theory as process data can lead to later difficulties. One subsequent difficulty is that if the espoused theory and the theory-in-use are not congruent, findings from the impact evaluation may be confusing or misleading. Implementation of the program may be inconsistent, leading to nonstandardized interventions. This makes it difficult to relate the health effects of the program to the program interventions. Corrective actions cannot be taken unless the theory-in-use has been identified through careful observation of program staff in delivering the intervention. The process evaluation of the intervention thus needs to take into account the possible sources of inconsistency in how the program intervention is delivered.

The inconsistencies among the three theories (effect theory, espoused theory, and theory-in-use) can be a source of decision drift. Although a decision is made as a milestone in the planning process, over time the decision can evolve, resulting in decision drift among planners and program staff. Decision drift is a natural process in long-term health programs, but it can also occur within short spans of time, even within single meetings. Decision drift is detrimental only if it results in a program that lacks coherence or that no longer addresses the health problem. Through process evaluation, the extent to which decision drift has occurred can be assessed and the specific areas in which the decision drift occurred can be pinpointed. Knowing that decision drift has occurred provides a basis for either revising the decisions or modifying the program and objectives to be more in line with the current decisions. Which action to take will depend upon whether the decision drift has resulted in a more or a less efficient and effective health program.

QUANTIFYING OUTPUTS OF THE SERVICE UTILIZATION PLAN

During a process evaluation of each of the service utilization plan outputs, one of the first decisions to be made is what time frame will be used. Because seasonal fluctuations can affect many health programs, the time frame used is significant. For some programs, annual measures will be more reasonable, whereas for other, shorter programs, the end of the program will be sufficient. Ideally, the evaluation of the service utilization plan outputs occurs as close to "real time" as possible, rather than being retrospective, to ensure that programmatic changes are made in a timely fashion. The four service utilization plan outputs discussed here are coverage, units of service, service completion, workflow, and materials produced. Again, these are assessed with regard to the extent that corresponding process objectives have been achieved.

Measures of Coverage

Monitoring the degree of participation in a health program is a basic aspect of monitoring evaluation. All funding agencies and program managers want assurances that the program had participants. The mechanism for tracking the numbers must be in place before the process evaluation begins. Measures of coverage require having accurate data on the number of program participants at or within a given time period. Collecting data on a frequent or periodic basis allows for ongoing monitoring and still makes possible the aggregation of the numbers to get totals for a given time period. For example, if immunization clinics are offered three times a month, collect the number of participants per clinic and then add the three clinics to have a total number of participants per month.

Coverage is assessed with regard to undercoverage and overcoverage. Data from the needs assessment are required regarding the numbers of individuals in need and not in need of the program. These data, along with the actual number of individuals served by the program, form a matrix of undercoverage, ideal coverage, and overcoverage (Exhibit 8.9). Undercoverage is measured as the number of individuals in need of the service who received the service divided by the number of individuals in need. Undercoverage occurs when the program is not delivered to a large portion of the target audience. On the other side of the coin, overcoverage occurs when the program is being used by individuals not in the target audience. Overcoverage is the number who are not in need of the service but who receive the service divided by the number who receive the service. There is one more coverage measure; it is coverage efficiency (Exhibit 8.10). Coverage efficiency is calculated as 100% multiplied by the undercoverage plus overcoverage. Taken as a set, the coverage measures are useful as indicators of the extent to which efforts to enroll individuals into the program are effective, and they are also useful from the perspective of managing and tailoring the program. In addition, they provide some information regarding whether the target audience was reached. A narrative example of coverage measures is shown in Exhibit 8.11a, with the corresponding data in Excel shown in Exhibit 8.11b.

While the measures of coverage provide information about the extent to which the program is reaching the target audience, they do not provide information on the extent to which the program is meeting its goals. For this the efficiency index is needed; it is calculated as the number in need minus the number in need served divided by the target set in the program objective times the number in need. This is another way for program managers and staff to determine whether the program is reaching its objectives. The efficiency index can be applied to the program as a whole by summing the efficiency indices for each program component and dividing this sum by the number of program components. The number crunching and math involved is simple and yields a great deal of information about which program component needs attention due to undercoverage. The coverage information that reflects high coverage also can be used to market the program to funding agencies.

Exhibit 8.9   Table of Undercoverage and Overcoverage

	Not Served	**Served**
No Need	Ideal coverage	*Overcoverage*
Need	*Undercoverage*	Ideal coverage

Exhibit 8.10 Formulas for Coverage Measures

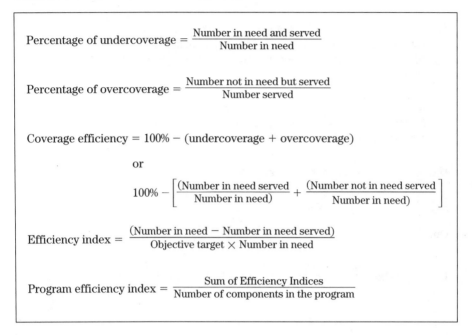

$$\text{Percentage of undercoverage} = \frac{\text{Number in need and served}}{\text{Number in need}}$$

$$\text{Percentage of overcoverage} = \frac{\text{Number not in need but served}}{\text{Number served}}$$

$$\text{Coverage efficiency} = 100\% - (\text{undercoverage} + \text{overcoverage})$$

or

$$100\% - \left[\frac{(\text{Number in need served}}{\text{Number in need})} + \frac{(\text{Number not in need served}}{\text{Number in need})} \right]$$

$$\text{Efficiency index} = \frac{(\text{Number in need} - \text{Number in need served})}{\text{Objective target} \times \text{Number in need}}$$

$$\text{Program efficiency index} = \frac{\text{Sum of Efficiency Indices}}{\text{Number of components in the program}}$$

Exhibit 8.11a Example of Coverage Measures

The state has established a funding stream for counties to provide an early childhood intervention program to families with infants diagnosed with a cognitive disability. The state set as the program standard that the county programs reach 90% of families in need. Two counties in the state applied for funds for the program and implemented the standardized early childhood intervention program. All programs were required to have three components: direct services to the infant, transportation as an enabling service for the parents, and support groups as an enabling service for the parents. In both counties, the community needs assessment data revealed that 1000 families were in need of the direct services component of the program. In both counties the need for transportation was found to be 500 families and the need for support groups to be 300 families. After one year, the programs reported the following program monitoring statistics on the implementation of their early childhood intervention program. The state is reviewing these programs with a goal of making recommendations to other counties interested in similar programs.

Exhibit 8.11a Example of Coverage Measures *(continued)*

In County A, the direct services component of the program had the following program statistics. Data on the number of participating families came from enrollment records, and data on the need for the program were based on a one-year follow-up screening and assessment.

Number of families served = number of participants = 400
Number of families in the program who needed the program = 300
Therefore, the number of families who did not need the program = 100

Direct services component coverage measures:

Percentage reached = $\dfrac{800}{1000}$ = 80%

Objective target = 90%

Undercoverage = $\left(\dfrac{1000 - 700}{1000} \right)$ = 0.30, or 30% of the families in need of the program did not get it

Overcoverage = $\dfrac{100}{800}$ = 0.13, or 13% of families in the program did not need the program.

Coverage efficiency = 100% − (30% + 13%) = 58%, or the program was 53% efficient in reaching the target population.

Efficiency index = $\dfrac{700}{1000 \times 90\%}$ = 78% efficient based on the state target.

Transportation component coverage measures:

Percentage reached = $\dfrac{450}{500}$ = 90%

Objective target = 90%

Efficiency index = $\dfrac{450}{500 \times 90\%}$ = 100% efficient based on the state target.

Exhibit 8.11a   Example of Coverage Measures *(continued)*

Support group component coverage measures:

Percentage reached $= \dfrac{100}{300} = 33\%$

Objective target $= 90\%$

Efficiency index $= \dfrac{100}{300 \times 90\%} = 37\%$ efficient based on the state target.

Program efficiency $= \dfrac{78\% + 100\% + 37\%}{3} = 72\%$, or overall, the early childhood intervention program in County A achieved the state target by 72%.

In County B, the direct services component of the early childhood intervention program had the following program statistics. Data on the number of participating families came from enrollment records, and data on the need for the program were based on one-year follow-up screening and assessment. The program in County B also used a basic screening or intake tool before enrolling families, and marketed the program to local pedestrians.

> Number of families served = number of participants = 900
> Number of families in the program who needed the program = 875
> Therefore, the number of families who did not need the program = 25

Direct services component coverage measures:

Percentage reached $= \dfrac{900}{1000} = 90\%$

Objective target $= 90\%$

Undercoverage $= \dfrac{1000 - 875}{1000} = 0.13$, or 13% of the families in need of the program did not get it.

Overcoverage $= \dfrac{25}{900} = 0.03$, or 3% of the families in the program did not need the program.

Exhibit 8.11a   Example of Coverage Measures *(continued)*

Coverage efficiency = 100% − (13% + 3%) = 84%, or the program was 84% efficient in reaching the target population.

Efficiency index = $\dfrac{875}{1000 \times 90\%}$ = 97% efficiency based on the state target.

Transportation component coverage measures:

Percentage reached = $\dfrac{400}{500}$ = 80%

Objective target = 90%

Efficiency index = $\dfrac{375}{500 \times 90\%}$ = 83% efficiency based on the state target.

Support group component coverage measures:

Percentage reached = $\dfrac{150}{300}$ = 50%

Objective target = 90%

Efficiency index = $\dfrac{150}{300 \times 90\%}$ = 56% effective based on the state target.

Program efficiency = $\dfrac{97\% + 83\% + 56\%}{3}$ = 79%, or overall, the early childhood intervention program in County B achieved the state target by 79.

Based on these measures of coverage, the state realizes that the standard of 90% for all three program components may not be completely realistic, particularly given the pattern of achieving the standards. Providing support groups for families seems the least well implemented of the three program components.

When thinking about the sources of data needed to measure participation, one must think in terms of target population and recipients. The number of individuals in need of the program—in other words, the size of target population—ought to have been determined through the community assessment. If the community needs assessment data do not include some estimation of the size of the target population, it becomes virtually impossible to determine

Exhibit 8.11b Example of Coverage Measure Using an Excel Spreadsheet

	A	B	C	D	E
1	*Early Childhood Intervention Program:*		*County A*	*County B*	*State Objective*
2	**Direct Services Component**				
3	Number in need of direct services		1000	1000	1000
4	Number served in need		700	875	
5	Number served not in need		100	25	
6	Number not served in need	C3−C4	300	125	
7	Total served		800	900	900
8		*FORMULAS*			
9	Percent reached	C7/C3	80%	90%	90%
10	Percent overcoverage	C5/C7	13%	3%	0%
11	Percent undercoverage	(C3−C4)/C3	30%	13%	0%
12	% in need served	(100−C11)	70%	88%	
13	Coverage efficiency	100%−(C10 + C11)	58%	85%	
14	Efficiency index	(C4)/(E9*E3)	78%	97%	
15					
16	**Transportation Program**				
17	Number in need of transportation		500	500	500
18	Number served in need		450	375	
19	Number served not in need		10	25	
20	Number not served in need	C17−C18	50	125	
21	Total served		450	400	450
22		*FORMULAS*			
23	Percent reached	C21/C17	90%	80%	90%
24	Percent overcoverage	C19/C21	2%	6%	0%
25	Percent undercoverage	C21/C17	10%	25%	0%
26	% in need served	(100−C25)	90%	75%	
27	Coverage efficiency	100%−(C25+C24)	88%	69%	
28	Efficiency index	(C18)/(E17*E21)	100%	83%	
29					
30	**Support Group Program**				
31	Number in need of support group		300	300	300
32	Number served in need		100	150	
33	Number served not in need		0	0	
34	Number not served in need	C31−C32	200	150	
35	Total served		100	150	270
36		*FORMULAS*			
37	Percent reached	C35/C31	33%	50%	90%
38	Percent overcoverage	C33/C35	0%	0%	0%
39	Percent undercoverage	C35/C31	67%	50%	0%
40	% in need served	(100−C39)	33%	50%	
41	Coverage efficiency	100%−(C38+C39)	33%	50%	
42	Efficiency index	(C32)/(E31*E37)	37%	56%	
43					
44	**Early Childhood Intervention Program Efficiency**	(C14+C28+C42)/3	72%	79%	

undercoverage and overcoverage. At best, these can then be estimated only from alternative data sources. The number of individuals actually in the program can be derived from participant sign-in lists, program records, participant tracking forms, billing or claims data, or client records.

Units of Service

For some programs, it will be important to distinguish between the number of program participants and the number of contacts. Outreach programs may be quite successful in making a high number of contacts with potential program participants, but the number of individuals who actually show up for the program may be a small fraction of that number. In this case, a decision must be made as to whether the number of individuals contacted is equivalent to the number of outreach recipients. These are gray areas, and each program will have a slightly different answer. The key is to make clear what is being counted and the definition on which it is based. The process objective should specify what is being counted.

The unit of service must be clearly defined and articulated before the count can begin. A unit of service (UOS) is a predetermined unit, such as number of contact hours, number of individual clients seen, number of educational sessions offered, or size of caseload. It is primarily used for programs at the direct or enabling services levels of the public health pyramid. For some programs the UOS is specified by the funding agency, in which case data for that UOS become a minimum of what is included in the process evaluation of services delivered.

Service Completion

Estimating the degree to which program participants completed the health program is the inverse of estimating the dropout rate of the program. One-shot programs, such as screening clinics, versus programs with longer-term involvement with the participants, such as substance abuse counseling, meals on wheels, or exercise classes, are likely to have different completion rates. For some enabling services, service completion is the achievement of the service plan or care plan. Counting the number of participants who have completed a service provides different information on the extent to which the intervention was implemented and the dosage received by the average participant. Service completion can be estimated only if there are good records of enrollment and attendance that are recorded on an individual basis. Drastic changes in completion rates may signal problems with program staff or with the design of the program. The process objectives should include a threshold for what is an acceptable completion rate.

Level of participation is a corollary of service completion. If the intervention or impact theories are predicated on a given level of participation, then data on the level of participation need to be collected as a means of determining whether participants received the appropriate "dose" of the intervention. For some health programs, level of participation might be a simple yes/no on attendance at, say, an immunization clinic, or a weighted calculation of the percentage of time during a set of sessions in which the participant was actively engaged with the group. The measure chosen will depend on the nature of the program and the target and indicator specified in the process objective. A low level of participation can result if program staff are not skilled in engaging participants (a managerial issue) or if the intervention is not appealing to the participants (a process theory issue).

Workflow

There is an interaction between the procedures used for managing waiting participants and the amount of work done by program staff. The process evaluation thus focuses on workflow as one indicator of the amount of work done by the program staff and the queuing of participants. Examples of workflow measures include minutes that participants spend waiting to be seen, number of days between signing up for the program and beginning the program, number of days between being referred to the program and being accepted into the health program, and amount of time required of program staff to complete a specific task. Of course, the amount of work done by program staff is influenced by the volume of program participants and the rate at which they participate in the program. For direct services health programs, the volume and queuing will greatly affect the workflow of program staff. For population-based programs, the level of cooperation from others, such as broadcasters, may affect the workflow of program staff—say, in delivery of a mass media campaign.

Data for both volume of participants and workflow come from a variety of sources. Observations of program staff, participant records, appointment logs, class sign-in sheets, and billing statements are common sources of data. For some programs it may be appropriate to develop specific data collection forms. If this is done, the program staff should be involved, as using the empowerment approach to planning increases the likelihood that optimal measures will be developed and used by program staff.

Materials Produced

Both the quantity and quality of the materials produced for the health program need to be considered in the process evaluation. Having data about the materials provides insights into the work done by staff and the extent to which the intervention was delivered in the manner planned. One managerial insight that emerges from tracking the production of materials is whether resources are directed more toward the materials than toward implementation of the intervention. Data about production of materials can be difficult to obtain and will be very program specific.

FROM DATA TO ACTION

The value of having data lies in its being used. The data collected can be compared to the targets set in the process objectives. The larger issue is how to transform the data from the process evaluation into information and subsequent actions. In addition, the process monitoring data can reveal which elements of the process theory may need to be modified in order to have appropriate coverage. Each of these topics is covered in this section.

Process Objectives Revisited

The conversion of data into information begins by comparing the results of the process evaluation with the targets stated in the process objectives. The efficiency index described earlier is one way to do that. However, each objective developed for the organizational plan and service utilization plan needs to be compared with the actual program accomplishments as revealed through the process evaluation. A simple tally of the number of process objectives met, exceeded, or not met is also a realistic approach. The extent to which the objectives were met could be a function of the objective targets not being realistic, in terms of being either unobtainably high or unnecessarily low.

If the comparison of the findings from the process evaluation to the objectives does not reveal any pattern or provide useful insights, the data could be used to compare the program to similar health programs. This process is called benchmarking. When the health program is compared to other known successful programs on a limited and relevant set of indicators, it is easier to determine the extent to which the program was successfully implemented. This approach has the advantage of not relying on potentially flawed targets for the process objectives. Other external sources of norms or standards on which to make comparisons are performance measures for health programs set by different federal health bureaus or departments. If they exist for the health program, they can be used as standards against which to draw conclusions regarding program implementation.

Process Evaluation Data as Information

Once the data collection phase of the process evaluation is complete, the data obtained from it need to be analyzed and interpretations constructed in ways that enable action to be taken that maintains or improves the program. Process evaluations are valuable only if the findings are used in a timely manner to make alterations in the program. In this way, process evaluations are similar to the continuous quality improvement (CQI) and total quality management (TQM) approaches, as well as other improvement methodologies. However, process monitoring data are more immediately useful as quality assurance information, which focuses on the level to which standards are met, hence assuring a minimum level of quality. Quality assurance is most easily understood as the setting of standards for laboratory testing of specimens or the production of medications. It is an important element of assuring that program interventions are delivered as planned and according to the program standards.

Corrective managerial actions generated from quality assurance tend to stress following procedures, rather than identifying larger, more systemwide program process improvements. Process evaluation data relevant to quality assurance lead to two possible avenues of action: managerial actions focused on implementation and subsequent planning focused on modifying the process theory. Before either type of action is taken, data from the process evaluation need be converted into information. Ideally, program staff are included in discussions about the degree of congruence found between the objectives and the actual accomplishments. Their insights can provide plausible explanations for gaps. It is possible that the cause of the gap was not addressed in the data that were collected as part of the process evaluation.

A report that describes how data were collected and that makes connections between the data and the program objectives is usually a product of the process evaluation. The report ought to address both organizational plan objectives and achievements as well as service utilization plan objectives and achievements. The report, or appropriate portions of it, ought to be shared with program staff as well as with funding agencies and other stakeholders. A periodic process evaluation that is shared with program staff can be used to identify factors that contribute to the "success" or "poor performance" of the program. Findings from the process evaluation can be shared in ways that maintain individual confidentiality but allow staff members to see their productivity in comparison to other staff. Reasons for higher and lower productivity that are amenable to managerial intervention might be identified. In addition, sharing the process evaluation data with staff provides an opportunity for them to express their concerns, challenges in complying with intervention specifications, and overall morale on the health program.

Once the areas of deficit or weakness or unachieved objectives have been identified, action is required. To the extent that the process evaluation is used for ongoing program improvements, feedback exists between the process evaluation and the process theory. Actions can be broadly related to either the organizational plan or the service utilization plan.

Action Focused on the Process Theory

Undercoverage or overcoverage may be a result of bias in program participation. Individuals can self-select into or out of a program for which they may be eligible and in need. When individuals in need of the program choose to not participate, undercoverage results; conversely, individuals self-selecting into a program that they do not need results in overcoverage. Understanding the reasons for bias in participation is tricky. It requires both a careful review of program procedures and a qualitative investigation into the perceptions of participants (especially those who are not in need of the program) and of program staff.

Undercoverage can result from a small program addressing a big problem. In this instance, documentation of undercoverage, along with documentation of program success in achieving the desired effects, can be used to seek funds to expand the program. If serious undercoverage is found in the process evaluation, the social marketing plan that was implemented ought to be reviewed and perhaps revised based on the available process evaluation data about the participants. In addition, it may be necessary to review the cultural acceptability of the program. Barriers to access, availability, acceptability, and affordability all affect who receives the program. These must be considered when reviewing the reasons for undercoverage.

Overcoverage is as likely to result from poor program administration as from the program inadvertently addressing an unrecognized need. Recruitment, screening, or enrollment procedures may be faulty or inadequate. These administrative issues can be addressed with staff training and revisions of the procedures. Overcoverage resulting from an unrecognized need is more difficult to assess. Consider an immunization clinic for school-age children. If many children who are already fully immunized are brought for immunizations, overcoverage exists. But the unrecognized need may be parental confusion regarding school immunizations or the lack of a centralized immunization tracking system. Another example of overcoverage would be more than the expected number of senior citizens attending a free lunch program. The unrecognized need may be for socialization opportunities for the seniors of the community, or the free ride to and from the luncheon site may be the only way for the seniors to get to a nearby mall. In other words, overcoverage can be thought of as a form of expressed needs. Thus, the reason for overcoverage, if not administrative, may lead to new programs.

If the program is provided to individuals who are not in the target group, and who hence would not benefit from the program, the intervention will appear to have no effect. Understanding of the degree of undercoverage or overcoverage is critical in determining the cause of program failure, should the impact evaluation show no programmatic effect on the participants.

Another consideration is the extent to which program components are provided. This is especially important for complex programs that entail interdependent program components. For example, a program for the severely mentally ill may include a transportation component as well as social activities and independent living education. If the transportation component is not provided, the other component will naturally fail to show any effects. It is through the process evaluation that these "flaws" in the delivery of the program are identified. Program components for which the effectiveness index is low alert program planners and managers to revisit the feasibility of the program, the degree to which the objectives were realistic, and the logic behind the interventions being used.

If the program has been ongoing for several years, and the indices of efficiency are declining, it may be time to fine-tune the program (Rossi & Freeman, 1993). This might entail updating the needs assessment, revising program objectives, altering the marketing strategy, changing the interventions offered, or adjusting the organizational plan.

Accountability

Accountability is being held answerable, or accountable, for the program delivery and consequences. Being accountable accompanies being responsible. There are several ways in which one can be answerable or provide an account of the program delivery and effect. The five types of accountability (Rossi, Freeman, & Lipsey, 1999) apply to the organizational plan, the service utilization plan, and the effect theory. In addition, for each type a set of indicators can be constructed (Exhibit 8.12). Three types of accountability relate to the organizational plan: efficiency, fiscal, and legal accountability. Efficiency accountability is the extent to which resources are used without waste or redundancy, and is measured in indicators such as the dollars spent, the cost per program participant, and the cost per unit of impact. In contrast, fiscal accountability is the extent to

Exhibit 8.12 Types of Program Accountability, with Definitions and Examples of Process Evaluation Indicators

Accountability Type	Definition The extent to which:	Indicators
Organization plan		
Efficiency	Resources are utilized without waste or redundancy	Dollars spent on the program; cost per client served; cost per unit of outcome
Fiscal	Resources are managed according to the budget	Budget categories; existence of receipts and bills paid; number of errors found during annual audit; percent variance from budget
Legal	Legal, regulatory, and ethical standards are met	Number of malpractice suits; number of investigations; number of personnel with current licensure
Service utilization plan		
Coverage	The target population is reached	Number of clients served; number of persons in need of service
Service delivery	The intervention is provided as planned	Number of units of service provided; number of breaches in intervention protocol; number of modifications to intervention
Effect theory		
Impact	Participants are changed because of the intervention	Very program specific; discussed in Chapters 9 and 10

which resources are managed according to the budget and is reflected in the percentage of expenditure variance from the budget, documentation of expenditures, and collections. Legal accountability is the extent to which legal, regulatory, and ethical standards are met. Indicators of legal accountability are the number of malpractice suits, investigations, and personnel with current licensure.

With regard to the service utilization plan, coverage and service delivery are the two types of accountability. Coverage accountability is the extent to which the target population is reached and participates in the program. Coverage accountability is documented with the calculation procedures described earlier. Service delivery accountability is the extent to which the intervention is provided as planned, and is indicated not only by the number of units of service provided but also by the number of times the program intervention protocol was not followed or the number of changes made to the intervention. Finally, there is impact accountability which is the extent to which program participants changed due to receiving the program. The indicators for impact accountability are highly tailored to reflect the effect theory of the program.

ACROSS THE PYRAMID

At the direct services level of the public health pyramid, program process evaluation and monitoring focus on the inputs and outputs of the organizational and service utilization plans (Exhibit 8.13). Indicators would, of course, be tailored to the specific program; nonetheless, a process evaluation for service utilization will include measures of the units of service that are individuals served and number of contact hours with individuals. Such measures are consistent with the nature of health programs designed for the direct services level of the pyramid.

At the enabling services level, as at the direct services level, process evaluations and monitoring efforts ought to address inputs and outputs of the organizational and service utilization plans. The indicators are likely to be similar to those used at the direct services level (Exhibit 8.13), but modified to reflect the specific program and the use of different sources of data.

At the population-based services level, as with the direct services and enabling services levels, program process evaluations and monitoring efforts also ought to address inputs and outputs of the organizational and service utilization plans. The units of service could be number of individuals served, number of agencies involved, or number of households reached.

At the infrastructure level, program process evaluations and monitoring efforts need to address inputs and outputs of the organizational and service utilization plans. If the health program is designed for one of the other levels

Exhibit 8.13   Examples of Process Evaluation Measures Across the Pyramid

	Direct Services	Enabling Services	Population Services	Infrastructure
Organizational Plan Input	Provider credentials, location	Provider credentials, physical resources (i.e., cars)	Provider credentials, managerial resources	Personnel qualifications, managerial resources, fiscal resources
Organizational Plan Output	Protocols and procedures for service delivery, data about individual participants	Protocols and procedures for service delivery, data about participants	Protocols and procedures for service delivery	Budget variance, fiscal accountability, data and management information systems
Service Utilization Plan Input	Wait times, characteristics of participants	Wait times, characteristics of participants	Characteristics of the population	Characteristics of the workforce
Service Utilization Plan Output	Measures of coverage	Measures of coverage	Measures of coverage	Materials produced, number of participants

of the pyramid, then the infrastructure becomes the source of the inputs and outputs of the organizational and service utilization plans. However, if the health program is targeted at the members of the infrastructure, then the infrastructure is more like a place, and the program is better considered in terms of whether it is a direct service, such as an on-site health education program, an enabling service, such as subsidizing membership in a health club, or a population-based service, such as a workplace safety program. For programs in which the infrastructure is considered the site, units of service could be the number of employees involved, and outputs might be the number of policy or procedure updates.

If the program is targeted at personnel within the infrastructure, then measures of job satisfaction might be considered, particularly of health practitioners such as nurses (Misener & Cox, 2001) or physicians (Beasley, Kern, Howard, &

Kolodner, 1999). However, they are best considered as measures of the effect of the intervention on the human resources—in other words, effect theory measures—in contrast to satisfaction measures, which are measures of the process theory. This same reasoning can be applied to programs that uses community coalitions, consortia, collaboratives, or interagency consortia to implement the health program. These groups would be comparable to the program personnel and thus are elements of the program infrastructure.

Interventions that are changes in health policy are also best considered at the infrastructure level. One infrastructure intervention in health services that has received considerable attention is the financing of health care. Just as customer satisfaction has been widely studied with regard to direct services, so has satisfaction been studied with regard to health care financing (Dellana & Glascoff, 2001). A careful examination of the satisfaction tools used, elements of both the organizational and service utilization plan are included. Because satisfaction data can be readily collected and analyzed, it has the potential to provide timely feedback data with regard to the effect of infrastructure-level interventions.

DISCUSSION QUESTIONS

1. Involvement of community coalitions and consortia in the implementation of health programs has become widespread. What would be possible and appropriate measures or indicators of having implemented community coalitions or consortia as part of the program delivery?

2. What would you suggest as methods and techniques to avoid the failure of interventions? Justify your ideas in terms of the ways interventions can fail.

3. In order to have accurate measures of coverage, what information systems and data collection methods need to be in place? What steps can assure that these are in place in a timely manner?

4. Process evaluation and program monitoring data are useful only when interpreted and used to make program changes. Outline a plan, with actions and stakeholders, for increasing the likelihood that the process data will contribute to accurate and responsible program delivery.

References

Armburster, C., Gale, B., Brady, J., & Thompson, N. (1999). Perceived ownership in a community coalition. *Public Health Nursing, 16*, 17–22.

Argyris, C. (1992). *On organizational learning.* Cambridge, MA: Blackwell Publishers.

Beasley, B. W., Kern, D. E., Howard, D. M., & Kolodner, K. (1999). A job satisfaction measure for internal medicine residency program directors. *Academic Medicine, 74*, 263–270.

Cox, L. E., Rouff, J. R., Svendsen, K. H., Markowitz, M., & Abrams, D. I. (1998). Community advisory boards: Their role in AIDS clinical trails. *Health and Social Work, 23*, 290–297.

Dellana, S. A., & Glascoff, D. W. (2001). The impact of health insurance plan type on satisfaction with health care. *Health Care Management Review, 26*, 33–46.

Drain, M. (2001). Quality improvement in primary care and the importance of patient perceptions. *Journal of Ambulatory Care Management, 24*(2), 30–46.

Gesell, S. B. (2001). A measure of satisfaction for the assisted-living industry. *Journal of Healthcare Quality: Promoting Excellence in Heatlhcare, 23*, 16–25.

Green, L. W., & Lewis, F. M. (1986). *Measurement and evaluation in health education and health promotion.* Palo Alto, CA: Mayfield Publishing.

Hays, C. E., Hays, S. P., DeVille, J. O., & Mulhall, P. F. (2000). Capacity for effectiveness: The relationship between coalition structure and community impact. *Evaluation and Program Planning, 23*, 373–379.

Higginbotham, N., Heading, G., McElduff, P., Dobson, A., & Heller, R. (1999). Reducing coronary heart disease in the Australian coalfields: Evaluation of a 10-year community intervention. *Social Science and Medicine, 48*, 683–692.

Horne, R., Hankins, M., & Jenkins, R. (2001). The Satisfaction with Information about Medicines Scale (SIMS): A new measurement tool for audit and research. *Quality in Health Care, 10*, 135–140.

Misener, T. R., & Cox, D. L. (2001). Development of the Misener Nurse Practitioner Job Satisfaction Scale. *Journal of Nursing Measurement, 9*, 91–108.

Mostyn, M. M., Race, K. E., Seibert, J. H., & Johnson, M. (2000). Quality assurance in nursing home facilities: Measuring customer satisfaction. *American Journal of Medical Quality, 15*, 54–61.

Paine-Andrews, A., Fawcett, S. B., Richter, K. P., Berkley, J. Y., Williams, E. L., & Lopez, C. M. (1996). Community coalitions to prevent adolescent substance abuse: The case of the "Project Freedom" Replication Initiative. *Journal of Prevention and Intervention in the Community, 14*, 81–99.

Parasuraman, A., Zeithaml, V. A., & Berry, L. L. (1985). A conceptual model of service quality and its implications for future research. *Journal of Marketing, 49*, 41–50.

Patton, M. Q. (1997). *Utilization-focused evaluation* (3rd ed.). Thousand Oaks, CA: Sage Publications.

Pellegrin, K. L., Stuart, G. W., Maree, B., Fruech, B. C., & Ballenger, J. C. (2001). A brief scale for assessing patients' satisfaction with care in outpatient psychiatric services. *Psychiatric Services, 52*, 816–819.

Raube, K., Handler, A., & Rosenberg, D. (1998). Measuring satisfaction among low-income women: A prenatal care questionnaire. *Maternal and Child Health Journal, 2*, 25–33.

Rossi, P. H., & Freeman, H. E. (1993). *Evaluation: A systematic approach* (5th ed.). Newbury Park, CA: Sage Publications.

Rossi, P. H., Freeman, H. E., & Lipsey, M. W. (1999). *Evaluation: A systematic approach* (6th ed.). Thousand Oaks, CA: Sage Publications.

Roush, S. E., & Sonstroem, R. J. (1999). Development of the physical therapy outpatient satisfaction survey (PTOPS). *Physical Therapy, 79,* 159–170.

Seibert, J. H., Brien, J. S., Maaske, B. L., Kochurka, K., Feldt, K., Fader, L. & Race, K. E. (1999). Assessing patient satisfaction across the continuum of ambulatory care: A revalidation and validation of care specific surveys. *Journal of Ambulatory Care Management, 22*(2), 9–26.

Sinacore, J. M., Connell, K. M., Olthoff, A. J., Friedman, M. H., & Gecht, M. R. (1999). A method for measuring interrater agreement on checklists. *Evaluation and the Health Professions, 22,* 221–234.

Steine, S., Finset, A., & Laerum, E. (2001). A new, brief questionnaire (PEQ) developed in primary health care for measuring patients' experience of interaction, emotion and consultation outcome. *Family Practice, 18,* 410–418.

Section 4

Evaluating the Impact and Outcome of Health Programs

CHAPTER 9

Planning the Methods for Evaluating Intervention Effects

In the daily work of implementing a program, evaluating intervention effects can seem like a luxury. The reality is that conducting an evaluation whose purpose is to identify whether or not the intervention had an effect requires considerable forethought regarding a broad range of issues, each of which has the potential to seriously detract from the credibility of the evaluation. Intervention effect evaluations deserve the same degree of attention during program planning as the development of the program interventions themselves and, ideally, ought to be designed concurrently with the program. Too often, attention is focused on developing the evaluation only after the goals and objectives are finalized and after the program is up and running. Well-articulated program outcome goals and impact objectives facilitate development of the evaluation, but insights about the program process can be gained from developing an evaluation plan. Thus, the placement of these chapters on evaluating intervention effects after the chapters on program development and monitoring ought *not* be interpreted as being when one should actually plan the intervention effect evaluation.

This chapter addresses the broad areas of data collection and evaluation rigor, within the context of the program theory and feasibility considerations. Information presented in this and the next chapters on designs and sampling is not intended to duplicate the extensive treatment of research methods and statistics provided in research textbooks. Basic research content is presented as background to the problems commonly encountered in conducting a health program intervention evaluation; and practical suggestions are provided for minimizing those problems. Because the focus is on practical solutions to real problems, the suggestions may differ from those usually found in research and statistics textbooks. Nonetheless, good research methods and statistics textbooks are invaluable resources and ought to be on the bookshelf of every program evaluator.

Planning the evaluation begins with deciding upon the evaluation questions and then proceeding to develop a detailed evaluation implementation plan, similar to the details of the program organization plan. Aspects of the evaluation plan related to data collection are discussed, namely levels of measurement and levels of analysis, as well as techniques for collecting data. Designs that can be used to conduct the evaluation and issues related to sampling are discussed in the next chapter. These elements of evaluations are closely aligned with research methodology, and achieving scientific rigor is the first yardstick used when planning the intervention effects evaluation. However, the first step in planning the evaluation is to decide what questions the evaluation must be able to answer.

DEVELOPING THE EVALUATION QUESTIONS

The assessment statement developed during the community needs assessment stage that articulated the risk of "x" among "who" became the basis for impact objective elements of "who" will do "what" "by when." Those same elements are used in the evaluation. The first place to start in developing the evaluation questions is with the logic model, the effect theory, and the impact objectives; they ought to be the basis for decisions about the focus and purpose of the intervention evaluation. The effect theory focuses attention on the specific aspects of the health problem that the program is addressing. An evaluation could address many aspects of the health problem and possible health outcomes, and novice evaluators and enthusiastic program supporters will be tempted to include as much as possible in the evaluation. Succumbing to this temptation will lead to higher evaluation costs, and an overwhelming amount of data to analyze and interpret, as well as generating distractions from the essence of the program. Thus, staying focused on key impact objectives minimizes the chances that the evaluation will become a fishing expedition. In other words, designing an evaluation can quickly lead to the development of a creative wish list of statements such as, "If only we knew x about the target population or recipients." The impact objectives become a sounding board against which to determine whether that "if only we knew" statement has relevance and importance to understanding whether the program was effective.

Why an evaluation is done and what is expected from the evaluation must be considered early in the evaluation planning. The obvious reason for doing an evaluation is to determine the effect of the program on recipients. Patton (1998) argued that the usefulness of evaluation information ought to be a major reason for doing the evaluation. But there may be other reasons to conduct an evaluation, such as to fulfill requirements of funding agencies. The need to respond to funding agency requirements can be an opportunity to engage program stakeholders and elicit their interests with regard to why an evaluation should be done. Information that stakeholders want from an evaluation, once made explicit, then can be incorporated into the evaluation. An aspect of the question of why an evaluation should be done involves asking who cares whether the evaluation is done and what it might find. There might also be a desire to "prove" that the program was the source of some beneficial change. Answering causal questions is the most difficult type of evaluation, but causality testing provides the richest information for understanding the validity of the effect theory.

Characteristics of the Right Question

Evaluations ought to be useful as well as scientifically sound and based on the program objectives (Patton, 1978, 1998). From the perspective of being useful, the "right" evaluation question has three characteristics (Patton, 1978), and evaluation questions with all of these characteristics will lead to useful and feasible evaluations.

One characteristic is that relevant data can be collected. For example, a community agency wanted to know if their program was having an effect on the substance abuse rates among school-age children. The stakeholders did not believe that data collected several years prior to their program from across the state were relevant to their community. Yet data could not be collected from children in grades 6 through 8 regarding their use of illegal drugs, because the school board refused to allow the evaluators into the schools. Thus, the evaluation question of whether the substance abuse prevention intervention changed the behavior of these children could not be answered. The program staff restated the question to ask whether children who had received the substance abuse prevention program had learned about the negative health effects of illegal substances. The school board was willing to allow the evaluators to collect data on this question from children.

Another characteristic of the "right" evaluation question is that more than one answer is possible. While this may seem counterintuitive, allowing for the possibility of multiple answers shows less bias on the part of the evaluator for arriving at the desired answer. Having multiple answers also may reveal subtle differences among participants or program components that were not anticipated. Compare an evaluation question such as "Did the program make a difference to participants?" with the question "What types of changes did participants experience?" The second question makes it possible to identify not only changes that were anticipated based on the effect theory, but other changes that may not have been anticipated.

The right evaluation question also leads to information that decision makers want and feel they need. Stakeholders as well ought to want the information from the evaluation and be interested in the answer to the evaluation question. Ultimately, the right question will produce information that decision makers can use, regardless of whether it actually is used in decision making. The test of usefulness of the information generated by the evaluation will help avoid the fishing expedition and, more importantly, could be a point at which developing the evaluation becomes feedback to the design of the interventions.

Having a clear purpose for the evaluation and knowing what is needed as an end product of the evaluation are the critical first steps in developing the evaluation. The nature of the evaluation depends upon the skill and sophistication of the evaluator and the purpose of the evaluation. One way to think about the purpose of the intervention effects evaluation question is to consider the degree to which the evaluation needs to document or explain the changes in program participants.

Impact Documentation, Impact Assessment, or Impact Evaluation

Evaluating the effect of the intervention can vary from the simple to the highly complex. At a minimum, an evaluation ought to document the impact of the program in terms of reaching the stated impact and outcome objectives. An impact documentation evaluation asks the question "To what extent were the impact objectives met?" Thus, an evaluation that is an impact documentation evaluation will use data collection methods that are very closely related to the objectives. The impact objectives that flowed from the effect theory become the cornerstone of an impact documentation evaluation.

The next level of complexity is an impact assessment evaluation, which seeks to answer the question "To what extent might any noticeable change or difference in participants be related to having received the program interventions?" An impact assessment goes beyond documenting that the objectives were met by quantifying the extent to which the interventions seem related to changes observed or measured among program recipients. Thus, the data collection for an impact assessment may need to be more complex and better able to detect smaller and more specific changes in program participants. Note that the impact assessment addresses only the existence of a relationship between having received the program and a change, not whether the change was caused by the program. This subtle linguistic difference, often not recognized by stakeholders, is actually enormous from the point of view of evaluation and research.

The most complex and difficult question to answer is "Were the changes or differences due to having received the program and nothing else?" To answer this question, an impact evaluation is needed. Because the impact evaluation seeks to attribute changes in program participants to the interventions, and nothing else, the data collection must be able to detect changes due to the program and other potentially influential factors that are not part of the program. This makes an impact evaluation the most like basic research, especially clinical trials, into the causes of health problems and the efficacy of interventions.

Thinking of the three levels of intervention effect evaluations (Exhibit 9.1) as impact documentation, impact assessment, and impact evaluation helps delineate the level of complexity needed in data collection, the degree of scientific rigor called for, and, as will be discussed in the next chapter, the design of the evaluation.

Exhibit 9.1   Three Levels of Intervention Effect Evaluations

	Impact Documentation	**Impact Assessment**	**Impact Evaluation**
Purpose	Show that impact and outcome objectives were met	Determine whether those in the program experienced any change/benefit	Determine whether participating in the program caused a change or benefit for recipients
Relationship to Program Effect Theory	Confirms reaching benchmarks set in the objectives that were based on the program effect theory	Supports the program effect theory	Verifies the program effect theory
Level of Rigor Required	Minimal	Moderate	Maximum
Data Collection	Data type and collection timing based on objectives being measured	Data type based on program effect theory; timing based on feasibility	Data type based on program effect theory; baseline or preintervention data required as well as postintervention data

Evaluation and Research

The distinction between evaluation and research can be ambiguous and is often blurred in the minds of stakeholders. Nonetheless, fundamental differences do exist (Exhibit 9.2), particularly with regard to purpose and audiences for the final report. There is much less distinction with regard to methods and designs; both draw heavily from methodologies used in behavioral and health

Exhibit 9.2   Differences Between Evaluation and Research

Characteristic	Research	Evaluation
Goal or purpose	Generate new knowledge for prediction	Social accounting and program or policy decision making
The questions	Scientist's own questions	Derived from program goals and impact objectives
Nature of problem addressed	Areas where knowledge is lacking	Assess impacts and outcomes related to program
Guiding theory	Theory used as base for hypothesis testing	Theory underlying the program interventions, theory of evaluation
Appropriate techniques	Sampling, statistics, hypothesis testing, etc.	Whichever research techniques fit with the problem
Setting	Anywhere that is appropriate to	Usually wherever one can access the question the program recipients and nonrecipient controls
Dissemination	Scientific journals	Internal and externally viewed program reports, scientific journals
Allegiance	Scientific community	Funding source, policy preference, scientific community

sciences. The differences between research and evaluation are important to appreciate for two reasons. One reason is that communicating the differences to stakeholders and program staff helps establish realistic expectations about implementing the evaluation and about the findings of the evaluation. As a consequence it will be easier to gain their cooperation and feedback on the feasibility of the evaluation. The other reason is that it can allay anxieties about spending undue amounts of time "doing research" that will take time away from providing the program, the primary concern of program staff.

Research, in a pure sense, is done for the purpose of generating knowledge, whereas program evaluation is done for the purpose of understanding the extent to which the intervention was effective. These are not mutually exclusive. That is, a good program evaluation can advance knowledge, just as knowledge from research is used in program development. Evaluation research is done for the purpose of generating knowledge about the effectiveness of a program and, as such, is the blending of research and evaluation. While these three terms are often used interchangeably or ambiguously, it is easiest to think of evaluation research as research done by professional evaluators, following standards for evaluation and using research methods and designs. Evaluation research is most often an impact assessment or an impact evaluation. In this regard, it tends to be more complex, more costly, and require more evaluation skill than most program staff have. None of this is to imply that a simpler impact documentation is not as valuable. The value always lies in asking the right question for the program.

Rigor in Evaluation

Rigor is important in evaluation, as it is in research, because there is a need to have confidence that the findings and results are as true a representation as possible of what happened. The deck is often stacked against finding any impact from a program, for programmatic reasons, such as having a weak or ineffective intervention, and for reasons involving the evaluation research methods, such as having measures with low validity or reliability. Rigor results from minimizing the natural flaws associated with doing evaluation or research, that would diminish the ability to identify the net effects of the program. The net effects are those that are attributable only to the program, whereas the gross effects are the total effects from the intervention without effects from other causes, plus any effects that are artifacts of the evaluation design. The purpose of the evaluation is to identify the net effects, and therefore, rigor is used to minimize the inclusion of nonintervention effects and design effects.

INTERVENTION EFFECT EVALUATION VARIABLES FROM THE PROGRAM EFFECT THEORY

During program planning, an effect theory was developed as the logic model. Based on that, impact and outcome objectives were developed that focus on what the program ought to achieve. Just as process objectives were useful in developing the program monitoring evaluation, the effect theory and the impact and outcome objectives are cornerstones that guide decisions regarding what to measure in the intervention effect evaluation. The effect theory is composed of (1) the determinant theory, which explains the relationship between the determinants of the health problem and the health impact; (2) the intervention theory, which specifies how the programmatic interventions change the determinants of the health problem; (3) the impact theory, which shows the relationship of the antecedents of the health problem to the determinants and the subsequent health impact; and (4) the outcome theory, which explains how the immediate health impacts become the longer-term health outcomes, given the presence of contributing factors to the health outcome. The intervention evaluation uses these theories to identify what gets measured, specifically with regard to the determinants of the health problem and the health outcomes. At a minimum, the determinants and health impacts specified in the theories need to measured.

In the following discussion and in the subsequent chapters, the convention used in research and statistics is used. The impact and outcome variables are designated as y, the dependent variable; and variables that precede the impact are designated as x, independent variables. Strictly speaking, any antecedent, determinant, intervention, or contributing factor is an independent variable. This nomenclature is shown in Exhibit 9.3. Labeling the variables as x and y at this stage of planning will help later during data analysis.

Impact and Outcome as Dependent Variables

The heart of any evaluation is *what* health or behavioral characteristic is assessed for impact. The "what" question ought to be answered directly from the "what" aspect of the impact objective, which in turn came from the "risk of x" portion of the community health statement. If a community health statement was that school-age children were at risk for elevated cholesterol, and the impact objective states that 90% of program participants will have normal cholesterol levels, then cholesterol is measured in the evaluation. The choice revolves around which cholesterol test to use, not whether to measure cholesterol or body weight.

The impact variable, called the dependent or y variable, is the same as was specified in the impact objectives. Similarly, the long-term health outcome variable is also a dependent variable, as specified in the outcome objective (Exhibit 9.4). The difference between these two dependent variables is a matter of what the evaluation question is. In the newborn health example, the impact variable as a dependent variable would be used for questions such as "Was the rate of neural tube defects lower among program participants?" In contrast, the outcome variable, the rate of birth defects, would be used for a question such as "Was having a state nutrition program related to a decrease in birth defects?"

Typically, health program evaluations assess the effect of programs in the seven domains of well-being: physical health, knowledge, lifestyle behaviors, cognitive processes, mental health, social health, and resources. These domains of health and well-being can also be related to the determinants, antecedents, and contributing factors to the health problem of concern. During development of the program effect theory and logic model, the role of those domains in the health problem was determined. In planning the evaluation, it will be crucial to refer back to those discussions and decisions as a means of deciding whether the health domain is the dependent or an independent variable in the intervention evaluation. At this juncture, during the discussion of what exactly the dependent variable is, it is possible that program staff and stakeholders could have new insights into their program and want to modify the logic model. This discussion, if it occurs before the program is implemented, can then become one of the feedback loops to program development or improvement. In any event, the impact objectives provide direct guidance and ought to specify what

Exhibit 9.3   Using Elements of the Effect Theory to Identify Evaluation Variables

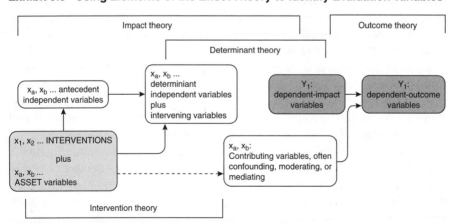

Exhibit 9.4   Evaluation Variables Based on the Effect Theory of Improving Newborn Health Status

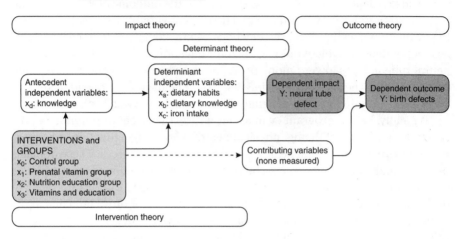

indicators, and subsequently which measures, to use in the evaluation. If the impact objectives fail to be helpful, this is another point at which developing the evaluation can become feedback to the program development.

If the program planners were enthusiastic, energetic, and perhaps overly ambitious, the list of impact objectives may have become extensive. The program evaluators then face choosing between measuring everything on the laundry list or selecting key impact objectives for measurement. Attempting to measure many impacts is another form of going on a fishing expedition. Remember that just by chance alone, there is a 5% probability that something will be statistically significant (if the p value is .05). Therefore, evaluators are wise to work with program planners and stakeholders to narrow the field from all possible impacts to only those impacts about which having information is critical. Also, just because something can be evaluated does not mean it is worth evaluating; don't evaluate the obvious (Patton, 1998). For example, there is no benefit to evaluating the antibody status of children who attended an immunization clinic and received the recommended pediatric vaccines.

For programs with multiple intervention components and multiple health impacts, at least one health impact per program component needs to be measured. Thus, it may be difficult to have a short list of dependent variables, especially if different outcomes are expected for each component. The intervention theory related to that component will help identify variables that are key or common across program components or are central to achieving over-all program success. Those dependent impact variables need to be measured.

The decision as to who is included in the evaluation is derived from the "among [target population]" portion of the community health statement and the "who" in the impact objectives. The delineation of "who" leads to consideration of the sample and to the appropriate sampling frame given who is thought to be affected by the program. At a minimum, the "who" includes program recipients who are assessed for degree of program impact. However, if the health program has the potential to reach and affect an audience beyond known recipients, as might happen with an educational campaign, then the issue of who to assess becomes more complex. The decision also leads to considering the use of a comparison group that did not receive the program. Deciding who ought to be in the comparison group is discussed in detail with regard to sampling in the next chapter.

Determinants as Independent Variables

A temptation is to include in the evaluation measures of various antecedent, determinant, and contributing factors to the health problem. Because the list of these can be extensive, decisions need to be made as to which factors are crucial in explaining the health impacts of the program. For impact documentation, these need not be measured; only the impacts as stated in the objectives are measured. But for impact assessment and especially for impact evaluation, measuring key antecedents, determinants, and contributing factors will be important. The program effect theory can help identify the specific variables in each category that will be important to measure. Specifically, the determinant factors become a set of independent variables that ought to vary with having received the intervention. This may seem like they are dependent variables, but they are independent relative to the health impact that is the true dependent variable. Whether the independent variables will be measured before and after the program or in the participants and control group is a design decision that is made based on available resources and the level of scientific rigor needed in the evaluation.

Determinants, as the key independent variables, are the first to be considered for measurement. Having data on the presence and strength of the determinants of the health problem can provide extremely useful information that helps evaluators understand how the intervention effect was manifested. For example, descriptive data on determinant factors can reveal patterns of intervention effects among different groups of participants and whether the interventions were mismatched to determinants found among the actual program participants.

Contributing and Antecedent Factors as Variables

Other factors can influence the effectiveness of interventions, such as moderating and mediating variables. A moderating variable is a variable that affects the strength or direction of the relationship between two other variables, whereas a mediating variable, sometimes called an intervening variable, is a variable that is necessary for the relationship between two other variables to exist (Donaldson, 2001). The difference among these types of variables is based on their role in the relationship between the independent and dependent variables (Donaldson, 2001). An analogy helps explain the difference between moderating and mediating variables. Suppose that there is only one road between the cities of Xanadu and Yessler, and that road goes through Medina. Medina is the mediating variable. The drive from Xanadu to Medina is affected by the condition of the road, and the drive from Medina to Yessler is affected by weather conditions. Both road conditions and weather are moderating variables in getting between the cities, and especially in getting safely to the dependent variable, Yessler. In evaluations of health programs, the logic model is likely to identify antecedents and contributing factors in terms of being moderators, and it is likely to identify the determinants as the mediator variable between the intervention and the health impact. Exhibit 9.5 shows the role of each of these variables. A change in the contributing and determinant factors can be viewed as support for the determinant or impact theory. But what is critical to the program evaluation is that the intervention theory is correct—in other words, that the interventions actually lead to the desired change in the determinants of the health problem.

While the effect theory used throughout this text as an example is comparatively simple, the reality is that antecedent and contributing factors, as well as determinants, can play complex roles in achieving the desired health impact. The value in distinguishing whether a factor functions as a moderating or mediating variable comes in deciding whether it is important to measure and, especially later, in data analysis and interpretation. The importance of identifying and including moderators and mediators in evaluations is stressed by Bauman, Sallis, Dzewaltowski, and Owen (2002), who were focused on understanding influences on the success of physical activity interventions. In an evaluation comparing two interventions to reduce alcohol consumption, Maisto et al. (2001) found that readiness for change had a moderating effect on the relationship between one of the interventions studied and alcohol consumption. Their study is an example of how having information on moderating and mediating variables provides more specific information about program effectiveness.

MEASUREMENT CONSIDERATIONS

When planning the effect evaluation, there are numerous qualities of the measures, the data collection, and the data that must be considered when designing the evaluation. These considerations are essentially research issues, but are discussed in the following sections as they relate to evaluating the effects of health programs.

Units of Observation

The unit that is observed or measured in the evaluation must match the level of the program. Suppose that a program is designed to reduce family violence through an intervention that involves the entire family. If the evaluation needs to assess the degree of change within the family, the questionnaire must be given to family members and must ask questions about the family members. If the questionnaire is given to only one individual within the family and asks questions about that individual's perceptions or behaviors, there is a mis-

---

Exhibit 9.5   Example of Possible Roles of Moderating and Mediating Variables in the Effect Theory

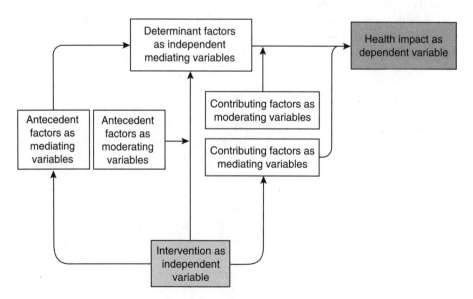

Exhibit 9.6   Advantages and Disadvantages of Using Each Type of Variable

Type	Examples	Advantage	Disadvantage
Nominal, categorical	Zip code, race, yes/no	Easy to understand	Limited information from the data
Ordinal, rank	Social class, Lickert scale, "top ten" list (worst to best)	Gives considerable information, can collapse into nominal	Sometimes statistically treated as a continuous variable, sometimes not
Interval, ratio: continuous	Temperature, IQ, distances, dollars, inches, dates of birth	Gives most information; can collapse into nominal or ordinal categories. Used as a continuous variable	Can be difficult to construct a valid and reliable interval variable

match between the level at which the intervention is targeted (the family) and the unit for which evaluation data are collected (the individual). The same rationale applies to evaluating community or neighborhood level interventions (Best, Brown, Cameron, Smith, & MacDonald, 1989).

Types of Variables (Levels of Measurement)

Another factor to consider is what type of variable to use in the evaluation, meaning how complex the information gathered by each variable is. Variables are classified according to the level of complexity of information, and each has advantages and disadvantages (Exhibit 9.6). Nominal variables are simplest, in that the information indicates only yes/no, absent/present, or a name. Nominal variables that only give yes/no types of information are also called dichotomous or categorical. Ordinal variables provide slightly more information by indicating an order, a sequence, or a rank. The most common ordinal variables are generated from a Lickert scale, such as good, fair, and poor. The most complex, rich, and complete information is provided by interval variables, in which the intervals between the values are equal. Generally, interval variables are continuous, with no practical starting or ending points to the values, like the number of miles across the universe. However, some interval variables do have limits, like the number of miles between the moon and planet Earth; these are considered discrete interval variables. In terms of statistical tests, whether a variable is an interval variable is less important than whether zero can be a starting point. In health care the issue of having a starting point, or zero value, is often quite relevant and can affect the subsequent statistical analysis. For example, the number of days that a patient is hospitalized is an interval variable with a valid zero value as the starting point for the variable.

For each domain of health and well-being, variables can be constructed at each of the three levels (Exhibit 9.7). Careful attention to the level of the measurement is crucial for several reasons. One is that the measurement level directly relates to the statistical tests that can be used with that level of measurement (as will be further discussed in Chapter 11). Basically, a higher level of measurement (interval or ratio) enables the use of a greater variety of statistics. Another reason to consider the level of measurement is that the level of measurement used needs to provide clinically meaningful information. In addition, the level of measurement must be sufficiently sensitive so that a distinction can be found among participants with regard to program effects (Green & Lewis, 1986).

Timing

The timing of the evaluation is guided by the "by when" portion of the impact objectives. The "by when" ought to have been determined based on the intervention theory and the determinant theory, which indicate the duration of the intervention effects and the amount of time needed to achieve a noticeable effect. It thus provides guidance as to (1) the earliest time at which an intervention effect ought to be found, (2) when the maximum intervention effect is expected to occur, and (3) the rate at which change in the health domain is expected to occur. All of this information is used in choosing methods, specifically with regard to when to collect data. However, the impact objectives, because they are about the program participants, do not take into account programmatic timing. For example, if a program has cycles, as with a series of classes, then the evaluation ought to occur after at least one group has received the full intervention. For this type of information, the process objectives need to be reviewed, along with the findings from the process evaluation, because at a minimum, the impact evaluation ought to be done after the program is sufficiently well implemented. An additional consideration with regard to the question of "when" is whether baseline or preintervention

Exhibit 9.7 Examples of Nominal, Ordinal, and Continuous Variables for Different Impact Domains

Impact/ Outcome (DV)	Nominal/ Categorical	Ordinal	Interval/Ratio (Continuous)
Physiological Impact Domain			
Childhood immunization	Yes/no up to date	None required, one immunization required, more than one required	Rubella titer
Physical abuse	Yes/no have experienced physical abuse; type of abuse	Level of abuse is same, more or less than last month	Rate of physical abuse in a county; number of times abused in past six months
Workplace injury	ICD-9 for injury	Level of severity of injury	Number of disability days per year in construction industry
Knowledge Impact Domain			
Understand how alcohol affects judgment	Agree/disagree	Three most common ways alcohol affects judgment	Score on test of knowledge about effects of alcohol
Behavioral Impact Domain			
Breastfeeding	Yes/no breast-fed	Category for how long breast-fed: 2 weeks, 3 to 6 weeks, more than 6 weeks	Number of days breast-fed
Smoking	Yes/no smoke	Number of cigarettes smoked per day	Nicotine levels
Readiness of change	Yes/no likely to change next week	Stage of change in terms of readiness	How likely (on 100-point scale) will change in next week

Exhibit 9.7   Examples of Nominal, Ordinal, and Continuous Variables for Different Impact Domains *(continued)*

Cognitive Process Impact Domain			
Legally competent	Yes/no; DSM IV code for mental illness	Level of mental incapacity	Score on standardized competency questionnaire
Mental Health Impact Domain			
Depression	Above/below clinical cut-off on score for depression	Rank of depression on list of prevalence of mental health problems	Score on standardized depression assessment scale, such as CES-D or Beck Depression Scale
Social Health Impact Domain			
Social support network	Yes/no have friends	Number of people in social support network	Degree of support from those in social support network
Resources Impact Domain			
Housing situation	Homeless or not	Housing autonomy (own, rent monthly, rent weekly, homeless)	Number of days have been living at current residence

data are needed as part of the evaluation plan. If baseline data are needed, then decisions will center around how far in advance of receiving the program it is reasonable and feasible to collect data.

Sensitivity of Measures

An interplay exists between the nature of the factor being measured and the measure itself. Of concern is that the measure is sensitive to variations and fluctuations in the factor such that minor changes can be detected. Measure sensitivity is the extent to which the difference among or within individuals can be detected. Fluctuations can be due to individual variations, changes over time, or the influence of other factors. The measure used to collect data on the factor thus needs to be carefully chosen. For many measures used in health care and health programs, publications exist describing evaluations or research on the measure or that used the measure. Such reports provide clues as to which measures will be sensitive enough to meet the needs of the evaluation.

The following examples illustrate this point. If one impact objective of the health program is to reduce anemia in pregnant women, then some blood samples are used to determine anemia. Different tests can be used; for example, if the program is focused on overall anemia, hematocrit is sufficient but will not be sensitive to underlying causes. If the program is focused on a specific cause of anemia, a more elaborate test is needed. The issue of sensitivity of the measure is one that has led to the development of almost innumerable measures, some of which have been compiled in books, such as Cohen, Underwood, and Gottlieb's (2000) compilation of social support measures or Bowling's (1997) review of quality-of-life measurement scales.

THREATS TO DATA QUALITY

No matter how good the planning or how much effort is put into having the best possible data, some problems are guaranteed to exist that will affect the overall quality of the data available for analysis. These problems include missing data, concerns about the reliability of the data, and issues involving the validity of the measures used.

Missing Data

A very common problem is missing data. Data can be missing on single items in a survey, or variables can be missing in existing records. It will be important to look at possible reasons for the missing data: was it a sensitive question, was the page skipped, was there no response category to capture a possible valid response, was the answer not known to the participant? If data are missing in a haphazard pattern, rather than in a systematic pattern, the occasionally missed item will not dramatically affect the analysis and subsequent findings. However, if there is a systematic pattern to the missing data, decisions will need to be made regarding the analysis plan. Systematic skips or extensive missing data will have a consistent effect on the results of analyses that include that item or variable. Once the data have been collected, it is highly unlikely that any missing data can be retrieved. Being proactive about training data collectors, surveyors, and data abstractors, as well as making the measurement tools as fail-safe as possible, are the best ways to minimize missing data.

Reliability Concerns

A threat to data quality is the reliability of the data. Reliability refers to the extent to which the data is free of errors. There are several sources of errors in data that diminish its reliability. One is the instrument, tool, measure, or test used to collect the data. Other factors also can lower the instrument's reliability, such as questions that are not age appropriate when children are the respondents (Hennessy, 1999). The reliability of the instrument can be statistically assessed as the alpha coefficient or the half-split coefficient (Pedhazar & Schmelkin, 1991), which can be readily performed using statistical packages and spreadsheets (Black, 1999). The extent to which the instrument consistently measures what was intended can be affected by the wording of the questions.

Another source of data error is the person providing the data—in other words, the test taker. An individual may vary from day to day on responses, mood, knowledge, or physiological parameters. The reliability of the instrument, regardless of such influences, can also be statistically tested using the test-retest approach, in which the same group of individuals takes the questionnaire twice. Higher correlations between those two scores indicate that the instrument was constructed so that the data collected are not affected by minor fluctuations within individuals.

An instrument also can be affected by differences across individuals. In such cases, the degree to which the individuals agree is assessed with the inter-rater agreement, sometimes referred to as the inter-observer agreement. It is particularly important to establish high inter-rater agreement, meaning between individuals, when abstracting data from medical or other records. Interpretations of what is being abstracted and what needs to be abstracted can vary across individuals without specific training. Having a high degree of inter-rater agreement increases the confidence that the data collected across abstractors is highly comparable. The simplest approach to calculating inter-rater agreement is a percent agreement, using, as the denominator, the number of items to be coded and, as the numerator, the number of items for which both had "correct" agreement. Alternatively, a statistical approach is to calculate the Kappa statistic (Cohen, 1960), which is a measure of agreement that takes into account not only the observed agreements but also the expected agreements. Kappa can be calculated using statistical software packages, such as SAS.

Another aspect of reliability is the quality of data-entry into the statistical software. Data need to be reliably entered. The problem of low-data entry reliability can be minimized greatly by training those doing the data entry, as well as by performing data-entry verification. Select a portion of the data to be double entered by a second data-entry person, and keep track of the percentage of data entered for which there was a discrepancy. At least a 95% accuracy rate is need-ed. On one research project that involved a large survey, female inmates from the state prison entered the survey data into a database. Being skeptical, the researchers performed data verification on 10% of the surveys. Their data-entry accuracy rate was 99.8%, which was above the minimum 95% accuracy rate.

Validity of Measures

Validity of measures is the degree to which the tool captures what it pur-ports to measure—in other words, the extent to which the tool measures what it is intended to measure. Note that the validity of measures is different from validity resulting from the study design, which is concerned with being able to say that the results generally apply to the population (generalizability of find-ings). A measure is valid if it truly measures the concept. Establishing the validity of a measure through advanced statistical analyses is more properly a research activity rather than an evaluation activity. However, validity can be more informally established as face validity. Face validity, in the simplest pro-cedure, involves asking a panel of experts whether the questions appear or seem to be measuring the concept. If the panel agrees, face validity has been established. Because face validity can be relatively straightforward, stake-holders and program staff can be involved and can help establish it.

Time and resources used to establish face validity can be saved if exist-ing instruments and questions are selected. Several books are available that specifically review the validity and reliability of heath-related instruments (cf. Bowling, 1997). Other sources for locating existing instruments include the published literature. Researchers who have developed instruments for specific constructs often publish information about the instruments in sci-entific journals. Another source is electronic databases of instruments, typi-cally available through major universities. The Health and Psychological Instruments database contains published articles using health and psycho-logical instruments, thus facilitating the search for an instrument applicable to a specific variable.

DATA SOURCES (METHODS)

Methods are the techniques used to collect data, whereas design is the overall plan or strategy for when and from whom data are collected. Design is discussed in the next chapter. Methods generally fall into primary data collec-tion, or the generation of new data, and secondary data collection, or the use of existing data. The evaluation method needs to be consistent with the purpose of the evaluation and the specific evaluation question (Stead, Hastings, & Eadie, 2002). The following discussion of methods and data sources focuses on the collection of both primary and secondary quantitative data. Methods to collect qualitative data are sufficiently different to warrant discussion in a separate chapter. The most common method of collecting primary data is through surveys and questionnaires. For each health and well-being domain, various sources of data can be used to generate information (Exhibit 9.8).

Surveys and Questionnaires

A survey is a method that specifies how and from whom data are collected, whereas a questionnaire is a tool for data collection. Typically surveys use questionnaires; for example, the United States census is a survey that uses a questionnaire to collect data. In most cases, residents complete the pen and paper questionnaire. However, in some instances, a census taker completes the questionnaire while talking with the individual. Although the distinction between survey and questionnaire is important for the sake of clear thinking, generally the word "survey" implies the use of a questionnaire.

Considerations for Constructing Questionnaires

Much has been written about ways to construct health questionnaires (e.g., Aday, 1991; Krosnick, 1999; Streiner & Norman, 1989), how to write individual questions on the questionnaire (Aday, 1991), and techniques to have sets of questions form a scale (Pedhazar & Schmelkin, 1991). Several key points can be drawn from these resources that are paramount to developing a good health program evaluation.

To the extent possible, use existing questionnaire items and valid and reliable scales, to avoid spending resources to reinvent the wheel. Examples of existing items include the US Census Bureau's race/ethnicity categories. These categories can be used instead of creating new ones. An advantage of using existing items is having some assurance that the items are understandable. Existing scales also can be used, with the possibility of later comparing evaluation participants with those on which the scale was previously used. However, if the target audience has a unique characteristic—say, a specific medical diagnosis—that is relevant to understanding the effect of the program, then comparison to existing scales may not be the optimal choice.

Instruments also need to be appropriate for diverse ethnicities and possibly multiple languages. In terms of instruments, cultural sensitivity has two dimensions: the surface structure, which consists of the superficial characteristics, and the deep structure, which consists of core values and meanings. Just as

Exhibit 9.8   Example of Data Sources for Each Health and Well-Being Domain

Health Domain	*Method*: Examples of Sources of Data
Physical health	Survey data: self-report Secondary data: medical records for medical diagnoses Physical data: scale for weight, laboratory tests Observation: response to physical activity
Knowledge	Survey data: self-report, standardized tests Secondary data: school records Physical data: not applicable Observation: performance of task
Lifestyle behavior	Survey data: self-report Secondary data: police records Physical data: laboratory tests related to behaviors, such as nicotine or cocaine blood levels Observation: behaviors in natural settings
Cognitive processes	Survey data: self-report, standardized tests of cognitive development and problem solving Secondary data: school records Physical data: imaging of brain activity Observation: problem-solving tasks, narrative
Mental health	Survey data: self-report motivation, values, attitudes Secondary data: medical records diagnostic category Physical data: self-inflicted wounds, lab values Observation: emotional bonding
Social health	Survey data: self-report, social network questionnaires, report of others Secondary data: attendance records of recreational activities Physical data: not applicable Observation: interpersonal interactions
Resources	Survey data: self-report Secondary data: employer records, county marriage records, school records Physical data: address Observation: possessions

these are taken into account when the health program is developed (Resnicow, Baronowski, Ahuwalia, & Braithwaite, 1999), they also influence the construction of survey questionnaires (Ferketich, Phillips, & Verran, 1993).

One type of scale that is likely to be discussed with regard to evaluating health programs is the use of client goals developed by staff and to be achieved by the client as a result of being in the program. MacKay, Somerville, and Lundie (1996) reported that this evaluation technique has been used since 1968. Staff of such programs may be inclined to count the number of client goals attained as an indicator of program success. The temptation is to consider this as impact data that are very readily available. However, this crude measure of client impact is highly problematic from an evaluation perspective. The main problem is that unless the goals are highly standardized for specific health problems, there can be great variability in the goals that are set. Similarly, unless there are strict criteria for determining whether a client goal was reached, biases among program staff may influence client assessments. The use of goal attainment scaling, in which a Lickert scale around each goal is used, still poses serious problems (MacKay et al., 1996), and therefore its use ought to be seriously curtailed.

To assess the readability, ease of completing, and overall appeal of the questionnaire, a pretest or pilot test is advised. Involvement of stakeholders in this activity is encouraged because it helps the evaluators have a better questionnaire to give to the target audience, and it helps stakeholders anticipate what the evaluation data will include. Key points are to keep the language simple, use an easy-to-follow format and layout, and break down complex concepts into more easily understood ideas. Even if evaluation participants are expected to be well-educated, people are more likely to complete questionnaires that are easily and quickly read.

Verify that what is in the questionnaire corresponds to the program impact objectives. There is an inclination to add just a few more questions because the opportunity exists, or because it might be interesting to know. A shorter questionnaire is better and more likely to be completed. A good rationale for going beyond the program objectives in what is collected is if those data are going to be used for subsequent program planning or for refinement of the current program.

Regardless of the care taken to construct a questionnaire, anything that can be misinterpreted or be done wrong will be done. For example, questionnaires that are copied back to back on single pages that are stapled together are guaranteed to have skipped pages. Unless the questionnaire is done by an interviewer who is well-trained, do not use "skip patterns" that direct respondents to skip questions based on a previous response. These quickly become confusing, and the well-intentioned respondent will answer all questions, including the items that ought to have been skipped. Thus, the use of skip patterns is really appropriate only for questionnaires used with interviewing.

Survey Considerations

A survey, whether done in person or via mail or e-mail, needs careful planning. The process by which the questionnaire is distributed and returned to the evaluator must be thoroughly planned in order to minimize nonresponse and nonparticipation. That process is as critical as the quality of the questionnaire to the success of the evaluation. One technique for having a well-crafted survey plan is to imagine and role-play each step in the process, and to follow the paper from hand to hand. Increasingly, collection of questionnaire data is done electronically, whether via agency computers, hand-held devices used in the field, Internet-based surveys, or client-accessed computers. The same advice about the need to have a carefully crafted data collection plan applies to the use of electronic data collection: follow the answers from the asker to the responder through data-entry to computer output. Each of these steps is needed to be able to accurately and feasibly collect the data.

Nonresponse. Even with a detailed and well-constructed survey design, there will be evaluation participants who do not provide data for any number of reasons. Efforts must be made to minimize nonresponse and increase the response rate. A basic response rate is calculated as the number of usable surveys divided by the number distributed, multiplied by 100; this yields a percentage response. This same formula can be used with slightly different numerators and denominators to provide more detailed information about response rates for different groups in the evaluation. Response rates typically range from a high of 80%, which is achieved with considerable effort and expense, to a low of less than 30% for a mail survey with minimal incentive provided. A low response rate, less than 50%, is important for two reasons. One reason is that those who reply may not be like those who do not reply, thus biasing the sample with subsequent consequences on the data and findings. The other reason is that it is costly to try to achieve the desired sample size by continually needing to identify and obtain data from "replacements."

Nonresponse may be due to attrition, meaning that program participants or control subjects are no longer in the evaluation or the program. Attrition may occur because participants no longer fit the criteria for being in the program or the evaluation, are lost to follow-up, have died, or decline or refuse to continue. Attrition is a normal part of the evaluation process, and the sample size must be based on the expected loss of 10% to 40% of participants. Attrition is particularly crucial for impact assessment and impact evaluation designs, because it affects the final sample size and can affect the balance of participants and nonparticipants sought through a carefully constructed sampling method.

The most obvious approach to minimizing nonresponse of evaluation participants is to make the provision of data by participants as easy and pleasant as possible. The realistic approach is to provide monetary incentives for participating in the evaluation. Although many individuals participate in research for humanitarian reasons (such as contributing to making life better for others), there is also a culture among program participants of "pay me to participate." Even those who participate in the evaluation of television programs by providing data for the Neilson ratings are given a monetary incentive to keep a record of their TV viewing during the two weeks of sweeps. Thus, it is likely that participants in evaluations of health programs will expect some monetary incentive. An extensive body of literature exists on the use of incentives in research (Huby & Hughes, 2001) and the monetary amounts that are most effective in increasing the response rate. This knowledge needs to be used along with common sense and a working understanding of the community standard for incentives for a comparable request of participants.

Designing the monetary incentive must take into account both the total amount and the payment schedule. The amount must not be so great that it would be perceived as coercive, nor so small as to not be an incentive. The payment schedule for providing evaluation data needs to be congruent with the frequency with which participants are asked to provide data. The rule of thumb is that incentives ought to be provided at each data collection point. Consider an evaluation of a six-week exercise class for older adults. If class participants are asked to complete a survey before the first class and at the end of the last class, then the incentive could be for the same amount at the time the surveys are returned. However, if the participants are asked to undergo physical testing before the class, then the incentive may need to be larger for that more extensive request or burden on the participant. If the evaluation is longitudinal, with data collection at six months and one year after the classes have ended, a slightly larger incentive may be needed for those time periods, as a way to keep participants' interest in the evaluation study.

Some individuals selected for the evaluation will be difficult to reach or to convince to participate in the evaluation. Aggressive recruitment efforts may be needed. This would involve multiple attempts to contact the individuals, using different media (telephone and letter) at different times by different voices. The number of attempts made to reach an individual needs to be carefully weighed against the possible appearance of harassing the individual and the extent to which repeated attempts and refusals will affect the quality of the data eventually obtained. In many situations, evaluators, particularly external evaluation consultants, have little or no control over who is in the program and little or no control over who is selected for the evaluation. In such instances, additional efforts are needed to address the program staff as key stakeholders in the evaluation and to train or educate them about recruitment and retention techniques. Actions of program staff with regard to how the evaluation is presented and supported can drastically influence the participation and response rates.

Response Bias. A threat to the quality of questionnaire data, especially self-report data from individuals, is response bias, the intentional or unconscious systematic way in which individuals select responses. The most common type of response bias is in favor of answering questions in accordance with what the individual thinks the interviewer wants to hear. This is called social desirability (Resnicow et al., 2001). But response bias can also occur as a result of the respondent getting into a pattern of just giving the same response, regardless of the question or his or her true opinion or feeling. Response bias can be difficult to detect and to prevent. Nonetheless, evaluators are wise to consider that both response bias and errors inherent in the way the variables are measured can interactively produce questionable or even totally undesirable data (Exhibit 9.9).

Secondary Data

Secondary data are data that have already been collected and are being used for a purpose that is secondary to their original purpose. Some sources of existing data are appropriately used to assess the effect of health programs. Each source of secondary data must be carefully considered with regard to whether the data are needed to answer the evaluation question as well as with regard to their quality.

Vital records, namely birth certificates, death certificates, and disease registries, are a major source of secondary data for health program evaluators. Birth records (Exhibit 9.10) have a wealth of information on prenatal variables, as well as delivery complications and infant characteristics. Birth records are usually not available for up to a year past the date of the birth of the infant. Thus, evaluations of prenatal programs that are designed to affect birth outcomes will not be able to include data from birth records immediately following the program. If the evaluation is longitudinal and focuses on trends, then birth record data may be useful. However, pinpointing the time of the programmatic intervention may be challenging. In addition, for community-based interventions, sampling comparable communities for a comparison of birth data will need to take into account how to select the two communities using the address information on the birth certificates. These same caveats for using birth record data apply to data from death certificates (Exhibit 9.11) or disease registries.

Exhibit 9.9   Interaction of Response Bias and Variable Error

		Variable Error	
		Low	High
Bias	Low	Ideal: high range of honest responses on good measure	Questionable but acceptable data from high range of honest responses on poor measure
	High	Questionable but acceptable data from skewed responses (i.e., toward socially desirable) on good measure	Unusable data due to skewed responses on poor measure

Medical records, case files, or insurance claims may contain information desired for the evaluation. However, data abstraction from these sources entails using a form to record the variables of interest. Several issues must be considered before embarking on data abstraction. First is the quality of the data as recorded and thus available for abstraction. Because the data in records is for clinical rather than evaluation purposes, the information can be inconsistent and vary by the practitioner recording the data. If the evaluator has reason to believe that the data in the record are reliably recorded, he or she must devise a reliable way to abstract the data. This will involve training individual data abstractors. If any interpretation of the recorded information is required, guidelines for what will be recorded and decision rules for interpretation must be understood and applied consistently by the data abstractors. Typically, there ought to be at least 80% agreement between any two abstractors on the coding of data from a single data source.

Another source of secondary data is national surveys, such as the National Health and Nutrition Expenditure Survey or the National Family Planning Survey. These and several other surveys are conducted periodically by various federal agencies with a health focus, including the Occupational Safety and Health Administration (OSHA). These data sets have been used for community assessment. For example, Formisano, Skill, Alexander, and Lippmann (2001) used OSHA's Occupational Exposure database to determine factors contributing to occupational exposures. Data from these surveys are publicly accessible through the Internet, and they can be used to evaluate population-level programs. Some data sets have restrictions or stipulations

Exhibit. 9.10a   Example of a Birth Certificate

U.S. STANDARD CERTIFICATE OF LIVE BIRTH

LOCAL FILE NO.   BIRTH NUMBER:

CHILD

1. CHILD'S NAME (First, Middle, Last, Suffix)		2. TIME OF BIRTH (24hr)	3. SEX	4. DATE OF BIRTH (Mo/Day/Yr)
5. FACILITY NAME (If not institution, give street and number)	6. CITY, TOWN, OR LOCATION OF BIRTH		7. COUNTY OF BIRTH	

MOTHER

8a. MOTHER'S CURRENT LEGAL NAME (First, Middle, Last, Suffix)	8b. DATE OF BIRTH (Mo/Day/Yr)
8c. MOTHER'S NAME PRIOR TO FIRST MARRIAGE (First, Middle, Last, Suffix)	8d. BIRTHPLACE (State, Territory, or Foreign Country)

9a. RESIDENCE OF MOTHER-STATE	9b. COUNTY	9c. CITY, TOWN, OR LOCATION	
9d. STREET AND NUMBER	9e. APT. NO.	9f. ZIP CODE	9g. INSIDE CITY LIMITS? Yes No

FATHER

10a. FATHER'S CURRENT LEGAL NAME (First, Middle, Last, Suffix)	10b. DATE OF BIRTH (Mo/Day/Yr)	10c. BIRTHPLACE (State, Territory, or Foreign Country)

CERTIFIER

11. CERTIFIER'S NAME:	12. DATE CERTIFIED	13. DATE FILED BY REGISTRAR
TITLE: MD DO HOSPITAL ADMIN. CNM/CM OTHER MIDWIFE OTHER (Specify)_____	MM / DD / YYYY	MM / DD / YYYY

INFORMATION FOR ADMINISTRATIVE USE

MOTHER

14. MOTHER'S MAILING ADDRESS: Same as residence, or: State:	City, Town, or Location:	
Street & Number:	Apartment No.:	Zip Code:

15. MOTHER MARRIED? (At birth, conception, or any time between)   Yes   No   16. SOCIAL SECURITY NUMBER REQUESTED FOR CHILD?   Yes   No   17. FACILITY ID. (NPI)

IF NO, HAS PATERNITY ACKNOWLEDGMENT BEEN SIGNED IN THE HOSPITAL?   Yes   No

18. MOTHER'S SOCIAL SECURITY NUMBER: 19. FATHER'S SOCIAL SECURITY NUMBER:

INFORMATION FOR MEDICAL AND HEALTH PURPOSES ONLY

MOTHER

20. MOTHER'S EDUCATION (Check the box that best describes the highest degree or level of school completed at the time of delivery)	21. MOTHER OF HISPANIC ORIGIN? (Check the box that best describes whether the mother is Spanish/Hispanic/Latina. Check the "No" box if mother is not Spanish/Hispanic/Latina)	22. MOTHER'S RACE (Check one or more races to indicate what the mother considers herself to be)
8th grade or less	No, not Spanish/Hispanic/Latina	White
9th - 12th grade, no diploma		Black or African American
	Yes, Mexican, Mexican American, Chicana	American Indian or Alaska Native (Name of the enrolled or principal tribe)_____
High school graduate or GED completed		Asian Indian
	Yes, Puerto Rican	Chinese
Some college credit but no degree		Filipino
	Yes, Cuban	Japanese
Associate degree (e.g., AA, AS)		Korean
		Vietnamese
Bachelor's degree (e.g., BA, AB, BS)	Yes, other Spanish/Hispanic/Latina	Other Asian (Specify)_____
Master's degree (e.g., MA, MS, MEng, MEd, MSW, MBA)	(Specify)_____	Native Hawaiian
		Guamanian or Chamorro
Doctorate (e.g., PhD, EdD) or Professional degree (e.g., MD, DDS, DVM, LLB, JD)		Samoan
		Other Pacific Islander (Specify)_____
		Other (Specify)_____

FATHER

23. FATHER'S EDUCATION (Check the box that best describes the highest degree or level of school completed at the time of delivery)	24. FATHER OF HISPANIC ORIGIN? (Check the box that best describes whether the father is Spanish/Hispanic/Latino. Check the "No" box if mother is not Spanish/Hispanic/Latino)	25. FATHER'S RACE (Check one or more races to indicate what the father considers himself to be)
8th grade or less	No, not Spanish/Hispanic/Latino	White
9th - 12th grade, no diploma		Black or African American
	Yes, Mexican, Mexican American, Chicano	American Indian or Alaska Native (Name of the enrolled or principal tribe)_____
High school graduate or GED completed		Asian Indian
	Yes, Puerto Rican	Chinese
Some college credit but no degree		Filipino
	Yes, Cuban	Japanese
Associate degree (e.g., AA, AS)		Korean
		Vietnamese
Bachelor¡s degree (e.g., BA, AB, BS)	Yes, other Spanish/Hispanic/Latino	Other Asian (Specify)_____
Master¡s degree (e.g., MA, MS, MEng, MEd, MSW, MBA)	(Specify)_____	Native Hawaiian
		Guamanian or Chamorro
Doctorate (e.g., PhD, EdD) or Professional degree (e.g., MD, DDS, DVM, LLB, JD)		Samoan
		Other Pacific Islander (Specify)_____
		Other (Specify)_____

DRAFT 09/18/2001

Mother's Name _____

Mother's Medical Record No. _____

26. PLACE WHERE BIRTH OCCURRED (Check one)	27. ATTENDANT'S NAME, TITLE, AND NPI	28. MOTHER TRANSFERRED FOR MATERNAL MEDICAL OR FETAL INDICATIONS FOR DELIVERY? Yes No
Hospital	NAME: _____ NPI:_____	IF YES, ENTER NAME OF FACILITY MOTHER TRANSFERRED FROM:
Freestanding birthing center		
Home Birth: Planned to deliver at home? Yes No	TITLE: MD DO CNM/CM OTHER MIDWIFE	_____
Clinic/Doctor's office	OTHER (Specify)_____	
Other (Specify)_____		

Exhibit 9.10b Example of a Birth Certificate

MOTHER	29a. DATE OF FIRST PRENATAL CARE VISIT ___/___/_____ M M D D YYYY □ No Prenatal Care	29b. DATE OF LAST PRENATAL CARE VISIT ___/___/_____ M M D D YYYY	30. TOTAL NUMBER OF PRENATAL VISITS FOR THIS PREGNANCY _____ (If none, enter i0".)

	31. MOTHER'S HEIGHT _____ (feet/inches)	32. MOTHER'S PREPREGNANCY WEIGHT _____ (pounds)	33. MOTHER'S WEIGHT AT DELIVERY _____ (pounds)	34. DID MOTHER GET WIC FOOD FOR HERSELF DURING THIS PREGNANCY? Yes No

35. NUMBER OF PREVIOUS LIVE BIRTHS (Do not include this child)	36. NUMBER OF OTHER PREGNANCY OUTCOMES (spontaneous or induced losses or ectopic pregnancies)	37. CIGARETTE SMOKING BEFORE AND DURING PREGNANCY For each time period, enter either the number of cigarettes or the number of packs of cigarettes smoked. IF NONE, ENTER I0". Average number of cigarettes or packs of cigarettes smoked per day.		38. PRINCIPAL SOURCE OF PAYMENT FOR THIS DELIVERY Private Insurance Medicaid

35a. Now Living Number ____ None | 35b. Now Dead Number ____ None | 36a. Other Outcomes Number _____ None

			# of cigarettes	# of packs	Self-pay
		Three Months Before Pregnancy	_____ OR	_____	Other
		First Three Months of Pregnancy	_____ OR	_____	(Specify) _____
		Second Three Months of Pregnancy	_____ OR	_____	
		Last Three Months of Pregnancy	_____ OR	_____	

35c. DATE OF LAST LIVE BIRTH ___/___ MM YYYY	36b. DATE OF LAST OTHER PREGNANCY OUTCOME ___/___ MM YYYY	39. DATE LAST NORMAL MENSES BEGAN ___/___/___ M M D D YYYY	40. MOTHER'S MEDICAL RECORD NUMBER

MEDICAL AND HEALTH INFORMATION	41. RISK FACTORS IN THIS PREGNANCY (Check all that apply)	44. ONSET OF LABOR (Check all that apply)	46. METHOD OF DELIVERY

MEDICAL AND HEALTH INFORMATION

41. RISK FACTORS IN THIS PREGNANCY (Check all that apply)
Diabetes
  Prepregnancy (Diagnosis prior to this pregnancy)
  Gestational (Diagnosis in this pregnancy)
Hypertension
  Prepregnancy (Chronic)
  Gestational (PIH, preeclampsia, eclampsia)
Previous preterm birth

Other previous poor pregnancy outcome (Includes, perinatal death, small-for-gestational age/intrauterine growth restricted birth)

Vaginal bleeding during this pregnancy prior to the onset of labor

Pregnancy resulted from infertility treatment

Mother had a previous cesarean delivery
  If yes, how many _____
None of the above

42. INFECTIONS PRESENT AND/OR TREATED DURING THIS PREGNANCY (Check all that apply)
Gonorrhea
Syphilis
Herpes Simplex Virus (HSV)
Chlamydia
Hepatitis B
Hepatitis C
None of the above

43. OBSTETRIC PROCEDURES (Check all that apply)
Cervical cerclage
Tocolysis
External cephalic version:
  Successful
  Failed
None of the above

44. ONSET OF LABOR (Check all that apply)
Premature Rupture of the Membranes (prolonged, 12 hrs.)
Precipitous Labor (<3 hrs.)
Prolonged Labor (20 hrs.)
None of the above

45. CHARACTERISTICS OF LABOR AND DELIVERY (Check all that apply)
Induction of labor
Augmentation of labor
Non-vertex presentation
Steroids (glucocorticoids) for fetal lung maturation received by the mother prior to delivery
Antibiotics received by the mother during labor
Clinical chorioamnionitis diagnosed during labor or maternal temperature ≥38 C(100.4 F)
Moderate/heavy meconium staining of the amniotic fluid
Fetal intolerance of labor such that one or more of the following actions was taken: in-utero resuscitative measures, further fetal assessment, or operative delivery
Epidural or spinal anesthesia during labor
None of the above

46. METHOD OF DELIVERY
A. Was delivery with forceps attempted but unsuccessful?   Yes   No
B. Was delivery with vacuum extraction attempted but unsuccessful?   Yes   No
C. Fetal presentation at birth
  Cephalic
  Breech
  Other
D. Final route and method of delivery (Check one)
  Vaginal/Spontaneous
  Vaginal/Forceps
  Vaginal/Vacuum
  Cesarean
  If cesarean, was a trial of labor attempted?   Yes   No

47. MATERNAL MORBIDITY (Check all that apply) (Complications associated with labor and delivery)
Maternal transfusion
Third or fourth degree perineal laceration
Ruptured uterus
Unplanned hysterectomy
Admission to intensive care unit
Unplanned operating room procedure following delivery
None of the above

DRAFT 09/18/2001

NEWBORN INFORMATION

NEWBORN	48. NEWBORN MEDICAL RECORD NUMBER:	54. ABNORMAL CONDITIONS OF THE NEWBORN (Check all that apply)	55. CONGENITAL ANOMALIES OF THE NEWBORN (Check all that apply)

48. NEWBORN MEDICAL RECORD NUMBER:

49. BIRTHWEIGHT (grams preferred, specify unit)
  _____ grams ____ lb/oz

50. OBSTETRIC ESTIMATE OF GESTATION:
  _____ (completed weeks)

51. APGAR SCORE:
Score at 5 minutes: _____
If 5 minute score is less than 6,
Score at 10 minutes: _____

52. PLURALITY - Single, Twin, Triplet, etc.
(Specify) _____

53. IF NOT SINGLE BIRTH - Born First, Second, Third, etc. (Specify) _____

54. ABNORMAL CONDITIONS OF THE NEWBORN (Check all that apply)
Assisted ventilation required immediately following delivery
Assisted ventilation required for more than six hours
NICU admission
Newborn given surfactant replacement therapy
Antibiotics received by the newborn for suspected neonatal sepsis
Seizure or serious neurologic dysfunction
Significant birth injury (skeletal fracture(s), peripheral nerve injury, and/or soft tissue/solid organ hemorrhage which requires intervention)
None of the above

55. CONGENITAL ANOMALIES OF THE NEWBORN (Check all that apply)
Anencephaly
Meningomyelocele/Spina bifida
Cyanotic congenital heart disease
Congenital diaphragmatic hernia
Omphalocele
Gastroschisis
Limb reduction defect (excluding congenital amputation and dwarfing syndromes)
Cleft Lip with or without Cleft Palate
Cleft Palate alone
Down Syndrome
  Karyotype confirmed
  Karyotype pending
Suspected chromosomal disorder
  Karyotype confirmed
  Karyotype pending
Hypospadias
None of the anomalies listed above

Mother's Name *Mother's Medical Record No.*

56. WAS INFANT TRANSFERRED WITHIN 24 HOURS OF DELIVERY? Yes No IF YES, NAME OF FACILITY INFANT TRANSFERRED TO: _____	57. IS INFANT LIVING AT TIME OF REPORT? Yes No Infant transferred, status unknown	58. IS INFANT BEING BREASTFED? Yes No

Source: www.cdc.gov/nchs/about/major/dvs/vital_certs_rev.htm.

Exhibit 9.11   United States Standard Death Certificate

DRAFT 11/01/2001

LOCAL FILE NO.   **U.S. STANDARD CERTIFICATE OF DEATH**   STATE FILE NO.

NAME OF DECEDENT
For use by physician or institution

To Be Completed/Verified By: FUNERAL DIRECTOR

1. DECEDENT'S LEGAL NAME (Include AKA's if any) (First, Middle, Last)
2. SEX
3. SOCIAL SECURITY NUMBER

4a. AGE-Last Birthday (Years)
4b. UNDER 1 YEAR — Months / Days
4c. UNDER 1 DAY — Hours / Minutes
5. DATE OF BIRTH (Mo/Day/Yr)
6. BIRTHPLACE (City and State or Foreign Country)

7a. RESIDENCE-STATE
7b. COUNTY
7c. CITY OR TOWN

7d. STREET AND NUMBER
7e. APT. NO.
7f. ZIP CODE
7g. INSIDE CITY LIMITS? ☐ Yes ☐ No

8. EVER IN US ARMED FORCES? ☐ Yes ☐ No
9. MARITAL STATUS AT TIME OF DEATH ☐ Married ☐ Married, but separated ☐ Widowed ☐ Divorced ☐ Never Married ☐ Unknown
10. SURVIVING SPOUSE'S NAME (If wife, give name prior to first marriage)

11. FATHER'S NAME (First, Middle, Last)
12. MOTHER'S NAME PRIOR TO FIRST MARRIAGE (First, Middle, Last)

13a. INFORMANT'S NAME
13b. RELATIONSHIP TO DECEDENT
13c. MAILING ADDRESS (Street and Number, City, State, Zip Code)

14. PLACE OF DEATH (Check only one: see instructions)

IF DEATH OCCURRED IN A HOSPITAL: ☐ Inpatient ☐ Emergency Room/Outpatient ☐ Dead on Arrival
IF DEATH OCCURRED SOMEWHERE OTHER THAN A HOSPITAL: ☐ Hospice facility ☐ Nursing home/Long term care facility ☐ Decedent's home ☐ Other (Specify):

15. FACILITY NAME (If not institution, give street & number)
16. CITY, TOWN, AND ZIP CODE
17. COUNTY OF DEATH

18. METHOD OF DISPOSITION: ☐ Burial ☐ Cremation ☐ Donation ☐ Entombment ☐ Removal from State ☐ Other (Specify):
19. PLACE OF DISPOSITION (Name of cemetery, crematory, other place)

20. LOCATION-CITY, TOWN, AND STATE
21. NAME AND COMPLETE ADDRESS OF FUNERAL FACILITY

22. SIGNATURE OF FUNERAL SERVICE LICENSEE OR OTHER AGENT
23. LICENSE NUMBER (Of Licensee)

To Be Completed By: MEDICAL CERTIFIER

ITEMS 24-28 MUST BE COMPLETED BY PERSON WHO PRONOUNCES OR CERTIFIES DEATH
24. DATE PRONOUNCED DEAD (Mo/Day/Yr)
25. TIME PRONOUNCED DEAD

26. SIGNATURE OF PERSON PRONOUNCING DEATH (Only when applicable)
27. LICENSE NUMBER
28. DATE SIGNED (Mo/Day/Yr)

29. ACTUAL OR PRESUMED DATE OF DEATH (Mo/Day/Yr) (Spell Month)
30. ACTUAL OR PRESUMED TIME OF DEATH
31. WAS MEDICAL EXAMINER OR CORONER CONTACTED? ☐ Yes ☐ No

CAUSE OF DEATH (See instructions and examples)

Approximate interval: Onset to death

32. **PART I.** Enter the chain of events--diseases, injuries, or complications--that directly caused the death. DO NOT enter terminal events such as cardiac arrest, respiratory arrest, or ventricular fibrillation without showing the etiology. DO NOT ABBREVIATE. Enter only one cause on a line. Add additional lines if necessary.

IMMEDIATE CAUSE (Final disease or condition resulting in death) ----→ a._____ Due to (or as a consequence of):

Sequentially list conditions, if any, leading to the cause listed on line a. Enter the UNDERLYING CAUSE (disease or injury that initiated the events resulting in death) LAST

b._____ Due to (or as a consequence of):

c._____ Due to (or as a consequence of):

d._____

PART II. Enter other significant conditions contributing to death but not resulting in the underlying cause given in PART I.
33. WAS AN AUTOPSY PERFORMED? ☐ Yes ☐ No
34. WERE AUTOPSY FINDINGS AVAILABLE TO COMPLETE THE CAUSE OF DEATH? ☐ Yes ☐ No

35. DID TOBACCO USE CONTRIBUTE TO DEATH? ☐ Yes ☐ Probably ☐ No ☐ Unknown

36. IF FEMALE:
☐ Not pregnant within past year
☐ Pregnant at time of death
☐ Not pregnant, but pregnant within 42 days of death
☐ Not pregnant, but pregnant 43 days to 1 year before death
☐ Unknown if pregnant within the past year

37. MANNER OF DEATH
☐ Natural ☐ Homicide
☐ Accident ☐ Pending Investigation
☐ Suicide ☐ Could not be determined

38. DATE OF INJURY (Mo/Day/Yr) (Spell Month)
39. TIME OF INJURY
40. PLACE OF INJURY (e.g., Decedent's home; construction site; restaurant; wooded area)
41. INJURY AT WORK? ☐ Yes ☐ No

42. LOCATION OF INJURY: State: City or Town:
Street & Number: Apartment No.:   Zip Code:

43. DESCRIBE HOW INJURY OCCURRED:
44. IF TRANSPORTATION INJURY, SPECIFY: ☐ Driver/Operator ☐ Passenger ☐ Pedestrian ☐ Other (Specify)

45. CERTIFIER (Check only one):
☐ Certifying physician-To the best of my knowledge, death occurred due to the cause(s) and manner stated.
☐ Pronouncing & Certifying physician-To the best of my knowledge, death occurred at the time, date, and place, and due to the cause(s) and manner stated.
☐ Medical Examiner/Coroner-On the basis of examination, and/or investigation, in my opinion, death occurred at the time, date, and place, and due to the cause(s) and manner stated.

Signature of certifier:

46. NAME, ADDRESS, AND ZIP CODE OF PERSON COMPLETING CAUSE OF DEATH (Item 32)

47. TITLE OF CERTIFIER
48. LICENSE NUMBER
49. DATE CERTIFIED (Mo/Day/Yr)
50. **FOR REGISTRAR ONLY**- DATE FILED (Mo/Day/Yr)

51. DECEDENT'S EDUCATION-Check the box that best describes the highest degree or level of school completed at the time of death.
☐ 8th grade or less
☐ 9th - 12th grade; no diploma
☐ High school graduate or GED completed
☐ Some college credit, but no degree
☐ Associate degree (e.g., AA, AS)
☐ Bachelor's degree (e.g., BA, AB, BS)
☐ Master's degree (e.g., MA, MS, MEng, MEd, MSW, MBA)
☐ Doctorate (e.g., PhD, EdD) or Professional degree (e.g., MD, DDS, DVM, LLB, JD)

52. DECEDENT OF HISPANIC ORIGIN? Check the box that best describes whether the decedent is Spanish/Hispanic/Latino. Check the INol box if decedent is not Spanish/Hispanic/Latino.
☐ No, not Spanish/Hispanic/Latino
☐ Yes, Mexican, Mexican American, Chicano
☐ Yes, Puerto Rican
☐ Yes, Cuban
☐ Yes, other Spanish/Hispanic/Latino (Specify) _____

53. DECEDENT'S RACE (Check one or more races to indicate what the decedent considers himself or herself to be)
☐ White
☐ Black or African American
☐ American Indian or Alaska Native (Name of the enrolled or principal tribe) _____
☐ Asian Indian
☐ Chinese
☐ Filipino
☐ Japanese
☐ Korean
☐ Vietnamese
☐ Other Asian (Specify) _____
☐ Native Hawaiian
☐ Guamanian or Chamorro
☐ Samoan
☐ Other Pacific Islander (Specify) _____
☐ Other (Specify) _____

54. DECEDENT'S USUAL OCCUPATION (Indicate type of work done during most of working life. DO NOT USE RETIRED).

55. KIND OF BUSINESS/INDUSTRY

on their use that must be addressed before they can be used. A drawback to using these surveys is that the most recent data can be two years old. Also, as secondary data sets, they may be of limited value in determining the effect of small-scale programs. However, they may be useful if the impact evaluation is of a population-level health program, such as a state program, and the timing is such that immediate information is not critical. The use of large secondary data sets for the evaluation of programs faces the challenge of overcoming conceptual issues, such as associating variables available in the data set to the program theory and determining the reliability and validity of the data. There are also other pragmatic considerations, such as the selection of subsamples and recoding data (Shepard et al., 1999). In addition, data from some national surveys may not generate results applicable to rural populations (Borders, Roher & Vaughn, 2000), while other data may be at the individual rather than the aggregate level (Best, 1999). Overall, the evaluator needs to be cautious and have a specific rationale for using large secondary data sets for impact evaluation.

Physical Data

Biological samples, anthropomorphic measures, and environmental samples are examples of physical data that may needed to evaluate a health program. Biological samples are items such as blood, urine, or hair; anthropomorphic measures are typically height, weight, and body mass index; and environmental samples range from ozone levels, and bacteria count in water supplies to lead levels in fish. The decision regarding the inclusion of physical data in the evaluation ought to be based on the health programs goal and objectives. The decision regarding the use of physical data ought to consider whether the intervention and determinant theories underlying the health program, are sufficiently well substantiated to justify the cost and effort needed to collect physical data, especially laboratory tests.

As with the collection of other types of data, physical data need to be collected in a consistent manner. Evaluators may not have control over laboratory processing, and hence they need some assurance that the laboratory results are reliable, need to be familiar with the laboratory standards for processing the samples, and must take steps to minimize factors that would lead to erroneous variation in results. Another consideration with regard to physical data, specifically biological data, is the cost involved in collecting, storing, and processing the data. Generally, the use of biological data in an evaluation can be quite costly, and evaluators need to be proactive in budgeting for these expenses.

CONSIDERATIONS DURING PLANNING

Several broad considerations can influence the impact assessment. Each of these considerations comes into play to varying degrees during the impact assessment.

Stakeholders

One consideration is the stakeholders of the program and the need to take into consideration who wants to know what from the impact assessment. Once the key impact evaluation questions have been posed, it is important to also ask stakeholders what they want to know about the program. Involvement of the stakeholders in the development of the impact evaluation has some real payoffs. Not only will they become invested in the findings, but they will be more likely to believe the findings. Neither programs nor stakeholders are not static. Thus, the impact objectives might have been developed by people who are no longer involved with the program. Hence the objectives may not be valued as highly by current stakeholders, nor viewed as relevant given current circumstances. If the ultimate goal of the impact evaluation is its use in future program or policy decisions, stakeholder involvement is imperative. Involvement of stakeholders can also result in an improved impact assessment. For example, involvement of family members as stakeholders in a mental health program led to improved data collection, according to Osher, van Kammen, and Zaro, (2001). Another benefit of stakeholder involvement is that expectations can be addressed; that is, if their expectations are unrealistic given resource limits or methodological constraints, those expectations need to be acknowledged, discussed, and made more realistic.

At the end of the evaluation, the intended users of the evaluation need to be able to judge the utility of the design and know the strengths and weaknesses of the evaluation. The intended users may have different criteria for judging the quality of the evaluation, and so they may need to learn about the methods used. A debate about the possible findings before the evaluation is complete can be helpful to uncover what would and would not be acceptable findings from the perspective of the stakeholders.

Having a long list of variables to be measured may be met with resistance and skepticism by stakeholders, particularly those who advocate for the protection of the participants. This reality reinforces the need for stakeholder involvement in the development of the effect theory and its evaluation. However, there may be circumstances in which it will be important to go beyond the objectives in data collection. For example, the evaluation can be an opportunity to collect information deemed necessary for future program refinement or to update aspects of the community health assessment. The data collected for these purposes are best kept separate, with separate analyses and reporting.

For each element of an evaluation, there are both scientific and programmatic considerations (Exhibit 9.12). These considerations have the potential to influence the ultimate design and implementation of the impact and outcome evaluations. Reviewing these differences and considerations with stakeholders can help establish realistic expectations, as well as identify points on which consensus is needed. Whatever choices are being faced, ultimately the planners will need to be flexible so that the evaluation can adapt to the realities that are encountered (Resnicow et al., 2001).

Budget

Another consideration is the budget, specifically the cost involved in doing the impact assessment and the feasibility of allocating such funds to the impact assessment. This is akin to avoiding the Robin Hood syndrome of robbing from the program implementation to pay for the evaluation. This may occur if the intervention evaluation was not included in the total program budget developed during the planning or implementation stage. A rule of thumb is that evaluation ought to be between 10% and 20% of the program implementation budget. This translates into reducing the dollars for the program by 10% to 20% up front, before the program begins. A budget for the evaluation ought to delineate the costs for evaluation expenses, such as personnel, participant incentives, copying and duplicating data instruments or fees for purchasing data, additional office expenses, statistical software license, data-entry costs, and consultant fees. While it is difficult to set a minimum amount for an evaluation, these expenses can easily exceed $5,000 for a straightforward impact documentation and can reach $50,000 and up for an impact evaluation that involves evaluation research. Once the evaluation budget has been negotiated and established, the logistics focus on staying within that budget.

Ethics

One more consideration is the ethics inherent in conducting impact assessments. Ethical considerations can affect not only the criteria for eligibility as program participants, but also eligibility for evaluation participants and procedures in the evaluation. From the perspective of some health agencies, program eligibility, not just participation in program evaluation, to those in need may be a moral as well as an ethical issue. In other words, the ethics of program eligibility need to be addressed during the program development stage, and those decisions will affect the subsequent ethics concerning who is included in the evaluation.

Recent attention by the federal Office for Human Research Protection (OHRP) on health programs receiving federal funds has led to the need for evaluators to participate in efforts to comply with federal regulations. One area of great concern is obtaining informed consent, as discussed in Chapter 14. The regulations are complex, particularly if one is new to research. Resources that can be used are consultants and the OHRP web site (http://ohrp.osophs.dhhs.gov/polasur.htm).

These caveats and considerations can create circumstances in which an ideal impact assessment is not possible, despite efforts to make it as scientifically rigorous as possible. Recognizing this early in the process and working with it as a limitation is a strength. The solution is to focus on creating not a "perfect" assessment but a "good enough" assessment; good enough impact assessments use the best methodological design given the realities. One reason that a "good enough" impact assessment is acceptable is that intervention effect evaluations are different from research (Exhibit 9.12). The differences between research and evaluation can get blurry for some health program impact assessments, but recognizing the differences can help develop a strong, "good enough" intervention evaluation. Stakeholders may not understand these differences well, and therefore, education about how the evaluation will be different from research can help them have greater trust and confidence in the evaluation. A good enough evaluation needs to have the same characteristics as the criteria discussed earlier for all evaluations—namely, a feasible design that produces credible, believable, and potentially important findings.

Evaluation Standards

The criteria for a good evaluation were established by the American Evaluation Association. Patton (1998) discussed these criteria in terms of four issues. One criterion is the process by which decision making occurs regarding the evaluation. That is, a good evaluation is generated from a decision process that is inclusive and thoughtful. Another criterion is that stakeholders need to be able to believe the evaluation results and the evaluator. The third criterion is that they need to be able to trust the evaluation as being scientifically and ethically conducted and trust the evaluator as a person who will do what is ethical and scientifically sound. The last criterion is that the most feasible and reasonable design must be used, given the constraints and resources of the health program.

Exhibit 9.12 Summary of Evaluation Elements

Elements of Effect Evaluation	Scientific Considerations	Program Considerations
What to evaluate	Impact and outcome variables most likely to demonstrate strength of evidence for effect theory	Highest-priority impact and outcome objectives, variables that meet funding agency requirements
Who to evaluate	Representativeness of sample and comparability to nonparticipants, ethics of assignment to the program or not	Accessibility of program participants, availability of easily accessed target audience members
When to evaluate	Onset and duration of effect	Convenience and accessibility of program participants
Why evaluate	Scientific contributions and generation of knowledge	Program promotion, refinement of program, funding agency requirements
How to evaluate	Maximize rigor through choice of measures and design and analysis	Minimize intrusion of evaluation into program through seamlessness of evaluation with program implementation

ACROSS THE PYRAMID

At the direct services level of the public health pyramid, the evaluation of the impact is the most straightforward, although not necessarily the easiest. It is straightforward in terms of the impact on individuals who receive the service. At this level, it is always individuals who complete questionnaire data, and about whom data are collected via secondary sources. Thus, the major considerations are how to construct the questionnaire and collect secondary data.

At the enabling services level, the same issues apply as those at the direct services level—namely, those of constructing sensitive and valid measures and the reliability of gathering secondary data. In addition, there is the issue of how to identify program participants, given that enabling services are likely to be embedded within other services and programs. At the enabling services level, the unit of observation is more likely to become a point of consideration.

At the population-based services level, the major issue is one of aggregation of data and the unit of observation. The inclination is to say that the population is the unit, but in actuality, it is most often an aggregation of individual-level data. A true population measure would be the GNP or population density. Data cannot be collected from an entire population, except by census. Sampling is paramount, as is developing a plan for construction controls, as is discussed more fully in the next chapter. Some researchers have attempted to use data from existing data sets to develop a single measure of community health, but they caution that more work is needed because such measures fail to explain across a variety of health outcomes (Studnicki, Luther, Kromrey, & Myers, 2001). This hints at the difficulty and challenge of evaluating impacts and outcomes at this level of the pyramid, particularly impact evaluations. Often health programs at the population services level address public knowledge, public opinion, or community outcomes. Stead, Hastings, and Eadie (2002) suggested that for such outcomes, methods ranging from surveys, focus groups, document reviews, and audits could be appropriate, depending on the specific evaluation question.

At the infrastructure level, the evaluation itself is an infrastructure process. But if the program was intended to affect the infrastructure, then impacts are measured as related to the infrastructure. If the skills of public health employees (capacity building) are the program intervention focus, then individual-level data are needed about changes in their skills. However, if the intervention impact of an infrastructure change is at another level of the pyramid—say, physical education to change a specific direct service practice—then the impact is measured as it relates to the other pyramid level. If the program is intended to have an impact at the infrastructure level, a major challenge is to construct measures that are at the infrastructure level. Although Halverson and others from the Centers for Disease Control and Prevention (Corso, Wiesner, Halverson, & Brown, 2000; Halverson, 2000) have been working to develop infrastructure measures, these global assessments of the public health infrastructure may not be useful unless the programmatic intervention has sweeping policy impacts that would be measurable throughout the infrastructure.

DISCUSSION QUESTIONS

1. Develop a working plan for how you would involve stakeholders in the development of the intervention evaluation plan. How does your plan address timing and budget constraints? In what ways does it include attention to interactions and group processes? What strategies will be used to address the four criteria for having a good evaluation question?

2. Select a health program with which you are familiar. Construct a levels of measurement table, similar to Exhibit 9.9, for one impact (dependent) variable in three different health or well-being domains.

3. What are the major problems in using secondary data sources, such as birth or death certificate data? What, if anything, can the evaluator do about these problems?

4. How do the steps in instrument development apply to making surveys cross-culturally appropriate? What effect might you expect in the data and subsequently in the data interpretation if surveys are not culturally appropriate?

References

Aday, L. A. (1991). *Designing and conducting health surveys.* San Francisco: Jossey-Bass.

Bauman, A. E., Sallis, J. F., Dzewaltowski, D. A., Owen, N. (2002). Toward a better understanding of the influences on physical activity: The role of determinants, correlates, causal variables, mediators, moderators, and confounders. *American Journal of Preventive Medicine, 23*(Suppl. 2), 5–14.

Best, A. E. (1999). Secondary data bases and their use in outcomes research: A review of the area resource file and the Healthcare Cost and Utilization Project. *Journal of Medical Systems, 23,* 175–181.

Best, J. A., Brown, K. S., Cameron, R., Smith, E. A., & MacDonald, M. (1989). Conceptualizing outcomes for health promotion programs. In M. T. Braverman (Ed.), *Evaluating health promotion programs* (pp. 19–32). San Francisco: Jossey-Bass.

Black, T. R. (1999). *Doing quantitative research in the social sciences: An integrated approach to research design, measurement and statistics.* London: Sage Publications.

Borders, T. F., Rohrer, J. E., & Vaughn, T. E. (2000). Limitations of secondary data for strategic marketing in rural areas. *Health Services Management Research, 13,* 216–222.

Bowling, A. (1997). *Measuring health: A review of quality of life measurement scales* (2nd ed.). Philadelphia: Open University Press.

Cohen, J. (1960). A coefficient of agreement for nominal scales. *Educational and Psychological Measurement, 20,* 37–46.

Cohen, S., Underwood, L. G., & Gottlieb, B. H. (2000). *Social support measurement and intervention: A guide for health social scientists.* Oxford: Oxford University Press.

Corso, L. C., Wiesner, P. J., Halverson, P. K., & Brown, C. K. (2000). Using the essential services as a foundation for performance measurement: An assessment of local public health systems. *Journal of Public Health Management and Practice, 6*(5), 88–92.

Donaldson, S. I. (2001). Mediator and moderator analysis in program development. In S. Sussman (Ed.), *Handbook of Program Development for Health Behavior and Practice.* Newburg Park, CA: Sage Publications.

Ferketich, S., Phillips, L., & Verran, J. (1993). Focus on psychometrics: Development and administration of a survey instrument for cross-cultural research. *Research in Nursing and Allied Health, 16,* 227–230.

Formisano, J. A., Jr., Skill, K., Alexander, W., & Lippmann, M. (2001). Application of statistical models for secondary data usage of the US Navy's Occupational Exposure Database (NOED). *Applied Occupational and Environmental Hygiene, 16,* 201–209.

Green, L. W., & Lewis, F. M. (1986). *Measurement and evaluation in health education and health promotion.* Palo Alto, CA: Mayfield Publishing.

Halverson, P. K. (2000). Performance measurement and performance standards: Old wine in new bottles. *Journal of Public Health Management and Practice, 6*(5), vi–x.

Hennessy, E. (1999). Children as service evaluators. *Child Psychology and Psychiatric Review, 4,* 153–161.

Huby, M., & Hughes, R. (2001). The effects of data on using material incentives in social research. *Social Work and Social Sciences Review, 9,* 5–16.

Krosnick, J. A. (1999). Survey research. *Annual Review of Psychology, 50,* 537–567.

MacKay, G., Somerville, W., & Lundie, J. (1996). Reflections on goal attainment scaling (GAS): Cautionary notes and proposals for development. *Educational Research, 38,* 161–172.

Maisto, S. A., Conigliaro, J., McNeil, M., Kraemer, K., Conigliaro, R. L., & Kelley, M. E. (2001). Effects of two types of brief intervention and readiness to change on alcohol use in hazardous drinkers. *Journal of Studies on Alcohol, 62,* 605–614.

Osher, T. W., van Kammen, W., & Zaro, S. M. (2001). Family participation in evaluating systems of care: Family, research, and service system perspectives. *Journal of Emotional and Behavioral Disorders, 9,* 63–70.

Patton, M. (1978). *Utilization evaluation.* Beverly Hills, CA: Sage Publications.

Patton, M. (1998). *Utilization focused evaluation.* Newberry Park, CA: Sage Publications.

Pedhazar, E. J., & Schmelkin, L. P. (1991). *Measurement, design, and analysis: An integrated approach.* Hillsdale, NJ: Lawrence Erlabum Associates.

Resnicow, K., Baronowski, T., Ahuwalia, J. S., & Braithwaite, R. L. (1999). Cultural sensitivity in public health: Defined and demystified. *Ethnicity and Disease, 9,* 10–21.

Resnicow, K., Braithwaite, R., Diloria, C., Vaughn, R., Cohen, M. I., & Uhl, G. (2001). Preventing substance abuse in high risk youth: Evaluation challenges and solutions. *Journal of Primary Prevention, 21,* 399–415.

Shepard, M. P., Carroll, R. M., Mahon, M. M., Moriarty, H. J., Feetham, S. L., Dedrick, J. A., & Orsi, A. J. (1999). Conceptual and pragmatic considerations in conducting a secondary analysis: An example from research of families. *Western Journal of Nursing Research, 21,* 154–167.

Stead, M., Hastings, G., & Eadie, D. (2002). The challenge of evaluating complex interventions: A framework for evaluating media advocacy. *Health Education Research, 17*, 351–364.

Streiner, D. L., & Norman, G. R. (1989). *Health measurement scales: A practical guide to their development and use.* Oxford: Oxford University Press.

Studnicki, J., Luther, S. L., Kromrey, J., & Myers, B. (2001). A minimum data set and empirical model for population health status assessment. *American Journal of Preventive Medicine, 20*, 40–49.

CHAPTER 10

Choosing Designs for Impact Evaluation

Of the many factors contributing to the scientific rigor of an impact evaluation, design and sampling are key. In a health program evaluation, evaluators, as compared to researchers, may not have the same degree of control over sample construction, timing of data collection, or amount of exposure to the intervention. Such constraints and realities contribute to impact evaluations being different from pure research. Much of the evaluation literature discusses design from a research perspective and is geared toward maximizing the scientific rigor of the evaluation. While this is needed and appropriate if there is sufficient funding, most small health programs will not have such resources. Most agencies are more focused on and have expertise related to providing or delivering the health program. Personnel in such programs understandably can become lost, confused, and overwhelmed when faced with designing an evaluation. Therefore, this chapter is devoted to discussing designs and sampling from the perspective of evaluators and program managers who must address issues posed by program realities.

Underlying the discussion in this chapter are several assumptions. One is that regardless of the program or agency, there is a design that is both scientifically the best option and realistically feasible for the program. Another assumption is that program personnel would choose the best scientific option if it was clear and easy to identify. Thus, designs and sampling strategies are covered with respect to their feasibility for small, local, direct services programs as well as large-scale population-based programs. There is one other assumption: that there is a programmatic need to demonstrate that the participants have changed more than might happen by chance. This assumption means that merely collecting data on whether the impact objectives were met is not sufficient to meet the needs of stakeholders, including funders. Choosing the right design becomes critical in showing that changes to participants were not by chance or that one intervention is more effective than another.

The design of the evaluation consists of the grand scheme of when and from whom data are collected. There are many types of designs, such as experimental, quasi-experimental, and epidemiological. Qualitative designs, another type of design, are reviewed in Chapter 12. The methods used in the evaluation indicate the way in which the data are collected and typically involve strategies such as surveys, interviews, or observations. Designs can be very simple or extraordinarily complex. Most research textbooks cover designs and methods in considerable depth from a research perspective in which the researcher has a great deal of control over factors affecting the choice of a design. However, impact evaluations of health programs face circumstances that complicate the choice of a design.

CHOOSING AN EVALUATION DESIGN

Before we begin, a word about terminology is in order. Health program evaluation can be done from the perspective of a number of different disciplines, each with its own terminology for describing design (Exhibit 10.1). The social sciences typically focus on individuals and use experimental and quasi-experimental language to describe the major classification of designs. Health education mostly uses social science terminology for designs. Epidemiology is another discipline from which to drawn upon when developing the evaluation plan, particularly when program recipients or target audiences are populations. Historically, epidemiology designs have been classified into observational and intervention designs, as will be discussed later in this chapter. A third discipline that is relevant to the evaluation of health programs is health services research, which uses terminology drawn heavily from economics and social sciences. A given design for evaluating a health program can draw upon the strengths of each of these disciplines and can adapt the evaluation question, the design terminology, and the actual design to fit the purpose of the evaluation.

Throughout this chapter, the terminology used is a blend of social sciences and epidemiology, but because epidemiological designs have only recently been applied to the evaluation of health programs (Handler, 2002; Rosenberg & Handler, 1998), specific attention is given to understanding and applying those designs. In addition, this chapter uses the terms "pre-test" and "post-test," adopted from social sciences. When we apply these terms to health programs, two points are worth stressing. First, "pre" and "post" refer to the sequence of when data are collected; "pre" is anytime before receiving the program intervention, and "post" is anytime after receiving the program intervention. The precise timing of data collection depends, of course, not only on logistical

Exhibit 10.1   Contribution of Disciplines to Health Program Evaluation

Discipline	Typical Impact or Outcome Question	Typical Design Terminology
Social sciences	Are outcomes for individuals in the program (recipients) different from those in the comparison or control group (nonrecipients)?	Experimental, quasi-experimental
Epidemiology	Are cases (individuals who have the impact characteristic) less likely to have had exposure to the program than controls (individuals without the impact characteristic)?	Observational
Health services research	Does differential utilization of services (participation or not) by enrollees (target audience) and nonenrollees (nontarget audience) lead to differential outcomes?	Experimental, quasi-experimental, clinical trial

Adapted from Handler (2002) with permission.

issues but, more importantly, on the expected timing of the first program effects and the duration of those effects as articulated in the program effect theory. The timing of the pre-test and post-test data collection also ought to have been specified in the "by when" element of the impact objectives. Second, "test" is a convenient, shorthand term that refers to the measures being used to quantify the program effect. In other words, it is equivalent to the measurement of the specific impacts and outcomes. The pre-test can also be called the baseline data, as is more usual in epidemiology and health services.

Considerations in Choosing a Design

One consideration in choosing a design is whether it is important to determine if there is a cause and effect, or causal relationship, between receiving the health program and the outcomes. Some designs are better suited to establishing a causal connection. Another consideration is the need to balance the design with the skill and resources available to the health program personnel. A creative evaluator or evaluation team may devise a complex, scientifically rigorous design that would provide sound evidence for the effectiveness of the program, but unless there are resources for personnel, data collection expenses, consultants, and incentives for participants, the design will not be implemented. Therefore, there will always be an element of the ideal being adapted to reality when conducting impact evaluations. There is a direct relationship between the ability to show causality and the costs and complexity of the design (Exhibit 10.2), such that the costs and complexity increase along with the ability to show causality. Thus, these two factors become the first considerations in choosing a design.

Exhibit 10.2 Types of Design Complexity and Ability to Show Causality

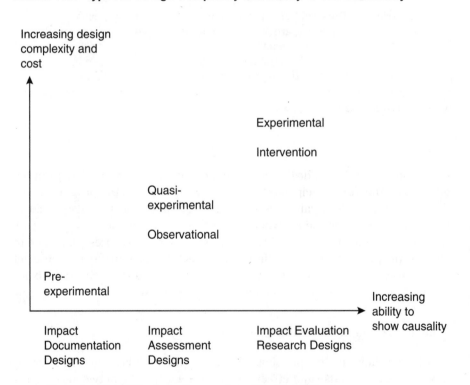

The choice of an evaluation design is also influenced by the need to have a design that is as free of bias as possible given the realities of the evaluation. Bias in design refers to the extent to which the design is flawed and consequently is more likely to lead to an inaccurate conclusion about the effectiveness of the health program. The flaws are categorized based on whether they affect the ability to generalize the findings to other samples (external validity) or whether they affect the ability to say that the intervention made a difference (internal validity) (Campbell & Stanley, 1963). Understanding the flaws that constitute threats to the internal and external validity of each design helps in choosing a design that is as free of bias as possible, given the evaluation question and the circumstances. In general, a design with fewer flaws is more complex and costly and better able to show causality.

There is one other major consideration in the choice of a design: whether data are collected retrospectively or prospectively. Retrospective designs entail gathering data from the point of intervention backward in time. In other words, participants will have received the program before any baseline data are gathered. Prospective designs entail gathering data forward in time, beginning from a point prior to the beginning of the intervention. If the evaluation is planned during the development of the health program, a prospective design is possible. Retrospective designs limit the options for measurement and for the selection of comparison groups, whereas prospective designs require that evaluation resources be obtained prior to the start of the program.

In practice, the process of choosing a design happens simultaneously with the process of identifying participants and nonparticipants in the program. Most research textbooks discuss designs separately from sampling. Because the choice of an evaluation design is influenced by the options for who can be participants and nonparticipants—in other words, sample groups—this chapter discusses designs for evaluation in conjunction with corresponding sample needs, considerations, and related issues.

The aim in choosing a design is to come as close as possible to an ideal design. An ideal design has (1) a comparison group of nonrecipients (called the control or unexposed group) who are as similar as possible to the program recipients (called the experimental or exposed group), (2) measurement of the impact variables before and after the intervention, and (3) minimal threats to internal and external validity. Such ideal designs, while not possible for some health problems (such as birth weight addressed with epidemiological designs), do allow the evaluator to make statements that attribute differences found between the program recipients and nonrecipients to the intervention and only the intervention.

Intervention and Observational Designs

Historically, study designs used to assess health problems and health outcomes have been divided into two groups. One group of designs is intervention studies: designs in which the exposure to the program or intervention is manipulated by the health professional, as typically occurs with health programs delivered to individuals and groups. Manipulation implies that those providing the program have some degree of control over choosing who among those eligible receives the program. Intervention designs are called clinical trials in the fields of epidemiology and clinical medicine and are called experimental designs (with random assignment to groups) or quasi-experimental designs (without random assignment to groups) in the social sciences.

Observational designs, which come from the field of analytic epidemiology (Fos & Fine, 2000), were initially developed for situations in which exposure to the program is not manipulated by the program staff but is more simply observed as it naturally occurs. Observational designs are typically used to study what constitutes environmental or lifestyle risks. The major observational designs are cohort and case-control study designs. Historically, these observational designs were reserved exclusively for examining health risk factors and outcomes. However, as epidemiologists have become more active in health services research and in conducting program evaluations, they have begun to use observational designs to examine the relationship between receiving health programs and health outcomes. When these designs are used for program evaluation, they are no longer purely "observational." The fact that a program was created and delivered, and that an exposure to the program occurred, similar to an exposure to a toxin, amounts to a de facto manipulation of the exposure. Hence, it is no longer purely an observation of the exposure. The manipulation, the delivery of the program, may have occurred at the policy or population level and thus might not have been directly under the full control of the evaluator or program staff, but manipulation has occurred nonetheless. Based on this logic, manipulation of the exposure to the program is no longer used to define the difference between intervention and observational epidemiology designs (Handler, 2002; Rosenberg & Handler, 1998).

Two conditions must exist for the use of observational designs in program evaluation. Obviously, one condition is that an intervention or program has taken place. The other condition is that it is possible to collect data on outcomes only after the delivery of the health program. Related to this condition is that it is impossible to collect baseline data on the same individuals due to the nature of the anticipated impact. Thus, these designs are used when the program impacts and outcomes are health status outcomes, such as low birth weight, adolescent pregnancy, or death, that have no natural baseline value (Handler, 2002; Rosenberg & Handler, 1998). For example, women in a prenatal health education program cannot provide baseline information on the birth weight of the infant in the current pregnancy; the birth weight outcome can occur only "after" the program.

Evaluation questions that ask whether the intervention has had an impact on whether the outcome occurs are best answered by observational designs. Observational designs can be thought of as analogous to post-test only designs in the social science language of experimental/quasi-experimental design. In the social sciences, post-test only designs, particularly those without random assignment (as will be discussed later), are considered some of the weaker designs. They are considered weaker because these designs do not control the bias or threats to internal validity that occur due to differences that might exist in the impact variables prior to the intervention. However, some health program effects can occur only once to the same individual, as happens with physical health outcomes such as birth weight. In comparison, some program effects can occur more than once, as happens in other health domains, such as mental health or behaviors. For program effects that can occur only once after the program, observational designs are particularly relevant, since there are, in effect, no baseline or pre-test differences to account for; all individuals in the evaluation have the same status prior to the intervention. In this context, concern about the weakness of the post-test only or observational design is unwarranted. In addition, epidemiological methods allow for the consideration of other variables that might explain differences in the outcome between those exposed and those not exposed to the program intervention (Handler, 2002; Rosenberg & Handler, 1998).

Given that a health program has been delivered and there is a recipient group with an outcome related to having received the program, choosing between an intervention and observational design rests on whether the outcome can be measured at two points in time. In experimental and quasi-experimental designs, the outcome variable can be measured at two points in time: pre-program or baseline data and post-program. Whether data are actually collected at both time points from the same program participants—individuals, clinics, or communities—becomes irrelevant.

In program evaluation, experimental and quasi-experimental designs can be used when four conditions exist. One is that information or data on the impact variable must exist before the program is delivered. Two, impact information must actually be collected from or on members of at least two groups. Three, an intervention must take place and be received by members of one of the groups. And, four, after delivery of the intervention, impact data must be collected from or on the same members of the groups as was collected from pre-program.

Evaluation questions that ask whether the intervention changed the impact variables are best answered through experimental and quasi-experimental designs (Handler, 2002; Rosenberg & Handler, 1998).

The following is an example (Handler, 2002; Handler & Rosenberg, 1998) of how both intervention and observational designs might be used for different components of a health program. The scenario is that at one Women, Infants, and Children (WIC) nutrition site, women receiving WIC also participate in a multicomponent program with a variety of interventions intended to change prenatal behaviors. Two of the program components are being evaluated for their effect on certain behaviors of the pregnant women. One program component is a household budgeting workshop and the other is a breastfeeding workshop. For the household budgeting workshop, the impact being evaluated is the purchasing behaviors of the WIC women. At the beginning of the first budgeting session, women could provide information on their current budgeting and purchasing practices. The same women could also provide impact data (their purchasing behaviors) at their next WIC visit some weeks later. The possibility that the same women would provide both pre- and post-program data on their behaviors permits the program evaluator to choose from among a set of experimental or quasi-experimental designs.

The situation is different for the evaluation of the breastfeeding workshop, which is provided to women who are pregnant for the first time. The impact being evaluated for this component is breastfeeding, and the mothers in the program have no prior breastfeeding behavior. Thus, theoretically, it is not possible to collect pre-test or baseline program data on actual breastfeeding behavior because the women in the breastfeeding workshop have not yet had the experience of breastfeeding. Consequently, the only choices for program evaluation design are the observational designs. For this intervention, an observational design, such as a two-group prospective cohort study (described later) is ideal, because data can be collected after delivery from women in the program (exposed) and from a group of women not in the program (unexposed) and "observe" their breastfeeding behaviors. The collection of data from two groups after the intervention may seem like a quasi-experimental design; the distinction rests on whether it is possible to have pre-test or baseline data on the health outcome of interest. That observational designs are used for outcomes, such as birth weight, that cannot have a baseline contributes to their being used more widely in evaluations of prenatal programs.

Identifying Design Options

Intervention designs include experimental and quasi-experimental designs. Campbell and Stanley (1963), in their classic book, identified and described 16 different intervention designs, of which 3 were pre-experimental, 3 were truly experimental, and the remaining 10 were quasi-experimental. While this classification system is widely used, it does not readily lend itself to the real-world application of program evaluation, nor does this classification include the observational designs from epidemiology. The complexity of factors affecting decisions regarding evaluation of health programs, particularly large-scale or population-based health programs, may require a different framework for making the design choices (Habicht, Victora, & Vaughan, 1999).

From the point of view of health program evaluation, designs can be more easily understood if we think of them as having three levels of ability to attribute effects to the program (Exhibit 10.2), yielding three groups of designs: impact documentation, impact assessment, and impact evaluation. These three levels correspond to the trade-offs and choices that program administrators and evaluators must make in choosing a design. In keeping with the terminology used for the effect theory, "impact" rather than "outcome" is used. It is more important for the effects of the intervention theory to be assessed than the outcome theory, because, unless the determinants are changed by the intervention and the health impacts achieved, the longer-range health outcomes will not occur. This chapter reviews only the most common designs, with particular attention to selecting an optimal sample for that design and the types of bias that are likely to occur with that design.

Ideally, feasible and possible design options can be identified before the program begins, to assure that the strongest, most rigorous design possible can be implemented for the effect evaluation. Most of the stronger program evaluation designs must be implemented *before* recipients receive the program, necessitating that the evaluation be ready for implementation well before program implementation. Thus, the placement of this chapter after the chapters on program implementation and monitoring is somewhat misleading and must not be interpreted as indicating when planning for the evaluation of program effect should occur.

Overview of the Decision Tree

To assist with the choice of an evaluation design, Exhibit 10.3 gives a flow diagram of the key questions that need to be asked. Each of the designs discussed in this chapter is shown in the decision tree. At each branch, a yes or no response to the key question leads either to a design or to a subsequent choice. At each choice branch, the program evaluator and the program staff need to confer and agree on which branch to follow. The designs shown in the decision tree are the ones most likely to be used in the majority of program evaluations, although more-complex designs exist, such as the Solomon four

Exhibit 10.3   Decision Tree for Choosing an Evaluation Design

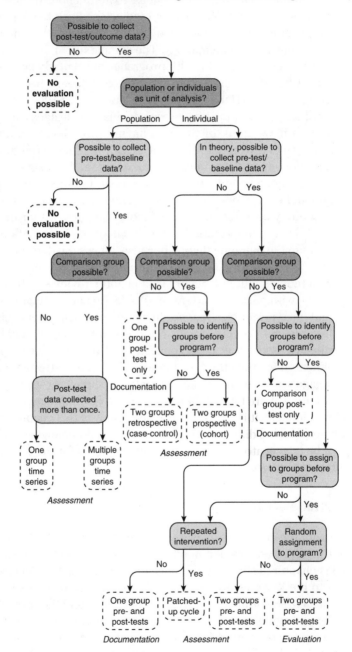

group design. However, such designs are more likely to be used in evaluation research, and thus they are not discussed or covered in this text. Also, the use of more than one comparison or control group or the collection of post data more than once (except for time series) is not reflected in the list of designs. These are considered modifications to the basic designs that do not intrinsically alter their structure or rigor.

As can be seen in the decision tree, the questions of whether a comparison group is possible and whether the group members can be identified before the program begins are critical to determining the design. If the answer to both questions is yes, the resulting possible designs tend to be stronger. There is one question that is rarely asked explicitly: whether the program is repeated. A yes response to this allows for the possibility of the patched-up cycle design.

It is important to note that the first decision question is whether it is possible, either theoretically or practically, to collect any post-test or impact data from program participants. The potential data can be obtainable either directly from individual participants or indirectly from secondary sources, such as medical records or vital records. If the answer is no, then it is not possible to determine whether the program had any effect, and an evaluation is not possible. The second branch in the tree focuses on whether the program, and hence the evaluation, is delivered to a population or to individuals. For population-based evaluations, it is necessary to have pre-test or baseline data on members of the population in order to have an evaluation. If it is not possible to have such data, an evaluation is not possible. An underlying assumption is that there is some means of knowing that an individual or individuals received the program. For population-level programs, such as a seat belt law or a mass media campaign, exposure to the program can be assumed for all members of the population, although it is sometimes possible to obtain measures of coverage. For programs at the direct services or enabling services level of the public health pyramid, indicators of having received the program can be obtained more directly.

Designs for Impact Documentation

At a minimum, an evaluation ought to document the impact of the program in terms of reaching the stated impact and outcome objectives. Focusing on documenting an impact from the point of view of the objectives often results in using designs that are called pre-experimental in social sciences terminology. These designs all involve collecting data after program implementation, or post-intervention. This theoretically allows post-test data to be compared to either the stated impact and outcome objective targets or to pre-test data.

These designs are actually used frequently because they are not complicated and are comparatively inexpensive. Their simplicity also contributes to their wide intuitive appeal, and sometimes to their unintentional use. It is important to understand that these designs are quite weak in terms of being able to attribute change or differences to the program. Because of their weaknesses, these designs are appropriately used to document the level or degree of reaching the target stated in the impact objective, remembering that these designs do not allow the evaluator to attribute any causality to the program. These designs can answer the evaluation question of whether there was any noticeable change or difference but they cannot attribute the change to the intervention.

One Group, Post-Test Only

An evaluation that collects data on the impact variable only from program participants and only after the program takes place is using a one-group, post-test only design. A post-test only design involves providing the intervention and then collecting data only on or from those who received the intervention. This design is inexpensive and simple to understand and so is often used in smaller programs with limited budgets, or by staff with minimal training in program evaluation. It may be the only option if the program is underway before the evaluation can be started. It would also be the only design option if there is no access to members of the target audience who did not receive the program.

Findings based on the data from this design can be misleading because the design has two major biases, or threats to the internal validity of the evaluation: history and maturation. History threats are specific events that happen to participants between the beginning and the end of the program, and these events might also explain the findings. Maturation threats are due to participants maturing physically or emotionally between the beginning and the end of the program. Because in the post-test only design there is no information about participants except at one point in time, there is no way of knowing whether external historical events or internal maturational processes affected the outcomes; hence the minimal usefulness of this design in determining the effect of the program.

One Group, Pre-Test and Post-Test

An evaluation that collects impact data only on or from participants before receiving the program and again after receiving the program is using a one-group, pre-test and post-test design. This design involves collecting data from program participants once at any time before and once at any time after they have received the program. It can readily be implemented by many direct services programs that collect data on a set of indicators at baseline or intake and again at exit from the program. This would be the case for substance abuse rehabilitation programs or occupational therapy programs. A major advantage of this design is that data can be analyzed for indications of the amount of change in program participants. The difference between the before and after program scores or levels for the impact variable is usually easy to calculate and to understand. In addition, because there is no expense involved in finding and gathering data from nonparticipants, the cost of this design remains relatively low.

The disadvantage of this design, as with the post-test only design, is that both history and maturation can affect the data. There are three additional threats or problems with this design. One is called a testing effect and occurs when the process of being involved in providing the pre-test data in some way affects the post-test data. For example, a questionnaire about exercise given at baseline may lead program participants to exercise more, such that on the post-test data they may report more exercise because of the questionnaire, not the program. Another possible threat is instrumentation. In this case the concern is with any possible changes or alterations to how or what data are collected for the post-test data as compared to the pre-test data collection. Unless exactly the same information is collected, the findings can be influenced by the data collection, rather than the program.

Comparison Groups, Post-Test Only

An evaluation that collects data on or from participants as they complete the program, as well as from a group of nonparticipants from the target audience, is said to use a post-test only with a comparison group. This is the third pre-experimental type of design. In this design, data are collected once from both program participants and another group that did not receive the program. Liller, Craig, Crane, and McDermott (1998) used this design to evaluate the effect of a poison prevention program on children ages 5 to 9 in three schools. After providing the educational program, they interviewed children who had received the program at the intervention schools and a comparable group of children from three schools that had not received the program. They were able to show that the children in the intervention schools had "better" scores on poison knowledge than the comparison group.

The simplicity of this design keeps the cost low, especially if the nonparticipants are recruited from a readily available source, such as a companion program or clinic. Like the one group, post-test only design, this design may be the only option available if the evaluation was started late. Usually, the difference between the scores or levels for the impact variable for the two groups is easy to calculate. Unfortunately, the difference may be incorrectly interpreted as an actual program effect, whereas in a stricter sense it may only suggest a program effect.

Although this design reduces the likelihood of instrumentation and testing threats, it is vulnerable to other threats, namely selection bias and program attrition. Selection bias refers to the fact that program participants may differ significantly from those not in the program. Unless more extensive data are collected from everyone in the evaluation, the extent to which they differ in fundamental ways will never be known. A difference in impact between the groups, if seen, may be attributable to factors other than the intervention. For example, suppose that WIC has initiated a breastfeeding education campaign, and the program evaluator plans to compare breastfeeding knowledge and attitudes of postpartum women in WIC to those of women not in WIC. However, the group of women in WIC might differ in fundamental ways from the group of women not in WIC, including factors that influenced their decision to be WIC recipients. It is possible that a difference in the breastfeeding knowledge and attitudes of the two groups of women might be due to those factors that influenced their decision to participate in WIC, rather than to the prenatal breastfeeding program.

Another example of a comparison-group, post-test only evaluation from the literature is informative. Klassen and associates (2002) matched women who attended a mammography program with friends and neighbors. They called the friends and neighbors "controls," connoting that they were not program participants. Data collection was done only once, after the program and from both groups, making it a comparison-group, post-test only design. However, they incorrectly called this another type of design, a case-control design. This example highlights the potential confusion over correctly describing and labeling designs, and hence the potential challenges program evaluators face when discussing designs with relevant stakeholders. They also claimed to have "matched" the program participants with their friends. It is worth noting that matching is done infrequently because of the cost involved in identifying and recruiting individuals who are completely like the program participants. Nonetheless, their use of a convenient and accessible comparison group highlights the potential for thinking creatively about how to arrive at the best possible design and sample.

Designs for Impact Assessment

If more resources are available for understanding the degree of effect from the program, then more complex and costly designs can be used. In general the quasi-experimental designs fall into this category, along with some observational epidemiology designs.

The designs for impact assessment answer the evaluation question of whether any noticeable change or difference seems related to having received the program. All of these designs are considered "stronger" than the impact documentation designs because these designs, to varying degrees, attempt to minimize possible differences between groups that may be related to some effect from the program.

These designs involve at least post-program or intervention data collection, plus the use of a comparison group. The comparison groups in these designs are nonequivalent, meaning that the groups being compared are not necessarily statistically similar or matched. Nonequivalence occurs because membership in the comparison group is influenced by the factors that influence the choice of being in the program or not. Those choosing to receive the program may be different from those not receiving the program, and without extensive data on both groups it may not be possible to know what those differences are. Thus, claiming that the program was the cause of differences in the impact variable between the groups remains problematic.

Three observational epidemiology designs can be used for impact assessment. Generally, the observational epidemiology designs are appropriate when the outcome being measured precludes the collection of baseline data, or when the intervention is a population-based intervention that precludes collecting data directly from program recipients. Designs for impact assessment are described in terms of their use in program evaluation and their commonly used names. For each design, the biases inherent in that design are discussed. Again, the trade-offs involved in choosing one design over another need to be weighed in view of the specific program characteristics and the evaluation needs of the program staff, stakeholders, and funders.

One Group, Time Series

As shown in the decision tree in Exhibit 10.3, the one-group, time series design is one of two designs that can be used if an entire population is the unit of analysis for the program evaluation. It can be used if data have been collected for the same group at several time points before the program, and the same data have been collected at several time points after the program. This design is also known as a single time series design because only one group is used, or as an interrupted time series design because the baseline value of the impact variable is interrupted by the program. The one-group, time series design might be one of the few options available if the program is delivered to or received by an entire population, such as seat belt laws, water fluoridation, or health insurance for underinsured children provided through state health insurance programs. Because the unit of analysis is the population rather than individuals, there is no assumption that exactly the same individuals contributed to the data at each time point. A time series, because it does not require following individuals, is often used in public health for evaluating policy effects on a population. It is also useful in evaluating programs that are delivered to only one distinct aggregate, such as a school, that will be included in the program and evaluation, and on which the same data have consistently been collected over time. The population focus of this design makes it very useful.

The key in choosing this design is the number of time points before and after the program at which data were collected and are available. For a variety of statistical reasons, the optimal number of time points to have would be five before and five after the intervention (Tukey, 1977). For a large population program, like seat belt laws, having five years of highway fatality data before and after the law may not be a problem. In other programs, such as a school-based program, where the data collection tools about students, such as the standardized tests, may change, having the same metric for five years before and after a program may be problematic. A reasonable rule of thumb, when the ideal is not possible, is to have a minimum of three years of data before and three years after the program. Fewer than three years makes it extremely difficult to statistically assess for the presence of a trend before and after the program.

This design has intuitive appeal, is easy to plan, and has a relatively low cost if the data already exist. An additional attractive feature of this design is that data other than physical health outcomes can be used. For example, Conrey, Grongillo, Dollahite, and Griffin (2003) used the rate of redemption of WIC coupons for produce at farmers' markets in New York as the impact variable for a program designed to increase the use of farmers' markets by women in WIC. This is an example of how existing data from social services might also be appropriate for population-focused health programs. Campbell and Russo (1999) pointed out that usually only effects from sudden and dramatically effective interventions can be identified and distinguished from the background, normal variations that occur over time. This is because the design has several biases, of which history is the major problem. The other threats—maturation, instrumentation, selection, and regression—tend to be less problematic and have less effect on the conclusions. One major disadvantage of this design is the challenge in interpreting the amount of change in relation to when the intervention occurred. It is possible that the change did not occur immediately and only after the program. The different patterns of the intervention–change relationship become evident only during the data analysis.

Multiple Groups, Time Series

If data have been collected about potential program participants and a comparison group at several time points before the program, and the same data have been collected at several time points after the program on the same groups, a multiple-group, time series design is possible. The addition of at least one comparison group that did not get the intervention is the most obvious way to improve on the one-group, time series design, so long as the data are from the same time frames for all groups. The classic example of this design is the comparison of two states, one with a seat belt law and the other without such a law. The annual mortality rates for motor vehicle accidents in both states are plotted across several years before and after enactment of the law. The rates in the two states are compared to determine whether the mortality rate in the state with the law declined more after the enactment compared to the mortality rate in the state without the law. Because this design requires collecting data on or from at least two groups many times before and after the program, it is generally used with large aggregates, such as schools, or with populations.

The major advantage of this design is that there are few biases that seriously affect the ability to draw conclusions regarding the program effect. In other words, this is a very strong design to use with population-focused health programs. A major disadvantage of the design is that the same impact variable data must have been collected on all groups being compared. If an impact variable such as mortality is the outcome of interest, then the data are likely to be similar across groups. In contrast, if the amount of prenatal care is the impact variable of interest, the states may use different indices for adequacy of prenatal care, such as the Kessner Index or the Kotelchuck Index. Thus, the similarity of data across groups, in this example states, could be problematic. Another disadvantage of both time series designs is the need for more-complex statistical analysis, which may require the use of a statistical expert.

Two Groups, Retrospectively Constructed (Case Control)

If it is possible to identify individuals with and without the program outcome and to review their historical, existing data to determine which individuals received the program and which did not, a retrospectively constructed, two-group design is possible. This observational epidemiological design is called a case-control design. It is used when, for whatever reason, the program evaluation is done after the program has started or has concluded and access to the individuals for data collection is limited. In this design, those with the outcome are compared to those without the outcome, with regard to whether they were exposed to, meaning received, the program.

The retrospective two-group design is useful because the degree to which the program improved the likelihood of the desired outcome can be statistically calculated by comparing those with the outcome to those who do not have the outcome for whether they were exposed to the program. The exposed/not exposed and the outcome/no outcome relationships are often represented by a two-row by two-column table, called a 2x2 table. In the retrospective two-group design, knowing who falls into which of the four cells in the table is possible only after the program and after the outcome has occurred, through a review of existing records that contain both program participation data and impact variable data. Thus, this design is possible only if there is access to those records and the information in those records includes data on both exposure to the program and the impact variable.

A point of clarification is in order. The retrospective case-control design is generally used when the "outcome" can be measured only once, as in dead or alive, or breastfeeding or not in first-time mothers, or when the outcome is measured as a simple dichotomous variable, as in yes or no low birth weight. In other words, this design can be used when it theoretically is not possible to collect baseline or pre-test data on the outcome. For impact variables that occur only once, the retrospective two-group (case-control) design is quite robust, meaning it is a strong design (Handler, 2002; Rosenberg & Handler, 1998). The unique feature of this design is that individuals are identified post hoc who have and do not have the outcome of concern, and they are then compared with regard to whether they received the program. In this sense, the evaluation is retrospectively assigning individuals to exposure groups.

The major advantage of the retrospective two-group design is that it can be used any time after the program has been implemented because it is not necessary to know before the beginning of the program who will be in the evaluation. Like other evaluation designs that are implemented after the program, it may be one of the few choices available if the evaluators were not involved in creating or choosing an evaluation design earlier in the planning cycle. The design does have disadvantages. One is the costs associated with the time and human resources needed to determine exposure to the intervention through a record review that requires abstraction of data. A related major limitation of this design is the ability to obtain high-quality data on exposure to the program, including whether the individual received the program. Although data warehousing by health care organizations has been increasing, there is no guarantee that the variables needed for the evaluation will be available nor that they will have been collected in a consistent and reliable manner. The cost associated with the retrieval of existing data, which is necessary in retrospective designs, will be lower if a comprehensive and stable management information system has been used for recording the data that need to be abstracted for the program evaluation. However, if budget constraints and data retrieval difficulties pose severe limitations on the number of individuals for whom adequate retrospective data are available, then the size of the sample can be a concern. A small sample size will affect the statistical conclusions that can be made about the effectiveness of the program. In addition, although the retrospective case-control design is robust, selection bias can be present. There is no way to know whether any apparent program effect might have been due to a selective preference for receiving the program. Another major issue with the case-control design is recall bias—that is, inaccurate memory— particularly if the participants are asked about their having received the program. Recall bias can be circumvented if there are records documenting the participants' participation in the program.

Two Groups, Prospective (Cohorts)

If the target population is distinct and clearly defined, and can be followed forward in time as a group (cohort), then a prospective design is possible. Like the retrospective two-group design, the prospective design is used if there is no theoretical possibility of collecting pre-test data because the outcome can be measured only once, as in the dead/alive, breastfeeding/not scenarios (Handler, 2002; Rosenberg & Handler, 1998). Prospective cohort designs are widely used in the evaluation of health services when the outcomes of interest are health impacts that occur only once for an individual. There are two versions of the prospective cohort design; they differ based on whether it is possible to know at the outset of the evaluation who will receive the program. In Version I, it is not possible to know beforehand who will participate in or receive the program. The members of the target population are followed forward in time (prospectively) as a group (a cohort) for a given time period, and some individuals are exposed to the program and some are not. The evaluators determine who received exposure to the program at the end of the evaluation. In Version II, it is known before the program begins who will and will not participate in or receive the program. Both groups are followed as a cohort forward throughout the duration of the evaluation. The difference between the designs rests in the nature of the impact variable being measured. In both versions of the prospective cohort design, at the end of the time period, the impact variable is measured to determine whether the outcome is present among those exposed.

Suppose there is a home visitation program for women who are pregnant for the first time, and the goal of the program is to prevent child abuse. It is possible to use a two-group, prospective cohort design. One group would be women in the program, and they would be followed for a year; at the end of the year, the evaluators would assess whether or not child abuse had occurred as the outcome variable. The other group would be pregnant women, perhaps from a waiting list or from a list of women who had refused the program, who do not receive the program and are followed forward in time, with child abuse measured at one year. At one year, the rate of child abuse for each group of new mothers is compared. This would be a Version II prospective cohort study.

The prospective cohort design is appealing because data can be collected on key variables, such as relevant antecedent and contributing factors, from members of the target audience before exposure to the program. In this regard, this design does not rely on existing data, as the retrospective two-group design does. Also, if Version I is used, this design does not require knowing who will receive the program. The exposed and unexposed groups are identified at the end of the time period, based on data collected over the duration of the evaluation. If data collection occurs over a long time period, this potentially allows more individuals to develop the outcome from the program intervention. This is an important feature for programs with a potentially long time lag between intervention and evidence of impact, such as programs aimed at changing substance abuse behavior, long-term weight loss programs, or a long-term medical treatment.

The major disadvantages of a prospective design are the need to track individuals for a substantial time frame, and the need to collect follow-up data on the impact variable. Maintaining contact with the individuals in the evaluation for a period of time can be costly as well as frustrating, particularly if they do not have stable lives or their whereabouts are not reliable. Loss of participants due to attrition does have consequences for the validity of the design and the statistical conclusions that can be drawn. Although attrition of those in the evaluation can be addressed and thus lowered through a variety of strategies (Resnicow et al., 2001), these strategies are costly and labor intensive.

Often it is not possible to actually determine who will be exposed to the program before the program begins. When program records are used to establish exposure but the analysis proceeds from the exposure forward in time (the prospective element) to the outcome, then the design is best called a retrospective cohort design. An example of this design is an evaluation of five types of providers of prenatal care services: public hospital clinics, health department clinics, community clinics, private physicians' offices, and private hospital clinics (Simpson, Korenbrot, & Greene, 1997). All women on Medicaid from specific geographic regions were included in the evaluation of the association of prenatal care provider type with pregnancy outcomes. The medical records of all women in the study regions who gave birth during the evaluation time period were reviewed. The evaluators noted where the women had received prenatal care, and then they compared the outcomes of the pregnancies across the types of providers. Despite the fact that the groups were retrospectively constructed, the design is prospective in that it followed the women forward through their pregnancy and reassessed the one-time-only outcome variables of birth weight and preterm delivery.

Patched-Up Cycle

If only post-test data are available from a first group of program participants (a one-group, post-test only design), but the program is being repeated, then a patched-up cycle design is possible. This design is a technique for patching up the one-group, post-test only design by adding a new group. Each time the program is offered, there is the possibility of collecting data from participants before and after the program. The patched-up cycle design, also called the institutional design, allows the post-program data from participants in the first cycle to become the comparison group for the pre-program data for the next cycle of program participants. It is patched up because the first cycle is a one-group, post-test only design, the second cycle is a one-group only, pre-test and post-test design, and the third cycle is a comparison-group only, post-test design. The cycle can be repeated as many times as the program is offered, and thus there can be more than three cycles. The patched-up cycle design is another design that is used if the first program was offered before the evaluation was started, but it is not too late to collect post-test data on the first set of program participants.

This design can be useful for health programs, such as health education programs, in which waiting for the program does not have serious health consequences. This allows for the collection of the pre-test data from the members of cycle 2. The advantage of the patched-up cycle design is that statistical comparisons can be done between those in each cycle of the program and data collection. Specifically, the cycle 1 post-test data are compared to the cycle 2 pre-test data. Then the cycle 2 pre-test data are compared to the cycle 2 post-test data, and, finally, the cycle 2 post-test data are compared to the cycle 3 post-test data. This set of comparisons allows the patched-up cycle design to compensate, to some extent, for the weaknesses of the design. The patched-up cycle design can be viewed as comprising of three designs: the one-group, post-test only design of cycle 1, the one-group, pre-test and post-test design of cycle 2, and the post-test only with a comparison group. Thus, the biases and weaknesses of each of these three designs are present in the patched-up cycle design, specifically maturation, regression, and history.

Two Groups, Pre-Test and Post-Test

An evaluation that collects impact variable data on or from program participants and nonparticipants, both before the program and once after the program,
uses a two-group, pre-test and post-test design. This design is more formally
called a nonequivalent two-group control-group design. It adds to the post-test
only design discussed earlier by adding the collection of data from both program participants and nonparticipants before receiving the program. In other
words, pre-test and post-test data are collected from both program participants
and nonparticipants on similar dates. This design has intuitive and practical
appeal because data are collected only twice and because the statistical comparison of the two groups is relatively simple and straightforward.

In using this design, evaluators must attempt to assure that the groups are
as alike as possible, by carefully selecting the nonparticipants, the control
group. However, without random assignment there is no assurance that the
groups will be alike, hence the nonequivalence. Selection bias is a major
threat in the two-group, pre-test and post-test design. If sufficient information
about those in both groups has been collected, such as demographic variables
and relevant antecedent variables, the differences between the groups can be
adjusted for in the statistical analysis. Another threat to this design is regression to the mean. Regression refers to the tendency for the scores of different
groups to become more alike over time. Thus, the longer the time period
between the intervention and the collection of the post-test data, the more
likely the two groups are to have no differences on the impact variable. This
suggests that the design is best used with impacts that are expected to occur
relatively soon after the intervention, and the post-test data should be collected at that time point.

Designs for Impact Evaluation Research

This last set of designs is the most costly and complex, but they enable
evaluators to show that the program was truly the cause of the effect. These
designs answer the evaluation question of whether the change or difference
can be attributed to having received the program. Experimental designs
involve a program, an outcome measure, and a comparison from which
change due to the program or intervention can be inferred. Only one of the
several experimental designs is discussed, specifically the two-group, pre-test
and post-test design with random assignment. The other experimental designs
are essentially variations on this design and, because they are more complex,
are used only in evaluation research. Experimental designs are expensive in
terms of the number of evaluation participants needed to reach statistically

sound conclusions and in the amount of time required to track those in the evaluation sample. Methods for determining the number of evaluation participants needed are discussed later in this chapter in terms of sample size and power. The distinguishing feature of all the experimental designs is the use of random assignment.

Random Assignment

Random assignment is the process of randomly determining who receives the health program intervention and who does not. This is not to be confused with random selection, which refers to the random identification from the target population of who will be in the evaluation. The advantage of using random assignment of participants to either the experimental/participant or control/nonparticipant groups is that it creates comparison groups that are theoretically equivalent. In other words, by assigning evaluation participants to either the experimental or control group on a random basis, the possibility of the two groups being different is no greater than the differences one might expect by chance alone. This is critical, as it eliminates design biases that stem from groups not being alike; with random assignment, the two groups are as alike as is theoretically possible, and so subsequent differences found in impact variables can logically be attributed to the effect of the intervention. Random assignment is, essentially, done using either a table of random numbers or the flip of a coin, so to speak, although more sophisticated methods of arriving at random assignment do exist. Random assignment is the basis for designs used in clinical trials, to use epidemiological or related terminology, or in experimental designs, to use social science language.

A reality for many health programs is that ethical concerns often preclude the use of random assignment to receive or not receive the program. In the WIC example given earlier, it might be ethically acceptable to randomly assign women to the household budgeting program, but it would not be ethically acceptable to randomly assign women to breastfeeding education. In highly vulnerable populations or communities, experimental designs may not be ethically realistic or even acceptable to stakeholders. For example, random assignment has been widely used in school-based interventions, but not without major ethical and policy issues (Metcalf, 1997). The objection of stakeholders is that not all who need the program are able to receive it, due to the random assignment. For example, a community agency may have a moral objection to not offering a health promotion program to all who are at high risk. However, if a new program is compared to the standard program, then health program evaluators might choose an experimental design that allows the unexposed group members either to receive the standard program or to receive the new program after the exposed group receives it. These approaches to random assignment help minimize ethical concerns yet maintain rigor in the evaluation.

Other practical issues exist with experimental designs. One is that the target population needs to be sufficiently large to have both an experimental group and a control group. Also, the program interventions must be robust, meaning having a statistical probability of having an effect. Experimental designs are thus not appropriate if any element of the effect theory is poorly substantiated or the intervention theory predicts only a small change in the impact variable. An evaluation of an educational intervention with older African-Americans (Walker, 2000) may have failed to find any program effect due to both of these challenges to an experimental design. The intervention for the experimental group consisted of spiritual and hypertension-related messages delivered by programmed telephone calls, and the control group received only the spiritual messages via the programmed telephone calls. Both groups also received pamphlets and home visits by a health educator. Thus, the only difference between the experimental and control group interventions was that hypertension-related messages were provided to the experimental group. It is likely that receiving such messages would produce only a small change in hypertension management behaviors. In addition, there were only 43 people in the experimental group and 40 people in the control group. This would be considered a small sample size, especially for attempting to find the small effect from the hypertension-related messages provided to the experimental group. The strong experimental study design might have been undermined by having a weak intervention and a small sample size. In other words, the choice of design must be considered in light of the whole program and the evaluation plan.

Another issue in the use of experimental designs is that logistically the evaluation team and budget must be able to accommodate the large number of evaluation participants needed in order for random assignment to work as intended. This is because when random assignment is undertaken with too few participants, it is possible that the two assigned groups will not be theoretically equivalent. For these reasons, random assignment, as an approach to the construction of control groups, is rarely, if ever, used in health programs that are not research projects.

Two Groups, Pre-Test and Post-Test with Random Assignment

If individuals from the target audience are randomly assigned to receive the health program or not, and data are collected from those who received the program (experimental) and those who did not (controls) both before and after receiving the program, then a two-group, pre-test and post-test with random assignment design was used. This design is very similar to the two-group, pre-test and post design described earlier, except that random assignment is used. Although technically incorrect, to some extent, the term "experimental group" is used in the health and evaluation literature instead of "cases" as a way to denote that random assignment to receive the program or not was used. This design is often called a randomized clinical trial and is often considered the "gold standard" in medical treatment research. Because it is the most rigorous of the designs, there are innumerable examples of this design being used, especially in the evaluation of medical treatments and pharmaceuticals. It is easiest to think of this design with regard to individuals and medical treatment, but the same design can be used with aggregates, such as schools (i.e., Nicklas & O'Neil, 2000), or with populations, such as geographically distinct communities. When applied at levels greater than the individual, the design is more likely to be called a community trial.

Biases associated with this design are minimal because of the use of equivalent groups. The major bias is the differential attrition that results if underlying but unknown causes exist for members of either the experimental or control group to drop out of the evaluation. This then results in a systematic difference between the groups, which affects the ability to attribute causality to the programmatic intervention. To avoid problems associated with differential attrition, evaluators need to carefully follow both groups and determine who is and who is not still in the groups at the end of the intervention. As was mentioned earlier, the greatest disadvantage of this design is the logistics involved in using random assignment.

SAMPLING

Sampling is the scientific and logistical process of choosing who will be included in the evaluation and whether they will be in the intervention or control groups. For program evaluations there are realities of constructing a sample from or on whom to collect impact data that need to be considered. Approaches to sample construction are based on science and have become well established. These are discussed in terms of impact assessments and evaluations. A critical issue in evaluation is the question of how many need to be in the sample in order to have a rigorous evaluation. This question is addressed in the section on sample size determination.

Sampling Realities

Devising a plan for selecting who will actually be included when evaluating the effects of the program is often a creative endeavor, albeit technical.

There are basically two steps (Rossi, Freeman, & Lipsey, 1999). The first step is to identify program participants and the target population. This step applies in some way to all designs. For impact evaluation designs, the second step is to develop a plan to select an unbiased sample from the target population and from among program participants. This overly simple description of sampling belies the complex procedures and intellectual challenges that are inherent in each step. When discussing sampling, statisticians use the term "population" to refer to the group from which a sample is selected. This may or may not be the same as the larger target population of the program.

It is important to remember that the approach chosen for constructing a sample, along with the design choice, has implications for the ability to draw statistical conclusions. The more carefully the evaluation needs to compare program participants (exposed/experimental) to nonparticipants (unexposed/control), the more careful the selection needs to be in terms of making the groups as alike as possible. In such cases, the random assignment approach is an important element of the evaluation plan. For example, if the program being evaluated has a novel intervention and the evaluation borders on research, then attention to random assignment becomes relevant. However, for most health programs, the efforts and resources required to accomplish random assignment are beyond the scope of what is need or expected by stakeholders.

Unlike sampling for research projects that are under the control of investigators, sampling for evaluations places several constraints upon evaluators. The foremost constraint is the number of people who can or did participate in the program. If the health program was a small health education class, then including all program participants in the evaluation sample may be feasible. In contrast, if the health program was delivered to the population at large, such as a public awareness campaign or passive protection through policy implementation, then it becomes necessary to select individuals from within the population for the evaluation. An alternative to selecting individuals to participate in the evaluation is to use a time series design, especially if the program is population based. A corollary constraint to the number of program participants is the size of the target population which can vary from a nation, if a national health policy is being evaluated, to a small, discrete group, such as adults between the ages of 75 and 80 with glaucoma who live within a small geographic location. Because nonparticipants in the target audience become controls, the number of potential controls needs to be taken into account.

The second sampling constraint is that it is not always clear who was a member of the target audience and, more importantly, who was a participant. This results from either unclear eligibility or limited documentation. Unless the program has clearly delineated criteria for membership in the target population and for designating a participant, it may not be possible to know who ought to have received the program and who actually received it. This fuzziness can make it difficult or impossible to know who is appropriately classified as a member of the exposed/experimental group versus the unexposed/control group. Hence, there is a need to have developed clear eligibility guidelines and procedures as part of the process theory. Ambiguous group membership may also result if the evaluator has limited access to or ability to identify program participants. This could occur if the program has poorly maintained records or if it is provided anonymously on a drop-in basis. A lack of such information makes it difficult to classify who was or is in the exposed/experimental group and unexposed/control group, which in turn has implications for design choice as well as sampling strategy. Just as being able to delineate program participants begins with the process theory, having information about who the program participants are can be addressed during the development of the process theory.

A third constraint involves how participants are classified by the program, meaning what criteria are used to assign participants to the experimental or control group. In some programs, participation in the program is not a clear-cut, dichotomous variable. This is particularly true for programs with multiple components that may be provided by multiple providers, or programs that are implemented over an extended time. For example, Manalo and Meezan (2000) were interested in evaluating family support programs that varied with regard to actual content. They found that the typology used to classify the family support programs (the unit of analysis) was problematic when they attempted to evaluate across programs, which limited their ability to draw conclusions about the effectiveness of different types of programs. Thus, part of the sampling strategy must be the development of a definition of "participation" in the program. This may be the same as the definitions developed for the process evaluation and may be based on a wide variety of criteria, ranging from hours of intervention received to membership in a health policy target audience.

Sample Construction

There are two broad classifications of sampling approaches: probability and nonprobability sampling (Black, 1999; Green & Lewis, 1986). Within each of these two approaches are sample types based on increasingly complex methods used to derive the sample. If each member of a population has an equal chance of being chosen to participate in the program, then the sample is said to be a probability or random sample, depending on the discipline. In other words, a probability sample, in theory, allows the evaluator to create equivalent groups. This type of sample is recommended if the evaluation is seeking to demonstrate that the program, and only the program, was responsible for the outcome—in other words, causation. Thus, ideally, probability samples are used with impact evaluation designs, specifically experimental or intervention designs.

The other approach to sampling does not rely on members of the population being equally likely to be selected to participate in the evaluation, and so it is called a nonprobability or nonrandom sample, depending on the discipline of the evaluator. Nonprobability samples are used with impact documentation and impact assessment designs. None of the nonprobability sample types (Exhibit 10.4) enable evaluators to say that the samples in the evaluation are representative of the population at large.

Exhibit 10.4   Types of Nonprobability Samples, with Corresponding Descriptions and Techniques

Type of Sample	Description	Technique
Convenience, volunteer, accidental	Whoever is available	Ask for volunteers from among those present at any event
Purposive	Selectively invite based on having a specific characteristic	From a list of individuals with known characteristics, select those with the characteristic of interest
Quota	Collect data from a number with specific characteristics, such that the proportions with the characteristics are similar to the population at large	From a list of individuals with known characteristics, select a proportion of those with the characteristic of interest that matches the known proportion in the population at large
Snowball	A participant nominates someone else for participation	Current participants name others with a specific characteristic

Sampling for Impact Assessment

Using a nonprobability sample, as is done in impact assessments, tends to be simple and not costly (Exhibit 10.4). For many smaller, locally based, or agency-specific health programs, a nonprobability sample will be adequate for the evaluation. This type of sample allows for a statistical comparison of differences between program participants and nonparticipants.

A nonprobability sample can be constructed in several ways (Exhibit 10.5), each with its own name. These types of samples come from the social sciences. A convenience sample is constructed by inviting whoever is accessible or available to participate. It is an inexpensive method of obtaining a sufficient number of evaluation participants. A purposive sample is generally one in which the evaluation participants are chosen based on a specific characteristic, thus ensuring that the program participant and nonparticipant samples are balanced with regard to that characteristic. A quota sample also involves selecting participants based on a specific characteristic, but the proportion of evaluation participants having that characteristic is proportional to those in the population at large. For example, if age is important in the evaluation and 10% of the population of participants at large is over 80 years old, then the evaluation sample must meet a 10% quota of 80-year-old participants. A snowball sample, so named for the analogy of how to make a snowball larger, is achieved by asking current evaluation participants who have a specific characteristic to identify or nominate other individuals they know who also have the characteristic of interest. Snowball sampling is useful when a list of names of potential evaluation participants does not exist. As more evaluation participants name others, the snowball of evaluation participants grows.

Overall, these sampling strategies are easy to implement and explain to stakeholders and thus are likely to be used in program evaluations. Each varies with regard to the ease of implementation, the degree of representativeness of the larger population, and the sampling frame used—in other words, the basis for inclusion in the evaluation sample.

Sampling for Impact Evaluation

If it is crucial to demonstrate that the health problem was changed, presumably improved, in program participants, a probability sample is recommended. A probability sample is also necessary in a needs assessment if one purpose of the assessment is to accurately estimate the rate of a health problem in a population. A probability sample is one in which all potential members of the evaluation have an equal probability of being selected to participate in the evaluation.

Exhibit 10.5   Comparison of Types of Samples, with Regard to Ease of Implementation, Degree of Representativeness, and Complexity of Sampling Frame

Type of Sample	Ease of Implementation	Representative-ness of General Population	Sampling Frame
Convenience	Easiest	None assured, but may occur by chance	Willingness to participate in the evaluation
Purposive	Easy	None	Specific characteristics of interest
Quota	Moderately easy	None assured, but possibly representative of those with characteristics by chance	Specific characteristics of interest
Snowball	Easy	None, and likely to be biased	Network of initial participants

The major barrier to having a probability sample is that evaluators may not have control over who receives the program, especially if the impact evaluation is not designed during program development. Probability samples are used to increase the external validity of the evaluation; however, for the vast majority of program evaluations external validity is less of an issue than the biases and threats inherent in the design.

Achieving equal probability of selection involves randomly selecting potential participants. Several types of probability samples can be constructed, depending on the specific method used to identify and then select members of the evaluation sample. Random selection of evaluation participants, whether individuals, classrooms, or neighborhoods, from the entire population of possible participants can be done in one of several ways, each resulting in a different type of probability sample. A simple probability sample is constructed by using a table of random numbers to select individuals from a known list of possible participants. The other types of probability samples involve increasingly more complex selection procedures from increasingly more specific groups within the population.

The various probability sample types are explained in greater detail in most research and epidemiology textbooks. Most local or agency-based program planning efforts and evaluations are not likely to have the resources required to obtain these more complicated samples. The costs increase in proportion to the complexity of the probability sample because of increases in the number and qualifications of personnel needed to "find" the individual selected, and because of increases in the amount of time required to establish the sampling procedures and then to carry out those procedures. The sample type chosen may be influenced by the ease of implementing that technique, the degree of representativeness of the target population, and the complexity of the sampling frame.

Sample Size

The question of how many subjects, whether individuals, families, or communities, are needed in the evaluation quickly becomes a complex issue. There are practical considerations, such as fiscal limitations, logistics of data collection and management, and accessibility challenges. There are also statistical considerations. In a pure research study, the investigator first chooses a level of probability that a significant result might be found by the study. This is called the power, and it is usually chosen to be between 80% and 90%. The number of study participants needed to achieve that level of power is then calculated. When the power is set higher, meaning a higher probability that a significant result will be found, more subjects are needed. Also, when more variables are included in the analysis, more subjects are needed. One other element that is factored into the calculation of the sample size is the degree of difference that is expected, whether the difference is between pre-test and post-test data or between program participants and nonparticipants. This difference is called effect size. The statistical process of analyzing the relationships among the power of a study, the type of statistical tests to be done, the number of variables, the effect size, and the sample size is called a power analysis.

Black (1999) summarizes the issue by showing that there are four factors affecting the power of a statistical test: the sample representativeness and size, the quality of the measurement in terms of reliability and design, the choice of the statistical test, and the effectiveness of the intervention (Exhibit 10.6). For program evaluation, the power analysis may face a specific problem: the number of evaluation participants may already be determined, perhaps because of funding limitations or because the program has already been provided. In such circumstances, the sample, measurement, and design of the evaluation take on even greater importance in determining whether the possibility exists of finding a significant difference that might be related to the program.

Exhibit 10.6   Factors Influencing Sample Size

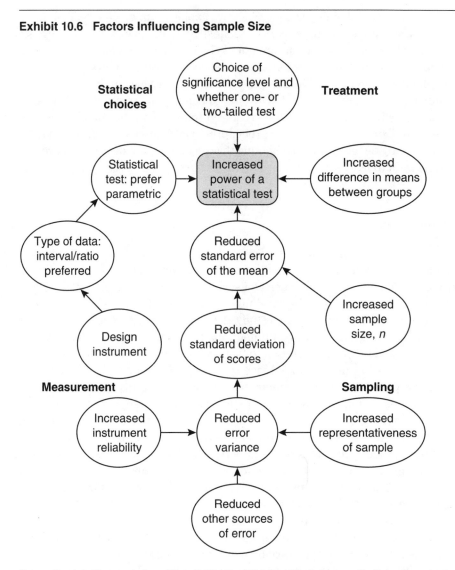

Source: Reprinted by permission of Sage Publications Ltd. from Black, Thomas R., *Doing Quantitative Research in the Social Sciences*, Copyright, (© Sage Publications, 1999).

Several software programs exist that can be used to do the calculations necessary for a power analysis. Many of these are available via the Internet. Whether freeware or copyright programs are used, the power analysis requires a clear understanding of the sample, the size of the anticipated effect of the program, and the statistical tests that will be used.

At the time the power analysis is done the evaluator can refine, modify, and solidify aspects of the evaluation design that are under the control of the evaluator in order to enhance the power. In addition, the power analysis may reveal that the possibility of finding a program effect is so unlikely as to make an outcome evaluation questionable, and thus an impact documentation or assessment design is better. The evaluator must then make a difficult choice regarding whether to proceed with the evaluation, search for alternative approaches to the evaluation or data analysis as assessed by the power analysis, or determine whether it is feasible to modify the evaluation in ways that will increase the power.

DESIGNS AND FAILURES

As was first mentioned in Chapter 5, there are two types of failure that program evaluators attempt to identify or avoid, to which a third type of failure can now be added (Exhibit 10.7). A summary of the strategies for avoiding each

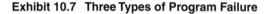

Exhibit 10.7   Three Types of Program Failure

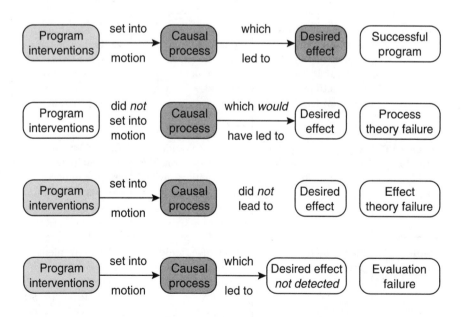

Source: Evaluation Research by Weiss, C. H. Copyright. Reprinted by permission of Pearson Education, Inc. Upper Saddle River, N. J.

type of failure is shown in Exhibit 10.8. One type of failure is process failure, in which the service utilization plan was not sufficiently implemented, thereby resulting in no or inadequate implementation of the intervention. Avoiding process theory failure involves careful program oversight and implementation. The process or monitoring evaluation, rather than the impact or outcome evaluation, provides insights as to whether a process theory failure occurred.

The second type of failure concerns the effect theory. If the program interventions did not lead to the desired program impacts and outcomes, then the rationale for choosing those interventions may have been flawed. If a high-quality evaluation found no effect and the process evaluation verified that the intervention was provided as planned, then an effect theory failure may have occurred. However, both the process evaluation and the impact evaluation must have been conducted and must have provided sufficient scientific data to draw a conclusion of effect theory failure. In particular, the impact evaluation

Exhibit 10.8   Approaches to Minimizing Each of the Three Types of Program Failure

	Process Theory Failure	Effect Theory Failure	Evaluation Failure
Definition	The interventions were not sufficiently implemented to (potentially) affect the health problem being targeted	The interventions did not or could not affect the health problem being targeted	The evaluation methods, design, or sample was inappropriate such that the true effects of the program were not detected
Design and methods considerations	Ability to link process data with effect data at an individual level	Ideally use random assignment; consider timing with regard to finding the maximum effect from the program	Tailor instruments to participants and specific impact expected; maximize internal and external validity
Sample considerations	Ideally include all program participants	Ideally use random assignment and random selection	Select equivalent intervention and control groups; have adequate sample size to achieve high power

must have been designed to assess for causality; this would have involved the use of experimental designs. Unless these were used, it will be impossible to conclude that there was an effect theory failure.

The third type of failure is directly related to the evaluation—namely, that it failed to correctly identify an effect that resulted from the interventions. If the evaluation was flawed with regard to the sample, the measures used, the design, or the statistical tests, then the findings regarding the success of the program are questionable. To prevent an evaluation failure it is necessary to adhere to the highest level of rigor possible given the programmatic realities (Exhibit 10.6). If there are adequate resources and the program is such that it is critical to greatly minimize the evaluation failure, there are steps that can be taken. However, these steps are costly and involve more stringent research methodologies. For example, if measurement is seen as a possible source of an evaluation failure, then additional, complementary, or redundant measures may be used to validate the measures used in the evaluation. To avoid evaluation failure due to inappropriate design choice, evaluators can use a decision flowchart, such as Exhibit 10.3.

ACROSS THE PYRAMID

At the direct services level of the public health pyramid, health programs are focused on individuals. Therefore, the sample frame is more likely to be accessible and knowable to the evaluators. If this is the case and the program is sufficiently large, a simple probability sample of the program participants is possible. However, getting a probability sample of nonparticipants may be more difficult. One technique that is used is to draw the controls from the list of those who refused to participate in the program. As one might imagine, there are major scientific and ethical difficulties with this approach. Another approach is to use a design in which the participants either become their own controls, as in a pre-test and post-test design, or future participants on a waiting list are used as controls. Overall, the impact evaluations of health programs at the direct services level can resemble or be straightforward research in terms of the sampling and design.

At the enabling services level, health programs are focused on groups of individuals and are provided in a wider range of contexts. Programs at the enabling services level will be most challenging to evaluate in terms of their impact, for several reasons. One is that the sampling frame is less likely to be knowable and accessible to the evaluators. This will necessitate that the evaluation sampling plan be creative and carefully tailored to the program realities. Some of the options may involve the use of statistically constructed control groups. Another reason that the impact evaluation will be more challenging is that health services programs at this level are probably not suited to experimental designs but may be appropriate for quasi-experimental designs. At a minimum, pre-test and post-test designs can be used. In addition, depending on the program, random assignment might be possible.

At the population-based level, health programs are provided to entire populations. Although this does not preclude the use of probability samples or experimental designs, it does limit the evaluation options to those sampling methods and designs that can reasonably be implemented with populations. Time series designs are especially useful for evaluating population-level programs.

At the infrastructure level, the program focuses on changing the working of the health care organization or the public health system. The impact evaluation question will determine whether the evaluation is about the changes in the infrastructure or the changes to the health status of clients. This distinction in turn influences the sample and the type of design that is needed to answer the intervention effect question. A time series would be appropriate if the focus is on a long-term change for which there are data across many time points, as might be the case for a policy analysis of funding for health departments. On the other hand, if the program is focused on the knowledge of individual workers, many of the designs that use pre-test and post-test data and comparison groups might be appropriate.

DISCUSSION QUESTIONS

1. Which designs are more appropriate for full coverage programs, and which are more appropriate for partial coverage programs? Justify your response.

2. Identify at least one sampling issue that would be particularly relevant at each level of the pyramid. What strategy could be used to minimize the problem?

3. Suppose the county board of supervisors has asked you, as an evaluation consultant, to evaluate a substance abuse prevention program delivered throughout the county. You have been asked to prove at least three options for how to evaluate the program, based on complexity and cost. What three designs would you propose and why?

4. Conduct an Internet search for power analysis software.

   a. From among the programs you found, select two (that are free-ware) and experiment with them. What information is required to conduct the analysis? In what ways does the need for that information affect how you would proceed with planning the impact evaluation?

   b. Now use the following information to determine the sample size needed. You plan on conducting a paired t test with program participants, using their pre-test and post-test data, alpha significance is set at 0.05, and the standard deviation on the outcome measure was reported in the literature to be 3.5 with a mean of 12.0.

References

Black, T. R. (1999). *Doing quantitative research in the social sciences: An integrated approach to research design, measurement and statistics.* London: Sage Publications.

Campbell, D. T., & Russo, M. J. (1999). An inventory of threats to validity and alternative designs to control them. In D. T. Campbell and M. J. Russo (Eds.), *Social experimentation.* Thousand Oaks, CA: Sage Publications.

Campbell, D. T. & Stanley, J. C. (1963). *Experimental and quasi-experimental designs for research.* Boston: Houghton Mifflin.

Conrey, E. J., Grongillo, E. A., Dollahite, J. S., & Griffin, M. R. (2003). Integrated program enhancements increased utilization of Farmers' Market Nutrition Program. *Journal of Nutrition, 133*, 1841–1844.

Fos, P. J., & Fine, D. J. (2000). *Designing health care for populations: Applied epidemiology in health care administration.* San Francisco, CA: Jossey-Bass.

Green, L. W., & Lewis, F. M. (1986). *Measurement and evaluation in health education and health promotion.* Palo Alto, CA: Mayfield Publishing.

Habicht, J. P., Victora, C. G., & Vaughan, J. P. (1999). Evaluation designs for adequacy, plausibility and probability of public health program performance and impact. *International Journal of Epidemiology, 28* (1), 10–18.

Handler, A. (2002). Lecture notes. *http://www.uic.edu/sph/mch/evaluation/index.htm* (accessed 7/14/03.)

Klassen, A. C, Smith, A. L., Meissner, H. I., Zobora, J., Curbow, B., & Mandelbatt, J. (2002). If we gave away mammograms, who would get them? A neighborhood evaluation of a no-cost breast cancer screening program. *Preventive Medicine, 34*(1), 13–21.

Liller, K. D., Craig, J., Crane, N., & McDermott, R. J. (1998). Evaluation of a poison prevention lesson for kindergarten and third grade students. *Injury Prevention, 4*, 218–221.

Metcalf, C. E. (1997). The advantage of experimental designs for evaluating sex education programs. *Children and Youth Services Review, 19*, 507–523.

Manalo, V., & Meezan, W. (2000). Toward building a typology for the evaluation of services in family support programs. *Child Welfare, 79*, 405–429.

Nicklas, T. A., & O'Neil, C. E. (2000) Process of conducting a 5-a-day intervention with high school students: Gimme 5 (Louisiana). *Health Education and Behavior, 27*, 301–212.

Resnicow, K., Braithwaite, R., Diloria, C., Vaughn, R., Cohen, M. I., & Uhl, G. (2001). Preventing substance abuse in high risk youth: Evaluation challenges and solutions. *Journal of Primary Prevention, 21*, 399–415.

Rosenberg, D., & Handler, A. (1998). Analytic epidemiology and multivariate methods. In A. Handler, D. Rosenberg, C. Monahan, & J. Kennelly, (Eds.), *Analytic methods.* Washington, DC: Maternal and Child Health Bureau, Health Resources and Services Administration, Department of Health and Human Services.

Rossi, P. H., Freeman, H. E., & Lipsey, M. W. (1999). *Evaluation: A systematic approach* (6th ed.). Thousand Oaks, CA: Sage Publications.

Simpson, L., Korenbrot, C., & Greene, J. (1997). Outcomes of enhanced prenatal services for Medicaid-eligible women in public and private settings. *Public Health Reports, 112*, 122–132.

Tukey, J. W. (1977). *Exploratory data analysis.* Reading, MA: Addison-Wesley.

Walker, C. C. (2000). An educational intervention for hypertension management in older African Americans. *Ethnicity and Disease, 10*, 165–174.

CHAPTER 11

Analyzing and Interpreting Evaluation Data

Patton (1997) suggested that during the development of the evaluation plan, evaluators develop a hypothetical data template: a set of hypothetical data that might result from the collection of evaluation data. Based on these hypothetical data, the evaluators then ask the stakeholders what they would want to know from that data and what actions or decisions they would make based on the findings. This mind exercise serves two functions. It allows the evaluator to educate the stakeholders with regard to the evaluation design, and it helps establish realistic expectations regarding the findings of the evaluation. Then, when data analysis is in progress and the stakeholders are involved in interpreting the data, they are better prepared to understand the data and its limitations. Patton's advice extends the involvement of the stakeholders from the program planning into its evaluation.

Needless to say, both stakeholders and evaluators will be focused on whether the program makes a difference. Program impact evaluations are essentially efforts to identify whether a significant degree of change occurred among program participants, compared to the rest of the target audience. Attention to the design of the impact evaluation, the sample selection, and the methods used to collect data provides the foundation for the subsequent statistical tests and the overall trustworthiness of the statistical findings. This chapter provides a rudimentary review of statistical tests and is not intended to duplicate material available in statistical textbooks. The focus is on the relationship of the statistical test to the design and sample, with an emphasis on understanding the implications of the statistical results in terms of program impact and outcome.

DATA ENTRY AND MANAGEMENT

If the evaluation method called for collection of data, those data will need to be computerized. If the data were collected on paper, as is often the case in survey methods, then the paper responses need to be entered into a computer database or spreadsheet in order to conduct statistical analyses. The software to be used for data analysis must be chosen before data entry begins. Be assured that given the computing capacity of today's computers and the size of computer memory, desktop computers can accommodate evaluation data sets of all but the largest and longest surveys. A consideration in the choice of statistical software must be the sustainability of the evaluation. If program staff and stakeholders are expected to be involved in the data entry and analysis, then their computer skills and interests need to be considered in choosing software. For the majority of program evaluations done by agencies, most of the widely used spreadsheets and database programs are adequate and convenient, particularly because such software is included in software packages like Microsoft Office or Lotus Office Suite.

The convention for entering data into a spreadsheet is that each row represents a person (a participant in the evaluation), and each column represents one variable. A variable, simply put, is one survey question, one item of data or information. Each column must contain no more than one discrete, distinct question. If a question contains several items with yes or no responses, each item is actually a question. In this way, the number of yes and no responses for each item can be counted. Setting up the spreadsheet is a crucial component of data management.

If the evaluation plan calls for outsourcing the data analysis, entering the data into a standard spreadsheet is recommended. The data files can then be read by more sophisticated commercial statistical software. The commercially available statistical software programs, such as SPSS©, Systat©, and SAS©, are increasingly user-friendly and marketed widely to larger organizations interested in ongoing evaluations and data management. These statistical software programs include components that facilitate highly complex statistical tests that are not built into the usual office applications. Another choice is to use free statistical shareware, such as EpiInfo. EpiInfo is downloadable from the Internet and is offered free through the Centers for Disease Control and Prevention. It is particularly helpful for program evaluations in which relative risks and odds ratios need to be calculated. Because it was designed to be used internationally and to be compatible with as many systems as possible, it will look a bit out of date to some users. However, its ease of use and inclusion of statistics needed for some health program evaluations can make it an appropriate statistical software choice.

Data management includes not only the choice of software but the management of the flow of paper and the oversight of the electronic files. The paper flow issues include tracking data entry, storing original paper questionnaires and consent forms, and destroying paper records. A rule of thumb is that paper ought to be kept for as long as the evaluation is active and until the final report has been distributed. This rule also applies to the electronic files. Of course, creating backup files and having a standard procedure for naming the files are mandatory.

A critical step that can take a noticeable amount of time and effort is data cleaning. This involves checking the data for obvious errors. Data cleaning is important because without good data, the statistical results are meaningless. Data cleaning can be minimized by good planning during the development of the instrument or questionnaire and careful adherence to the data collection procedures.

Data cleaning begins with reviewing the frequency distributions of all variables. First, look for values that do not seem reasonable or plausible, such as a participant's age being 45 when the program is for adolescents and is based in a regular high school, or a negative value for the number of days in a program that was calculated based on subtracting dates. If an unrealistic value is found, the next step is to review the data for the individual and determine whether the data were incorrectly entered, the value is plausible, or the value is so unlikely that the data ought to be considered as missing. Keeping an incorrect value can drastically alter the mean, standard deviation, and subsequent statistical tests.

The data also need to be reviewed for skip patterns, that is, systematic nonresponses to items on a questionnaire. If specific items have low response rates, then their use in subsequent analyses is called into question. As with unreasonable values, including an item with a low response rate has statistical implications. Including items that have missing data decreases the total number of respondents included in any analyses that include that item. This can result in distorted and unstable statistics.

Outliers

Outliers are those variables with reasonable and plausible but extraordinary values; they lie outside the normal, or at the extreme ends on the tails of a distribution curve. Outlying values can occur due to errors in the measures or instruments, data entry errors, or unusual but accurate data. A common example of outliers in health care is the one or two patients with extremely high hospitalization costs or lengths of stay, such as that for a very low birth weight infant or an individual with a rare but serious complication from a procedure.

Authors of statistical tests warn of the effects on statistical results when outliers are included (Kleinbaum & Kupper, 1978; Pedhazur & Pedhazur-Schmelkin, 1991). Outliers dramatically influence the statistical tests by shifting the mean and increasing the variance. Although there are complex statistical methods to correct for the effects of outliers, these methods are more than most program evaluations need to do. Essentially, evaluators need to decide whether to keep the outlier in the analysis or to exclude the outlier based on some defensible rationale. The rationale for exclusion is often based on determining some cut-off point for the values to be excluded. The decision to include or exclude an outlier is made on a case-by-case basis. One factor that can influence the decision is the sample size in the evaluation study. Statistics based on smaller samples will be more dramatically affected by outliers. For example, an evaluation of change in serum lipid levels studied 20 people. If one person had a decrease of over 50% while everyone else had a decrease of between 0% and 10%, the average percentage decrease would be larger than if that one individual was excluded. However, if data from 200 people were collected, with the same range in decrease, the one 50% individual would have less effect on the average decrease.

Linked Data

Linked data refers to the data set that results from collecting data from more than one source, such that a wide range of information is available on the subjects in the data set, whether the subjects are individuals, neighborhoods, or states. The types of data that are linked for health program evaluation can include survey data with survey data, vital records data with survey data, vital records data with population surveys, survey data with administrative data, or population survey data with population survey data. The use of linked data may be necessary if the evaluation question focuses on outcomes on which data exist from a variety of sources.

Linked data can be helpful throughout the stages of program planning and evaluation, from community assessment to outcome evaluation. The most common reason to use linked data is to connect program participation or impact data with outcome data. The study by Reichman and Hade (2001) is an example of linking participation data with outcome data; they matched a list of participants in a prenatal program with birth data from vital records in order to evaluate the outcome of the program. Another reason to use linked data is to associate program impact data with services utilization (process) data, as was done by Chamberlayne et al. (1998). There is one other reason to use linked data; to validate self-report responses. For example, Robinson, Young, Roos, and Gelskey (1997) linked heath insurance administrative data about individual patients with the self-report from those individuals regarding chronic health conditions. This strategy does, however, leave the evaluator with the dilemma of deciding which data to believe and use.

The basic steps involved in linking data are simple, although their implementation is often far from simple. First, the data sets to be merged need to be in compatible software files. As software has become more standardized, it has become easier to create data files that are compatible. Nonetheless, software compatibility must be checked before beginning. Second, it is necessary to have variables about the individuals that are the same in both data sets. In other words, there needs to be a set of variables that are the same in both data sets, and those variables must relate to only one individual. These are called the matching variables. Thus, each file needs to be checked for matching variables. Third, matching variables are used as the criteria for linking the data from each file and merging the data into one file.

There are two major issues associated with using linked data: confidentiality and accuracy. For the majority of health program evaluations, data about individuals will be linked. This requires that some unique identifiers of the individual exist in both data sets, such as date of birth, social security number, or medical record number. Having data that identifies individuals with their data can raise ethical concerns. There must be strict, comprehensive, and careful procedures to remove the unique identifiers after the data files have been merged. Accuracy can be an issue in terms of correctly linking the files so that all the data for a person are actually about that person. Achieving accurately linked files requires using a complex algorithm of matching variables. For example, if there are two Mary Smiths in the files, birth date and marital status may be needed to distinguish between them in order to accurately link the files.

SAMPLE DESCRIPTION

Once the data are clean, the statistical analyses can begin. Always begin the analysis with a careful examination of the sample or samples by reviewing frequency statistics on each group (participants only, control group only) for any obvious unexpected differences. If the frequencies appear to be as expected, proceed to statistical comparisons. If any frequencies are not as might be expected, the data need to be more carefully reviewed. For example, if the mean age for the participants looks considerably higher than for the control group, test whether there is a statistical difference. For more sophisticated program evaluations, the evaluator will want to statistically compare the participants and the control groups on basic demographic variables. This can be important as a means of convincing stakeholders and others that the differences found in the evaluation are not related to demographic differences—in other words, that the participants were representative of the population from which they were selected. This speaks to the generalizability of the results and the external validity of the evaluation. If there are statistically significant differences between the participants and the control group, they need to be acknowledged. This speaks to the trustworthiness of the evaluator. It may be important to then consider using those demographic factors in subsequent analyses in order to diminish their influence on the statistical findings about the effect of the program.

THINKING ABOUT CHANGE

A valuable starting point is to ask what constitutes change and which approach to finding change is indicated by the overall evaluation methodology. In terms of program impact evaluation, change is a measure of a difference, either between an initial state before and a designated final state after the program, or between the group that received the program and the group that did not receive the program (Exhibit 11.1). Essentially, the net program effect is the degree of intervention effect on participants compared to the

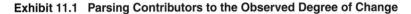

Exhibit 11.1   Parsing Contributors to the Observed Degree of Change

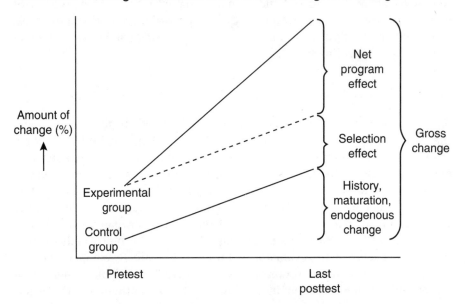

Adapted from Green, L. W., & Lewis, F. M. (1986). *Measurement and evaluation in health education and health promotion.* Palo Alto, CA: Mayfield Publishing.

effect on the comparison group, given the amount of error due to the design and measures used (all those validity issues). Under ideal conditions, there would be no design bias or measurement error, and thus the amount of difference between the participants and the comparison group would be the true amount of change from the program. However, real conditions make it more difficult to know the true and complete amount of change attributable to the program. There are knowable, and hence measurable, but not controllable factors that influence the amount of difference or change that is statistically found, such as growth or aging and recent media reports. In other words, media reports might influence study participants to change a behavior, in which case the change could not be attributed to the program. There are also unknowable or unanticipated, and hence unmeasured, factors that can influence the amount of difference or change that is statistically found, such as sudden disasters, epidemics, and policy changes. In other words, statistical findings are only as accurate and trustworthy as the design and measurement allow.

Limits of Finding Change

One particularly difficult problem, particularly for a population-focused program, is that behavioral change in the population follows the diffusion of innovation curve (Rogers, 1983). Innovations, as new and novel ideas or products, become adopted over time by a greater number of people. This process is referred to as the diffusion through the population of the innovation. The problem is that the higher the prevalence of the behavior before the program, the more difficult it becomes to increase the prevalence of the behavior. This seeming paradox is captured in the Effectiveness Index (EI) of Hovland, Lumsdaine, and Scheffield (1949) as cited in Green and Lewis's book (1986). This index compares the percentage of a population with the behavior after the program (% post) to the percentage of the population with the behavior before the program (% pre):

$$\text{Effectiveness Index (EI)} = \frac{\%\,\text{post} - \%\,\text{pre}}{100 - \%\,\text{pre}}$$

When the percentage after the program (% post) is higher than the baseline percentage (% pre), the index gives higher scores as the baseline percentage increases. In general, a higher EI is better. Take two communities in which the absolute change from pre-program to post-program is 10 units (Exhibit 11.2). In the community of Rosette, 30 percent have healthy behavior A after the program and 20 percent of the population had healthy behavior A—say, exercising—before the program, yielding an EI of (30 − 20 / 100 − 20), or 0.13. This is lower

Exhibit 11.2   Calculation of Effectiveness and Adequacy Indices: An Example

Category	Communities		Interpretation
	Rosette	**Blanchett**	
Pre-program	20	70	Baseline or control values
Post-program	30	80	Outcome values
Target rate or value	90	90	Value established as objective or desirable
Pre to post change	$30 - 20 = 10$	$80 - 70 = 10$	Unadjusted amount of change or difference
Effectiveness Index	$\dfrac{30 - 20}{100 - 20} = 0.13$	$\dfrac{80 - 70}{100 - 70} = 0.33$	Standardized measure of change; allows comparison of change across similar programs
Effectiveness Ratio	$\dfrac{30 - 20}{90 - 20} = 0.14$ or 14%	$\dfrac{80 - 70}{90 - 70} = 0.50$ or 50%	Ratio of actual to planned impact; reveals that the selection of the target rate influences interpretation of effectiveness
Target Adequacy Index	$\dfrac{30}{90} = 0.33$ or 33%	$\dfrac{90}{90} = 0.89$ or 89%	Level of adequacy in reaching target; reveals how close the community is to reaching the target value
Absolute Target Adequacy Index	$1 - \dfrac{90 - 30}{90 - 20}$ $= 1 - 0.86$ $= 0.14$ or 14%	$1 - \dfrac{90 - 80}{90 - 50}$ $= 1 - 0.50$ $= 0.50$ or 50%	Percentage gap between target and achievement addressed by program (Note: 0.86 and 0.50 reveal the amount of gap remaining to be addressed)

than in the community of Blanchett, where 80 percent exercise after the program and 70 percent exercise before the program (EI = 80 − 70 / 100 − 70 = 0.33). Higher baseline or pre-program percentages make it increasingly difficult to achieve a higher Effectiveness Index. This can be called a ceiling effect. The importance of this ceiling effect in terms of the adoption of behaviors in populations is that it becomes more difficult to get incremental proportions of a population to change as the behavior becomes more prevalent. In other words, programs become less effective at achieving change when the behavior is more prevalent before the program begins. One shortcoming of the Effectiveness Index is that it does not take into account the desired level, as might be reflected in the impact or outcome objectives.

Mohr (1992) addresses this issue. He argues that a simple difference score between the participants and nonparticipants (or between pre-scores and post-scores or rates) does not provide information on how effective the program was in terms of whether it was weak or strong. As an alternative, one might consider the Effectiveness Ratio:

$$\text{Effectiveness Ratio} = \frac{\text{post-score} - \text{pre-score}}{\text{target score} - \text{pre-score}}$$

The target score (or value) is the level that the program intended to achieve. This would be derived directly from the impact or outcome objectives. Thus, in Rosette, the exercise program reached 14% of its target, whereas Blanchette reached 50% of its target rate. The Effectiveness Ratio still does not help explain the extent to which the program addressed the health problem—in this example, the lack of exercising. For many health problems, the programs are designed to address gaps or disparities in health status. The aim of the program is to reduce the gap that exists. To estimate the extent to which the gap remains, the Absolute Target Adequacy Index can be calculated as follows:

$$\text{Target Adequacy Index} = 1 - \left(\frac{\text{target score} - \text{post-score}}{\text{target score} - \text{pre-score}} \right)$$

The shortcoming of such an approach is that it does not take into account the baseline (pre-score) rate. It does, however, facilitate reaching a standard target rate, such as the *Healthy People 2010* objectives, across programs and can highlight the absolute gap between the target and current levels of achievement.

An evaluator might want to describe how effective the program was in achieving healthy behavior A. This is estimated by subtracting the Adequacy Ratio from 1. This reveals that in Rosette, the program was 14% effective, whereas it was 50% effective in Blanchett. The point is that reducing gaps or disparities between the target value and the post-program value can be difficult. The evaluator might use this type of impact evaluation data to assist in revising target objectives and raising awareness of the difficulty in achieving the target objectives.

The effectiveness of a program can also be thought of in terms of the efficacy of the program. Abelson (1995) proposed that the causal efficacy of an intervention could be estimated as the effect size given the cause size. Stated as a formula that incorporates the effect size, the mean value of the dependent variable for both the experimental (mean e) and control/comparison (mean c) groups, given the causal size, the amount of the intervention for each group, is as follows:

$$\text{Causal efficacy} = \frac{\text{mean } e - \text{mean } c}{\text{amount of intervention } e - \text{amount of intervention } c}$$

The causal efficacy provides an alternative insight into the amount of effort for the amount of change observed. If there is a large effect size (50 − 20, for example) but little causal size (1 − 0), the causal efficacy is larger (30) than if the effect size is smaller (30 − 20, for example), but the causal size is larger (10 − 0). Thus, a higher causal efficacy index indicates more "bang for the buck" or amount of change for the amount of intervention. One might say that a "better" effect theory ought to lead to a higher causal efficacy index, and in this way the causal efficacy index helps interpret the overall usefulness or accuracy of the effect theory in light of some hard numbers.

Clinical and Statistical Significance

The presence of statistical significance does not necessarily equate to practical or clinical significance. An excellent example is the statistically significant increase in birth weight frequently found in a variety of prenatal programs. However, the amount of additional weight is often in the range of 5 to 10 grams, which is very minor and not clinically important. Statistical significance indicates the likelihood that one would get the result by pure chance, whereas clinical significance relates to the likelihood that the intervention will have a noticeable benefit to participants. Impact evaluations of health programs ideally seek to establish both the statistical and clinical significance of the program. Statistical significance also may not directly translate into practical importance, as is the case in making programmatic or policy decisions. For these reasons, the discussion of statistical analysis, and the associated tables located in Exhibits 11.7 and 11.8, distinguish between significance tests and tests that indicate the degree of effect due to the program.

ACROSS LEVELS OF ANALYSIS

Many health programs are designed to affect not individuals, but units of individuals, such as families, schools within a district, or work units within an agency. Data are then collected about the units such that questions on a questionnaire use phrases like "in our family," "in my school," or "in my department." In order to analyze the data collected from individuals about a unit, it is necessary to aggregate the data. Aggregation means summarizing data across the participants within one nested unit to create a variable at the unit level of analysis. The advantage of using aggregated data is that a different pattern exists for aggregates. Thus, the evaluator is able to describe the characteristics of the aggregates, make comparisons across aggregates rather than across individuals, and identify associations between characteristics of the aggregate and program or other variables. Epidemiological patterns can be more noticeable when comparisons of aggregates are done. For example, comparing data about different schools or work sites may provide more useful information than focusing on individuals. Although the aggregation of data is a fairly common community or public health approach, it can be viewed as being contrary to the clinical approach, in which each individual's data are most highly valued. In fact, however, neither aggregated nor individual-level analysis is right or wrong; each results in different information about programmatic impacts.

If the evaluation is focused on an aggregate, such as family, community, population, or work unit, the first step in aggregation is to analyze the data from the perspective of the within-unit variable. If those within the unit are more like one another than they are like the rest of the sample—in other words, if there is a low amount of variability among those within the unit— then it is acceptable to create a score per unit by aggregating their data to form a unit-level variable. The unit is then statistically considered to be one individual participant, one subject. Different statistical tests, such as the intraclass correlation (ICC) or the eta squared, are used to determine the validity of aggregating the data (Blise, 2000). The use and interpretation of these complex statistical tests will require statistical consultation and guidance. The important point is that statistical procedures for dealing with and analyzing aggregated data exist and may be appropriate for impact evaluations that are closer to the research end of the continuum.

If the analysis focuses on a health outcome and a characteristic of a unit (such as a school, a department, or a community), it is possible that it will find a higher correlation among the units than among the individuals. This is an ecological correlation. Black (1999) stressed that these ecological correlations are important to consider in terms of the intent of the research. The correlation between units is acceptable as a finding if the intervention was aimed at the unit and the impact being assessed was at the unit level. However, if the evaluation was intended to identify changes in participants across units, then the analysis should remain at the individual level.

In summary, statistical analysis of effect evaluation data follows all the conventions of statistical analysis of research data. Evaluators need to be ever cognizant of the interplay between how the health program is delivered, how the evaluation data are collected, and the choice of statistical tests. A word of caution is in order at this point. If much data have been collected and the statistical tests first used to assess for a change revealed no program effect, there will be an inclination to begin data dredging. Data dredging is the process of continuing to analyze the data in ways not originally planned—in other words, looking and looking and looking until some significant finding is unearthed. Data dredging will eventually yield statistically significant findings merely by chance. Therefore, unnecessary additional statistical tests ought to be avoided.

STATISTICAL ANSWERS TO THE QUESTION

Before statistical analysis is performed, it is important to review the program impact objectives and the purpose and questions of the impact evaluation. The impact evaluation questions help keep the analysis focused and thus minimize the inclination to go searching for significant findings. Staying close to the evaluation questions also assures that the concerns of the stakeholders are addressed first. Choosing the best statistical procedure and tests can quickly resemble a guessing game. This review is not intended as a comprehensive discussion of basic statistical principles; rather, it emphasizes the practical relationship between evaluation question and statistical test. The purpose of this section is to provide guidelines for choosing statistical tests and decreasing the guesswork involved. Given that spreadsheet and database software makes doing the mathematical calculations quite easy, it is imperative to have a framework for choosing the best and most appropriate statistical test.

Exhibit 11.3 lists a set of questions that need to be answered to arrive at an appropriate statistical analysis plan. At least three factors influence the statistical choice: type of design, level of measurement, and level of analysis. The interaction among these three dimensions is illustrated by the graphic representation of a cube (Exhibit 11.4). Based on the answers to these questions, a statistical analysis plan that takes into consideration complex and interactive factors can be developed. Unfortunately, two dimensions could not be shown on the cube. The fourth dimension is the level at which the programmatic

Exhibit 11.3   Factors that Affect the Choice of a Statistical Test: Questions to Be Answered

1. What is the focus of the evaluation question: comparison, association among variables, or prediction of outcomes?
2. What level of analysis will be used: individual, aggregate, or population?
3. What level of measurement was used for the dependent variables and for the independent variables: nominal, ordinal, or interval/ratio?

    3a. If interval/ratio measures were used, do the data have a parametric or nonparametric distribution?

4. What type of design was used: experimental, nonexperimental, quasi-experimental with one group, quasi-experimental with two or more groups, or quasi-experimental with other design?
5. Were data collected on a sample or a population?
6. What is the interest and capacity of the stakeholders with regard to understanding statistical analyses?

Exhibit 11.4   Three (of Five) Dimensions Influencing the Choice of a Statistical Test

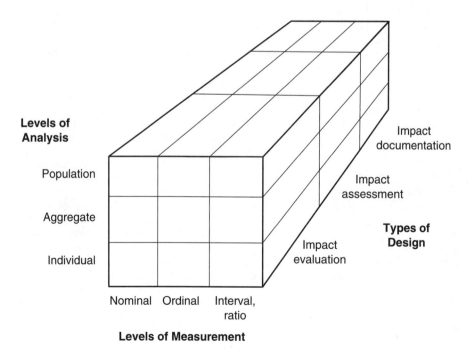

Levels of Analysis

Population

Aggregate

Individual

Impact documentation

Impact assessment

Impact evaluation

Types of Design

Nominal   Ordinal   Interval, ratio

Levels of Measurement

intervention was delivered, be that at the individual, aggregate, population, or infrastructure level. The fifth dimension is the complexity of the evaluation question in terms of the focus of the analysis. For the purposes of this discussion, the focus of the analysis refers to whether the impact evaluation is seeking to answer questions about a comparison of groups, associations among two or more variables, or the prediction of possible impacts and outcomes. This review of statistical data analysis is organized by those three dominant foci of impact and outcome evaluations.

With the level of intervention and level of analysis as two dimensions, the possible foci of analysis can be assigned (Exhibit 11.5). This table is based on the assumption that the evaluation data were collected at the same level as that of the program intervention. A careful look at Exhibit 11.5 reveals that

Exhibit 11.5   Analysis Procedures by Level of Intervention and Level of Analysis*

Level of Analysis (Effect)	Level of Intervention (Program)			
	Individual	Aggregate	Population	Infrastructure
Individual	Comparison tests Association tests Prediction tests	If individuals can be identified, then: Comparison tests Association tests	If individuals can be identified, then: Comparison tests Association tests	If individuals can be identified, then: Comparison tests Association tests
Aggregate	[not directly testable]	Comparison tests Association tests Prediction tests	If subgroups can be identified, then: Comparison tests Association tests	If subgroups can be identified, then: Comparison tests Association tests
Population	[not directly testable]	[not directly testable]	Comparison tests Association tests Prediction tests	Comparison tests Association tests Prediction tests
Infrastructure	[not directly testable]	[not directly testable]	Comparison tests Association tests Prediction tests	Comparison tests Association tests Prediction tests

* This table assumes that the data were collected at the same level.

statistical tests of comparison and association can be used widely and that prediction tests are recommended only when the level of intervention and the level of analysis are the same. In addition, analyses cannot be done at levels at which the data are more discrete (lower) than the level at which the programmatic intervention was delivered; hence, the blank cells.

In discussions of the types of statistical analyses that are appropriate for comparison, association, and prediction, a useful distinction is the difference between analysis procedure, measure of magnitude, and test for significance. This distinction is rarely emphasized in statistical textbooks. The essential question for impact and outcome evaluations is how much difference the program made, or how strongly the program was related to the effects. Measures of magnitude answer this question. In contrast, the question of whether the difference was more than would happen by chance is answered with tests of statistical significance. For each measure of magnitude, there is a corresponding test of significance. Both Aday (1991) and Newcomer (1994) draw attention to the importance of knowing both the magnitude and significance when evaluating programs.

Description

The first step in any statistical analysis focuses on description. Descriptive statistics, also called exploratory data analysis or univariate statistics, yield information of the most basic nature, such as frequency counts and percentages. Descriptive statistics can be generated with all types of data, regardless of the design. They answer evaluation questions such as, What were the demographic characteristics of program participants and comparison groups? How well did program participants do on the pre-test and on the post-test? and What percentage of the population benefited from the program? When the data are ordinal/rank and ratio/interval type data, descriptive statistics can include measures of central tendency (mean, mode, and median) and measures of variation (range, variance, and standard deviation). These measures were reviewed in Chapter 4 on community assessment. Spreadsheet and database software enable conducting descriptive statistics, and the results can be displayed easily with the associated graphics.

The central tendency and variation of variables need to be reviewed and understood because they are the foundation for further statistical analyses. The review of the variance needs to determine whether the variance is similar in the experimental and control groups. This information helps select the appropriate statistical tests for comparisons and correlations. Do not underestimate the power and information contained in simple descriptive statistics

(Tukey, 1977), nor the ease with which most stakeholders can understand them. Spend time reviewing the results of the descriptive statistics, because the distribution of values often gives the first understanding of a program's participants and effects. Also, because the statistics for each variable are reviewed, insights into unique characteristics of participants or unexpected distributions can be identified. Such observations may lead to additional, and sometimes unplanned, analyses.

Another reason to generate descriptive statistics is to assess whether the data are normally distributed. Data collected at the nominal or ordinal levels of measurement can be used only in nonparametric statistical tests. Data collected at the interval or ratio level of measurement and whose distribution follows the normal distribution curve are called parametric. However, if the interval or ratio level data are not normally distributed, nonparametric statistical tests must be used. Exhibit 11.6 summarizes the major nonparametric and parametric statistical tests that are used for comparison, association, and prediction. The type of evaluation design used is one factor in determining which types of tests are appropriate. Notably, prediction statistics are used with an impact assessment or, preferably, an impact evaluation design.

Exhibit 11.6   Types of Statistical Analysis by Type of Data and Complexity of Question Asked

Type of Data	Complexity of Question About Effect		
	Comparison	*Association*	*Prediction*
Parametric	Difference scores Tests of difference	Variance analyses (ANOVA, ANCOVA) Hierarchical analyses	Time series Regression analyses Logistic regression analyses
Nonparametric	Chi-square tests based on contingency tables	Odd ratio Relative risk Other (i.e., Sign test, Wilcoxon, Kruskal-Wallis)	Log linear regression analyses

Comparisons

Comparison questions typically ask for a within-group comparison: whether baseline (pre-test) scores are different from the follow-up (post-test). Comparison questions can also ask for a between-groups comparison: whether program participants are different from nonparticipants (control group). These comparison questions can be posed at the individual level of analysis as well as at the aggregate and population levels. Exhibit 11.7 summarizes the major types of comparison analysis procedures that are appropriate for each level of measurement. Of course, the level of analysis and whether the variables are parametric will influence the final choice of statistical procedure.

Comparisons between groups using only nominal data (for both the impact variable and any independent variable) are done with one of the various versions of the chi-square test, such as the McNemar or Cochran Q tests.

Exhibit 11.7   Main Types of Comparison Analyses Used, by Level of Analysis

Level of Measurement	Comparison-Focused Analyses		
	Tests of Differences	**Strength of Difference**	**Tests of Significance**
Nominal data	Difference scores Chi-square tests based on contingency tables (i.e., McNemar, Fisher exact)	% or mean difference Phi coefficient, Cramer's V, Lambda	*t* test
Ordinal data	ANOVA, ANCOVA	Eta	*Z* test *F* test
Interval data	*t* test (independent sample) Paired *t* test (related sample)	Eta	*Z* test

Whether the groups are related or matched and how many groups are compared (Black, 1999, p. 436) can make a difference in which statistic is optimal. Between-group questions addressed with such analyses involve some version of whether participants are statistically more likely to have characteristic x compared to nonparticipants.

If parametric data are available, and randomly assigned groups were used, then one of the analysis of variance (ANOVA) tests and corresponding F statistic is appropriate. ANOVA tests are used when the evaluation design involved random selection or assignment. The extent to which the groups vary from each other is assessed with one of the ANOVA tests. Evaluation questions that focus on whether groups differ significantly on independent variables, such as antecedent and determinant factors, and dependent variables, namely the health outcome of interest, can be answered using ANOVA. These tests are particularly germane to aggregate-level data and analyses.

Some questions in health program evaluations focus on comparing populations, such as the Behavioral Risk Factor Surveillance Survey (BRFSS) scores in different states or the percentage screened for cholesterol in the past month. These simple comparisons are done with the same statistical tests used with individual-level data. However, because the population rather than a sample is used, slightly different equations are involved.

Association

Most evaluations aspire to answer more than comparative questions. Questions about the relationship or association among variables are asked, such as whether receiving more interventions is related to a greater amount of change or whether the amount of change is associated with a specific characteristic of the program participants. Correlational statistics or other statistics of association do not provide information on the temporal sequence of variables and therefore do not provide information about causation. Instead, correlational analyses indicate the strength of the relationship and whether the relationship is such that the variables vary directly or inversely. An inverse relationship between the variables, such as increasing age and decreasing tissue resilience, is indicated by a negative correlation.

Exhibit 11.8 provides a summary of the main tests of association that are used. To choose the appropriate statistical test, one must consider the level of measurement, as always, along with the parametric character and the number of groups used in the analysis. Exhibit 11.9 provides an example of the tests of the strength of association that could be used with data at different levels of measurement. Based on a hypothetical program evaluation of a construction

Exhibit 11.8 Main Types of Association Analyses Used, by Level of Analysis

Level of Measurement	Association-Focused Analyses		
	Tests of Association	Strength of Association	Tests of Significance
Nominal data	Fisher's exact, x^2	Relative Risk, Cramer's V, Lambda	Confidence Intervals t test, F test
Ordinal data	x^2 Analysis of variance	Kruskal's gamma, Kendall's tau, Spearman rank correlation	F test F test
Interval data	Multiple regression analyses (independent samples), multiple regression of difference scores (related samples)	Pearson's correlation coefficient, biserial and partical correlation	F test Confidence interval

work-site safety program, the dependent variables are ICD-9 for injury, rank of number of injuries, and number of sick days, and the independent variables are the race of the workers, the rank in size of the construction site, and the number of hours of safety education. Exhibit 11.10 continues with the work-site safety example and shows how the design of the evaluation further affects the statistical analysis plan.

At the individual level, in addition to contingency table analysis procedures for nonparametric data, correlational analyses are possible with parametric data. When the correlational analysis includes a copious number of variables, the likelihood increases that some pairs will be significantly related. Therefore, is it wise to lower the alpha, from p <.05 to p <.01 or <.001, to provide a more conservative statement about what was statistically significant. One approach to reducing the number of variables in the analysis is to exclude variables on a logical basis, such as ones that could not be related (i.e., hair color and height), or that were not included in the program logic model.

Exhibit 11.9   Example of Statistical Tests for Strength of Association by Level of Measurement, Using a Work-Site Safety Example

		Nominal	Ordinal	Interval/ Ratio
	Examples of Variables	*ICD-9 for injury*	*Rank among construction sites in number of injuries*	*Number of disability days*
Nominal	*Race of workers*	Cramer's C (two or more categories) Phi φ (if two dichotomous), x^2	x^2, Mann-Whitney	Student's *t* test, ANOVA, Kruskal-Wallis
Ordinal	*Rank among construction sites for size of project*		Spearman's rho, Kendall's tau, Spearman's rank order, Eta coefficient	Spearman's rank, linear regression
Interval/ Ratio	*Number of hours of work safety instruction*			Pearson's *r*, Multiple correlation coefficient, linear regression

Prediction

Questions about how much of an effect a programmatic intervention might have on individuals, aggregates, or populations are basically questions of causation. Causal questions are the most difficult to answer, despite the fact that most stakeholders want an answer to the most fundamental causal question: Did our program cause the health improvement? Exhibit 11.11 provides a summary of key statistics that can help predict future outcomes.

Exhibit 11.10 Statistical Tests by Evaluation Design and Variable Type, Using the Example of Workplace Injury

	Variables	Nominal by Nominal	Interval by Interval	Interval by Nominal
	Examples of Variables	ICD-9 for injury by race	Number of disability days at the construction site by hours of work safety instruction	Number of disability days at the construction site by race
Designs	*Examples of Designs*			
One group (i.e., pre and post)	One work site (i.e., pre-post)	x^2, goodness of fit	*t* test, *z* test	Point biserial Coefficient
Two groups, independent	Two work sites, different cities and different types of jobs	x^2, *k* by 2 tables	*t* test, one-way ANOVA	x^2
Two groups, related/matched	Two work sites, same construction company and type of job	McNemar change test	*t* test for related/ matched sample	McNemar

To answer causal questions, it is absolutely necessary to have data from a rigorous quasi-experimental/impact assessment or true experimental/impact evaluation design. In other words, answering causal questions is a matter not only of statistical analysis, but of design. Unless a design has been used that enables the evaluator essentially to eliminate alternate causes, the cause and effect relationship between the program and health impact cannot be substantiated. The statistics used for causal evaluation questions are essentially the same as those used for relationships and associations, except that the findings can be interpreted as causal rather than only as a relationship.

Exhibit 11.11   Main Types of Prediction Analyses Used, by Level of Analysis

Level of Measurement	Prediction-Focused Analyses		
	Test of Prediction	Measures of Magnitude	Tests of Significance
Nominal data	Probit regression analyses	Correlation coefficient (r^2)	F test
Ordinal data	Trend analyses	Correlation coefficient (r^2)	F test
Interval data	Time series, Regression-discontinuity, mulitiple regression	beta	F test Confidence intervals

One major variation on the basic correlational analysis is regression analysis, sometimes called trend analysis (Veany & Kaluzny, 1998). Regression analysis allows for prediction, in terms of extrapolation and interpolation, based on a best fit line (Black, 1999; Pedhazur & Pedhazur-Schmelkin, 1991). As a tool, regression analysis answers evaluation questions such as, How much more improvement might occur with more intervention? and As participant characteristics x_1 and x_2 increase, how much change will occur in the health outcome? Regression analysis is based on the correlation of independent variables with the dependent variable and on the strength of the association among independent variables. It is used to predict a trend in the relationship, hence the infamous regression line.

Time series analysis requires having data collected on the same sample, using the same measure, at multiple time points. Time series analyses, based on the multiple regression model, can be used with data such as the annual number of motor vehicle accidents, the monthly number of Medicare enrollees, the weekly number of infants diagnosed with ear infections, or, protypically, the daily closing value of the New York Stock Exchange. If a health program was provided that was expected to affect any of these numbers, then a time series analysis would provide insights into whether a change was observed in the pattern across time.

There are many health program evaluation questions that focus on changes across time, rather than on change at a single point in time among participants. This is often the case for evaluations of full-coverage programs, in which there might not be a control group. Typical across-time evaluation questions are, To what extent is there a decline in the health problem from year to year? and To what extent was there a change in the health outcome from before and after the program? To answer such questions, the design for data collection must include data collected from the same individuals, on the same variables, at multiple points in time. Analysis of the repeated measures collected from the same sample becomes complex because there will be an underlying association between the individual and the data; each data set is not independent of the subsequent data set because the same people provided the data. If the level of measurement is at the interval level, then multiple regression analyses are appropriate.

INTERPRETATION

Patton (1997, p. 314) suggested using nonstatistical comparisons in program evaluation as a means of assessing programs. Comparisons can be done with the statistical findings and any of the following: the program goals, the impact objectives, benchmarks from other programs, results of similar programs, professional standards regarding the health problem, and intuition or educated guesses. These less scientific but practical comparisons do provide insights into the relative success of the health program and may highlight general areas of success and inadequacy.

In any study, spurious findings and surprises can occur. A spurious finding is one that is incidental to the evaluation question or that is an artifact of the factors that are not understood. Spurious findings are generally curiosities that can be discounted as the result of measurement error and random chance. Surprise findings are also not related to the evaluation questions but cause one to say, "Hmmm" (Abelson, 1995). Surprise findings can be either in support of the health program interventions or not, as well as leading to new descriptive insights. For example, if the evaluation measured x, but the finding is that the average value of x is considerably higher or lower than in the literature or than common sense would dictate, then the evaluator has a surprise. Surprises can be used as a basis for further exploration or for making revisions to the program or to the evaluation plan. While not common, surprises are important and need to be valued and acknowledged, as they may lead to further questions and new knowledge.

Four Fallacies of Interpretation

Green and Lewis (1986) suggested that there are four types of errors that can occur when interpreting evaluation data. One fallacy is that of equating effectiveness with efficiency. Effectiveness is the extent to which results are achieved, whereas efficiency is a ratio of the amount of effort or resources to the amount of effect achieved. Another way to think of this fallacy is in terms of the cost per unit of health improvement. There may be a point of diminishing returns in terms of additional resources, and further efforts may not result in large gains in effect. The issue is how much more is required in the organizational or service utilization plan for each additional unit of effect from the program.

Another fallacy is in assuming that a constant rate of progress or health improvement will occur or has occurred. There can be many reasons for the rate of change to be variable or sporadic. For population-focused services, particularly mass media awareness campaigns, the diffusion of innovation curve (Rogers, 1983) will be evident if population adoption of a new behavior is part of the effect theory. Change also occurs at a variable rate depending on the characteristics of the recipient audiences.

The third fallacy is in assuming ongoing improvement, the inexorable forward movement of change. Program impacts can be affected by time, such as relapse, lack of reinforcement or followup, memory failure, and program dropouts. Any one of these or similar factors can cause the health problem or condition to return. The extent to which it is possible to identify ongoing improvement can be influenced by the timing of data collection relative to the expected beginning of the impact or outcome. There are at least five ways in which there can be a lack of forward movement in the degree of change; each can be visualized graphically, as shown in Exhibit 11.12. In Exhibit 11.12a, the change over time reflects a delayed change called a sleeper effect. In Exhibit 11.12b, the program effect is seen following the intervention, but then a gradual return to the baseline rate, known as backsliding, occurs. Sometimes (Exhibit 11.12c) anticipation of the intervention leads to adopting the behavior before the program has actually started (trigger effect). If there are factors involved that influence the rate irrespective of the program, this is reflected in historical effects (Exhibit 11.12d). Finally, there can be a backlash due to the program being discontinued, such that the long-term rates are worse than before the program began (Exhibit 11.12e).

The fourth fallacy is in underestimating the complexity of the change process. Behavioral change within individuals involves multiple stages (Prochaska, DiClemente, & Norcross, 1992) and is influenced by multiple factors. Similarly, achieving physical changes can be complex, involving medications and procedures

Exhibit 11.12 Five Ways That the Rate of Change Can Be Affected*

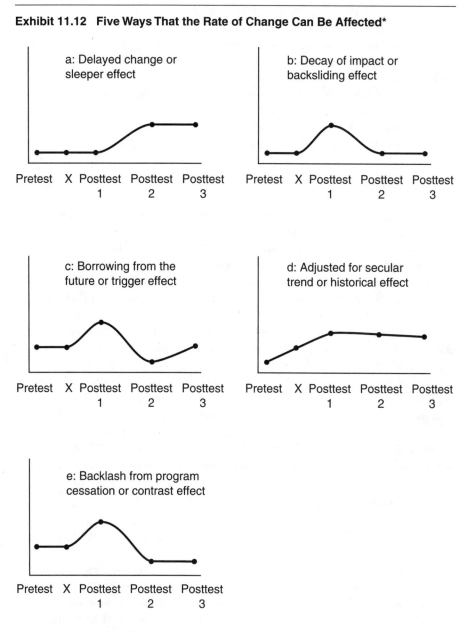

* X represents the point of program intervention.

Adapted from Green, L. W. & Lewis, F. M. (1986). *Measurement and evaluation in health education and health promotion.* Palo Alto, CA: Mayfield Publishing.

as well as behaviors. Underestimating the complexity inherent in achieving change in the target audience, whether individuals, families, communities, or organizations, can lead to oversimplification of the interpretation of the findings. In addition, what is noticed in the findings will be affected by what was articulated in the program effect theory, especially the theory of intervention, partially because the effect theory guides the decisions regarding what is measured and when. Therefore, better causal and intervention theories that explain or predict the change and possible factors contributing to either maintaining the status quo or changing are more likely to lead to an evaluation that can minimize this fallacy.

Ecological Fallacy

The ecological correlation mentioned earlier is not to be confused with ecological fallacy. Ecological fallacy has been an issue in program planning and evaluation for over twenty years (Milcarek & Link, 1981). It refers to the assumption that group characteristics apply to individuals within the group. For example, if a group of participants had an average of a high school education, the ecological fallacy would be to assume that any member of the group had a high school education. The ecological fallacy is one of interpreting the findings in a way that is not being completely truthful to the data. Within the group of participants, many may actually have college degrees and many may have only an 8th-grade education; this would yield an average of 12 years of school.

Richards, Gottfredson, & Gottfredson (1990) contrasted ecological fallacy with the individual differences fallacy, in which individual differences are assumed to apply to the group. Both fallacies stem from not being clear that data about one level of analysis do not translate exactly to data about other levels of analysis. Seiler and Alverez (2000) discussed ecological fallacy as it pertains to accurate risk assessment and to ecological studies of health effects.

ACROSS THE PYRAMID

At the direct services level of the public health pyramid, health programs are focused on individual change. Therefore, most of the analysis will revolve around identifying changes within subjects, such as changes in program participants, as shown in pre- and post-testing. Health programs at the direct services level are likely to be highly tailored and small. This leads to being concerned with having a sufficient sample size for statistical analysis. If the sample size is less than 30, the choice of statistical tests is affected. However, because it may be easier to identify nonparticipants in the program (controls), there may statistical tests that compare those groups.

At the enabling services level, health programs are focused on groups and changes evident in those groups. Issues related to levels of analysis begin to be of major importance at this level of the pyramid. If data from individuals within units, whether families, schools, social networks, or agencies, are to be aggregated, then statistical tests for within- and between-group variance need to be performed. Most of the data analysis needs to focus on identifying changes in the differences between groups based on aggregate data.

At the population-based level, it becomes more difficult to have nonparticipants. Therefore, it is more likely that statistical tests will involve trend analysis of population data or time series analysis. In some cases it may be possible to compare populations, such as counties or states. Because the population mean, and not just the mean of the sample, is known, a different set of statistical tests are possible.

At the infrastructure level, there are likely to be two major foci to the impact evaluation; one is on the change among participants who are part of the infrastructure, and the other is on the change in the population after the infrastructure change. In the first case, the statistical tests will depend on the design of the program. For example, public health workers in several different counties may receive the same training program. The analysis could be at the individual level of analysis and compare program participants with nonparticipants, or data from the workers might be aggregated to have a higher level of analysis, namely the county, and then compare participating counties with nonparticipating counties. If the impact evaluation was concerned with the health status of those served by the infrastructure, a trends analysis could be used to identify whether there was a change in the health status of county residents after the training program. These are just a few examples of the interaction between impact evaluation questions, design, and statistical analysis.

DISCUSSION QUESTIONS

1. What are the pros and cons of aggregating data to have a higher level of analysis? Under what conditions would aggregation be the preferred approach to handling the impact evaluation data?

2. Imagine that you have just been invited to become involved in an evaluation of a statewide health program. The program has components at each level of the public heath pyramid, such as a nutrition

program to increase fiber intake. The state has survey data from individuals who participated in a brief educational session, records data from a set of schools on the amount of high- and low-fiber foods that were purchased monthly for a year before and a year after the program was initiated, and rates of colon cancer. Develop a plan for the statistical analysis.

3. It is common for stakeholders to essentially ask, How can you prove that our program had an effect? What would be your standard, simple "sound bite" response to this question?

References

Abelson, R. P. (1995). *Statistics as principled argument.* Hillsdale, NJ: Lawrence Erlbaum Associates.

Aday, L. A. (1991). *Designing and conducting health surveys.* San Francisco: Jossey-Bass.

Black, T. R. (1999). *Doing quantitative research in the social sciences: An integrated approach to research design, measurement, and statistics.* London: Sage Publications.

Blise, P. D. (2000). Within-group agreement, non independence, and reliability. In K. Klein & S. Kozlowski (Eds.), *Multilevel theory, research and methods in organizations* (pp. 349–381). San Francisco: Jossey-Bass Publishers.

Chamberlayne, R., Green, B., Barer, M. L., Hertzman, C., Lawrence, W. J., & Sheps, S. B. (1998). Creating a population-based linked health database: A new resource for health services research. *Canadian Journal of Public Health, 89,* 270–271.

Green, L. W., & Lewis, F. M. (1986). *Measurement and evaluation in health education and health promotion.* Palo Alto, CA: Mayfield Publishing.

Hovland, C. F., Lumsdaine, A., & Scheffield, F. D. (1949). Experiments on mass communication. Cited in Green, L. W., & Lewis, F. M. (1986). *Measurement and evaluation in health education and health promotion.* Palo Alto, CA: Mayfield Publishing.

Kleinbaum, D., & Kupper, L. (1978). *Applied regression analysis and other multivariable methods.* Boston: Duxbury Press.

Milcarek, B. I., & Link, B. G. (1981). Handling problems of ecological fallacy in program planning and evaluation. *Evaluation & Program Planning, 4*(1), 23–28.

Mohr, L. B. (1992). *Impact analysis for program evaluation.* Newbury Park, CA: Sage Publications.

Newcomer, K. E. (1994). Using statistics appropriately. In J. Wholey, H. Hatry, & K. Newcomer (Eds.), *Handbook of practical program evaluation* (pp. 389–416). San Francisco, CA: Jossey-Bass Publishers.

Patton, M. Q. (1997). *Utilization-focused evaluation* (3rd ed.). Thousand Oaks, CA: Sage Publications.

Pedhazur, E., & Pedhazur-Schmelkin, L. (1991). *Measurement, design, and analysis: An integrated approach*. Hillsdale, NJ: Lawrence Erlbaum Associates.

Prochaska, J., Diclemente, C., & Norcross, J. (1992). In search of how people change: Applications of addictive behaviors. *American Psychologist, 47*(9), 1102–1114.

Reichman, N. E., & Hade, E. M. (2001). Validation of birth certificate data: A study of women in New Jersey's Healthy Start program. *Annuals of Epidemiology, 11*, 186–193.

Richards, J. M., Gottfredson, D. C., & Gottfredson, G. D. (1990). Units of analysis and item statistics for environmental assessment scales. *Current Psychology: Research and Reviews, 9*(4), 407–413.

Robinson, J. R., Young, T. K., Roos, L. L., & Gelskey, D. E. (1997). Estimating the burden of disease: Comparing administrative data and self-reports. *Medical Care, 35*, 932–937.

Rogers, E. M. (1983). *Diffusion of innovations* (3rd ed.). New York: The Free Press.

Seiler, F. A., & Alverez, J. L. (2000). Is the "ecological fallacy" a fallacy? *Human & Ecological Risk Assessment, 6*, 921–941.

Tukey, J. W. (1977). *Exploratory data analysis*. Reading, MA: Addison-Wesley.

Veany, J. E., & Kaluzny, A. D. (1998). *Evaluation and decision making for health services* (3rd ed.). Chicago: Health Administration Press.

CHAPTER 12

Qualitative Methods for Planning and Evaluation

Thus far, the approach to health program planning and evaluation has been essentially quantitative in nature. Numbers are used in the needs assessment, in budgeting and documenting the implementation of the service utilization plan, and to quantify the effect on individuals receiving the program. However, stories are equally valid and important in health program planning and evaluation. Therefore, this chapter presents qualitative designs and methods. Much has been written on ways to conduct qualitative research and on strategies to assure rigor in such research (Kirk & Miller, 1986; Lincoln & Guba, 1985; Strauss & Corbin, 1990), and there is no pretense of covering all that is currently known about it here. Like the chapters reviewing quantitative methods, this chapter reviews qualitative methods with particular emphasis on the use of these methods for health program planning and evaluation.

FUNCTIONS OF QUALITATIVE METHODS

The use of qualitative methods in planning and evaluation are appropriate throughout the planning and evaluation cycle. The six functions of qualitative methods, as summarized by Green and Lewis (1986), correspond to ways in which qualitative methods contribute throughout the health program planning and evaluation cycle. One way to use qualitative methods is to develop and delineate program elements before initiating a program—in other words, for program planning. Similarly, qualitative methods can help generate a theory, including a program theory, especially when a program theory is being developed based on existing program staff's theory-in-use. During the process monitoring phase, qualitative methods can take the place of quantitative methods, particularly for sensitive direct services type programs, and can broaden the observational field in terms of adding new types of information. During the impact and outcome evaluation phase, qualitative methods can enhance the explanatory power of quasi-experimental designs. Also, by providing analyses of processes and individual cases, qualitative data can help explain why or how impacts occurred. In other words, information from the qualitative data can be used to improve the effect theory upon which the program was based.

In addition, qualitative approaches give a voice, both literally and metaphorically, to stakeholders; this is important because they then feel valued. The act of speaking to someone and telling a story generates feelings that are substantively different from the feelings generated by responding to a survey questionnaire.

QUALITATIVE METHODS

The first challenge faced by evaluators and program planners is to select the best qualitative method to answer the questions at hand. Qualitative methods stem from various philosophical perspectives, each of which has influenced the development of the methodology. These underlying perspectives influence the evaluation questions that might be answered from that perspective (Exhibit 12.1). Thus, the choice of a qualitative method is based on whether it is the best method given the question being asked, with the understanding that several methods are applicable to more than one perspective (Exhibit 12.2). In the following sections, the major and most widely used qualitative methods are reviewed, with particular attention to how the method is useful in health program planning and evaluation. The benefits and challenges for each of the qualitative methods discussed here are summarized in Exhibit 12.3.

Case Study

A case study is an empirical inquiry into existing phenomena in their real-life contexts when the boundary between what is being studied and its context is not clearly evident. Typically, case studies use multiple sources of data (Yin, 1989). They also typically address questions of how or why something occurred, and there is no attempt to experimentally control what happens. The definition of a case is based on the question being asked, such that a case could be an individual, a classroom, an organization, a program, or an event. The case study methodology is particularly useful for getting insights into an entire program (Veney & Kaluzny, 1998) because the program is the unit of analysis, or case.

The methodology for conducting a case study was given by Yin (1989) and Stake (1995). They both argued that, as with any design, attention needs to be paid to the generation of the research question and rival hypotheses, and to

Exhibit 12.1 Comparison of Qualitative Perspectives with Regard to the Basic Question Addressed and Their Relevance to Health Program Planning and Evaluation

Perspective	Basic Question Addressed	Planning and Evaluation Relevance
Ethnography	What are the norms and values (culture)?	Participants' cultural patterns that contribute to the problem and acceptance of the program
Phenomenology	What does it mean to the person?	Participants' meaning of content and the problem being addressed
Critical analysis	How has power shaped it?	Participants' view of their ability to be in control of the health problem and the solutions; staff's view of their autonomy in improving the program
Grounded theory	What are the relationships (theory)?	Explanations that participants and staff have for the health problem and possible solutions
Content analysis	What themes are in the text?	Thoughts and perspectives revealed in the text and dialogues

the use of methods and techniques that enhance the scientific rigor of the study. Stake (2000) summarized the responsibilities of those doing case study research as being similar to the responsibilities involved in other qualitative methods, except that the first step in a case study is to circumscribe what is the case.

Generally, the issues of what constitutes the case to be studied are relatively straightforward for evaluators and planners. When one is considering the case study methodology for program process monitoring, the health program is the case. The issue of what constitutes a case becomes more complex in evaluations when multiple institutions or organizations are providing the intervention. This situation necessitates that the evaluator consider whether each organization is a case or whether the organization is the context for the

Exhibit 12.2   Comparison of Qualitative Perspectives with Regard to the Method Used

Perspective	Typical Method
Ethnography	Case study, participant observation, observations
Phenomenology	Individual in-depth interviews
Critical analysis	Individual in-depth interviews
Grounded theory	Individual in-depth interviews
Content analysis	Focus groups, survey with open-ended questions, narrative designs

program, thereby making each set of program staff and recipients the case. In contrast, for some impact evaluations, it may be important to view a select group of individual participants as cases, in order to refine the effect theory based on their experiences and processes of change.

A key feature of the case study methodology is the use of multiple sources of data. Typically, data collected as part of a case study include both primary data—generally interviews, observations of behavior, and survey data—and secondary data. Secondary data collection might include a review of agency or program documents, a review of existing data collected for other evaluation or program monitoring purposes, and a review of program-related materials, such as promotional materials, policies, and procedures. The case study then involves considering all these data to arrive at some answers to the evaluation question.

Examples of case studies used in program planning and evaluation can easily be found. From published reports, the value of case studies becomes evident. Goodman, Steckler, and Alciati (1997) used case study methodology to conduct a process evaluation of state agency programs that implemented the Data-Based Intervention Research program. This program was designed to build the state agency's capacity to translate research regarding cancer prevention into practice. Their decision to consider the four state programs as one case reveals the complexity of defining and selecting a case. Their report about capacity building around the implementation of cancer prevention and control programs also reinforces that program planning and evaluation occur at the

Exhibit 12.3   Summary of Benefits and Challenges to Using Qualitative Methods

Method	Key Benefits for Use in Planning and Evaluation	Key Challenges for Use in Planning and Evaluation
Case study	Allows for an understanding of context as an influence on the program or participant	Complex, overwhelming amount of data; definition of case
Observations	Can identify sequence of causes and effects; may identify new behaviors or events	Difficult to obtain reliable data unless one uses recording devices; sampling frame difficult to establish
Individual in-depth interviews	Provides rich insights into personal thoughts, values, meanings, and attributions	Identifying individuals who are willing to be open
Focus groups	Inexpensive given the amount and type of data; get collective views rather than individual views	Need training in managing the group process; need a good data recording method
Survey with open-ended questions	Very inexpensive method of data collection	Poor handwriting and unclear statements can make data useless
Narrative designs	Very inexpensive data collection; provides insights into social and cultural influences on thoughts and actions	Requires special training in data analysis; may not have credibility with stakeholders; difficult to select the most relevant texts to the health problem or program

infrastructure level of the public health pyramid. In a slightly different vein, Goodson, Gottlieb, and Smith (1999) reported using case study methodology to study the implementation of the Put Prevention into Practice program (PPIP). They interviewed all staff at the nine clinical sites where PPIP was implemented. Using structured interviews and open-ended questions with staff, they were able to identify site-specific problems with the implementation of the program. Again, their report is an example of how a case study is ideal for process monitoring evaluations and subsequent program planning, particularly at the infrastructure level.

Limitations are inherent in the case study methodology. As with all qualitative methods, the time and resources needed to carry out the research can be a major limitation. A limitation specifically of the case study methodology is that not all documents and key informants may be accessible to the evaluator, resulting in a systematic bias in the data available for analysis. In addition, the amount of data collected can be overwhelming and result in analysis-paralysis or delays in arriving at sound conclusions.

Observation

Using one's own eyes to collect data is another qualitative method. While one could look at and count things, when one is looking at the behavior of others and making interpretations about that behavior, the nature of the data becomes more subjective, more qualitative. Observational methods vary widely and range from nonparticipatory techniques, such as using rooms with one-way mirrors to observe parent and child interactions, to very participatory techniques, such as assuming the identity of a program participant to experience what they experience. Observations also occur across a wide variety of settings, from natural, such as a home or street corner in the neighborhood of the target audience, to less naturalistic, such as a clinic or laboratory.

Depending on the purpose of using an observational method, the specific procedures will vary. Nonetheless, there are some commonalities. First, training is needed with regard to what will be observed. For example, if the purpose is to assess the quality of interaction between program staff and participants, then dyadic or triadic actions and reactions will be the focus. If the purpose is to assess whether program participants have acquired a skill taught in the program, then the sequence of actions taken by the participant when in the situation requiring the skill will be the focus. In both the process monitoring and the impact evaluation examples, there are many other events, interactions, and factors occurring simultaneously that are not immediately relevant to the purpose and therefore are not recorded or noted during the observation.

Data collection can be done in several different ways. One is the use of audiovisual recordings. Although this data collection method is likely to capture all events or interactions of interest, it is also the most intrusive from the point of view of the one being observed. The advantage of using a recording is that data can be analyzed by several different analysts, and repeated viewings of the recordings can help assure that an important event or interaction of interest is not missed. Given that electronic equipment and recording devices are in wide use and increasingly less novel, and that they continue to decrease in size, a well-trained data collector can use these devices discreetly.

The other approach to collecting data involves coding events or interactions as they occur. The coding can be done on paper or using electronic aids. This approach has the advantage that the observer has recording equipment that may be less intimidating to those being observed. The disadvantage is that the quality of the data is dependent upon the accuracy of the observer's coding, and verifying the accuracy of the coding can be complicated and expensive.

The most qualitative approach to collecting observational data is making detailed notes and logs of occurrences and observations after one is no longer doing the observation. This method relies heavily on the recall accuracy and memory of the one who made the observations, and on the ability of that person to record what was observed with minimal interpretations in the description. While this approach to data collection is most susceptible to biases and inaccuracies, it is also the least intrusive.

An example of an observational method useful for community assessment is the Community Landscape Assessment Method (CLAM) (Issel, Searing, & Fleming, 2002). A team of observers from the community were hired and trained to walk around their neighborhood and record on paper forms the presence of key community factors. The problem of unreliable coding was minimized by having the observers work in pairs, so that there were duplicate data that could be used to assess the reliability of observation recording. They used sheets of paper that would generally be considered minimally intrusive. However, they reported that when they were at grocery stores to observe the presence of specific foods, they were treated with suspicion. In this case, they were making observations about the factors listed on their data collection sheets, but they were also making important observations of a more cultural nature about the openness of their communities. The CLAM thus provides both structured data as well as an opportunity to collect unstructured qualitative data from an open-ended field note.

Observational data can be analyzed as sequential data (Bakeman & Gottman, 1997), which means that the sequence in which interactions, behaviors, or reactions occurs is viewed as a pattern that is subject to specific statistical analytical procedures. Consider a situation on which an element of the process evaluation is focused, for instance the quality of staff and participant interaction. To study the interaction, the sequence of staff questioning and participant response are analyzed. Suppose program staff initiate a question (call it Q1) and the participant looks away (call it LA1), followed by the question being repeated (Q1). The Q1→LA1→Q1 sequence is what is analyzed. This approach to the analysis of observational data is a bit closer to a quantitative approach than if the observation data are collected as general categories of behaviors, events, and interactions. Using an impact evaluation example, suppose that a participant is observed in a real-life situation and context and is unaware of being observed. In this case, the data are more like field notes, and hence analysis is more likely to follow the approach used with other types of qualitative data, outlined later in this chapter.

Using an observational method has its advantages and disadvantages. Depending on the method used to record the observations, the data may be susceptible to recall bias and observational bias. This is particularly true if the observer is a participant observer who is not at liberty to record the observations as they actually occur. Another disadvantage is that deciding upon a sampling frame can be difficult. In other words, the number of observations needed for one to be confident that the behavior could have occurred at a usual rate and in a usual manner may not be readily knowable. As with most qualitative methods, the amount of time and resources needed can also be problematic. On the positive side, some behaviors and events might become known only through observation. The flexibility and variety of techniques that can be used to collect the data can be viewed as an another advantage.

In-Depth Individual Interview

The most widely known, and probably the most widely used, of the qualitative methods is the in-depth, open-ended questioning of an individual. Using questions that require more than a yes or no response, encouraging explanation, and allowing for storytelling lead to information that is detailed, personal, and often reflective. These types of data are preferred when meanings and attributions are the focus, and when new or fresh insights into a poorly understood phenomenon is sought. Typically, individuals who are interviewed are purposively selected based on a narrow set of criteria. They may be program recipients, stakeholders in the program, or members of the target audience.

In-depth interviews can be used throughout the planning and evaluation cycle. Kissman (1999) conducted in-depth interviews with homeless women, thereby identifying gaps in services to these women. This methodology, as compared with the use of a survey method, was particularly appropriate given that one of the obstacles identified by the women was their inability to read. In-depth interviews can also be used to understand the effects of the program. An example of using interviews to understand impacts is a study by Issel (2000). She interviewed women who had received prenatal comprehensive case management and learned from the women what they experienced as outcomes of having received that service.

Conducting in-depth interviews requires skill on the part of the interviewer. The interviewer needs to be sensitive to the cues of the interviewee with regard to when to stop the interview, as well as when and how to ask for clarification when the interviewee is either using slang or not providing an easily interpreted story. In-depth interviews can be done almost anywhere that the interviewer and the interviewee mutually feel comfortable and secure in terms of maintaining confidentiality. Interviews conducted in the office of the program staff would not be a good idea, particularly if information is sought from individuals who feel vulnerable or in a lower power position. More neutral territory is better, whether that is the interviewee's home or, for example, the local library.

Sometimes the interviewee is referred to as a key informant, denoting that the individual is unique in possessing information of a specific nature. Key informants are more likely to be useful during the community assessment and planning stages, as they would have knowledge of system processes and barriers to services and can draw upon a range of experiences to comment on generic issues that exist. Data collected from in-depth interviews with key informants are analyzed in the same manner as data collected from any other interviewee.

There are advantages and disadvantages to using in-depth interviews in program planning and evaluation. The time needed to collect and analyze the data is generally longer than that needed to conduct a simple survey. Also, the ability and skill of the interviewer is critical to getting a "good" interview that has sufficient details to make analysis less complicated and yet not disrupt the flow of ideas from the interviewee. One big advantage is that new ideas and information can be gained from in-depth interviews. Issel's (2000) study of impacts from prenatal case management revealed that, from the perspective of the women, the psychosocial benefits from interacting with the case managers were more salient than their medical outcomes. Such a finding can be used to modify the effect theory and possibly what is measured as an impact.

Focus Group

The focus group method of collecting qualitative data involves conducting an interview with a group of individuals, thereby taking advantage of the group dynamic that can lead to discussions and revelations of new information. For some individuals the group setting for interviews is less intimidating than a one-on-one interview. The steps involved in selecting focus group members, conducting the focus groups, managing the group process, and analyzing the data have been explicated by various authors (Krueger, 1994; Morgan, 1998;

Steward & Shamdasani, 1990). The types of questions posed to a focus group are constructed as open-ended ones. In order to maximize the data provided by the group members, the focus group leader actively directs the discussion by seeking clarification and eliciting views and opinions from those members who are more inclined to be quiet. Data are collected as either an audio recording or extensive written notes, and sometimes both; audiovisual recordings are only rarely used. The process of recording can be somewhat intrusive if the group members are not comfortable with a tape recorder or are distracted by the note taker. Thus, the physical location of the recorder and the note taker with regard to the focus group members becomes a conscious choice of how not to influence the interactions of the group members.

The efficiency aspect of the focus group method has led to its use in health program planning and evaluation. Clapp and Early (1999) used focus groups to study perceptions of outcomes from alcohol and substance abuse prevention programs. They were able to identify potential outcomes from such programs, as well as a program effect theory that was implicit in the understandings of the focus group participants. This is an example of using focus groups during the planning stage in order to refine the program effect theory and more accurately select potentially sensitive indicators of program impact.

Focus groups can also be used to develop the service utilization plan. For example, Shupe, Smith, Stout, and McLaughlin (2000) conducted focus groups with young adults who had recently experienced an unintended pregnancy. The focus group data led to programmatic initiatives at the community and direct services level designed to prevent unintended pregnancies. As these examples reveal, focus groups seem well suited for use during the community assessment and program planning phases. In contrast, focus groups may not be as useful for impact assessments because it may be inappropriate to ask individuals to reveal in a group setting what difference the program made to them. In some situations, focus groups can be appropriate as one method to collect process monitoring from data staff.

Individuals within a focus group can confirm or disconfirm the experiences and views of others. This contributes to the focus group method being somewhat more efficient than in-depth individual interviews that require a separate interview for the validation of interpretations. Data analysis follows the general steps used for analyzing in-depth interviews, as outlined later. Thus, those familiar with that data analysis procedure will be capable of analyzing focus group data. The difference is that the findings are not person-specific but are considered already validated during the group process.

The focus group method has limitations and challenges. The most immediately noticeable challenge is the logistics of scheduling a meeting with the 8 to 12 members of a focus group. Along these lines, it can be difficult to predict which combination of individuals will be optimal for producing insightful data. A balance between homogeneity and heterogeneity of group members is needed and can be difficult to anticipate. The selection of focus group members, the sampling strategy, ought to be guided by the notion that people who are alike are more likely to communicate with one another, and yet some degree of differences among the members stimulates discussions and promotes clarification. Capturing the data can also pose a challenge because people talk when others talk and often have voices that are difficult to identify on audiotapes, plus taking handwritten notes inevitably misses some comments. For this reason, more than one data recording technique is often used.

Survey with Open-Ended Questions

Sometimes surveys include an open-ended question or two to which respondents can provide qualitative information. Typically, questions such as, "Anything else?" "What was the best/worst?" and "What suggestions do you have?" are used. Such questions can be added to community assessment, process monitoring, or impact survey questionnaires. Because responses to such questions are generated by the individual, rather than the researcher, the responses are of a qualitative nature.

The major limitations of collecting qualitative data with written open-ended questions are that people often do not write legibly, are not articulate, or provide extremely brief responses. These factors can make it impossible to interpret their response, and hence render their data useless. Giving more explicit instructions and providing sufficient space to write detailed responses can help minimize these problems. However, if the information from the questions is considered crucial, then other methods for collecting the data ought to be considered. Nonetheless, open-ended questions on a survey can be beneficial. Such questions, compared to a survey of close-ended questions, provide respondents with an opportunity to express themselves, and thus they are likely to feel heard. Also, the response may provide sufficient information to generate an initial set of categories for a close-ended question. It becomes the discretion of the evaluator to decide whether the data are analyzable and useful. The analysis steps described later can be applied to this rather limited, but potentially fruitful, qualitative data.

Narrative Methods

A qualitative approach that is used rarely in health program planning and evaluation is the use of narrative methods. Narrative methods use text as the data. Text can come from personal sources, such as diaries, and from public or agency sources, such as existing agency records, memos, reports, videos, and newspapers and other print media. Narrative methods focus on the linguistics of the texts and often follow a more straightforward content analysis approach (Krippendorf, 1980).

Narrative methods can be helpful during the community assessment phase in understanding how a community presents itself through the local media and other writings. For process monitoring, narrative methods can be very helpful in tracking program drift as reflected in writings about the program or program procedures. They might also be useful for identifying outcomes of policy changes. Schram and Soss (2001) analyzed the discourse (narrative) about welfare to better understand perceptions of the welfare policy and how the narrative may shape future debates about welfare. A different type of narrative method was used by D'Emidio-Caston and Brown (1998). They conducted focus groups with children and selected the narrative stories found in the data for specific narrative analysis. The stories provided new insights into students' perceptions of substance abuse programs, and thus were valuable in assessing the program's impact. The authors further suggested that the insights might be useful in formulating policy.

The obvious limitation of a narrative method is the inherent limited nature of text sources and the lack of an opportunity to clarify meanings or intent. On the positive side, narrative methods can be less expensive than other qualitative methods, particularly if the texts are publicly and readily available. In addition, stories, as narrative texts, are easy to obtain during interviews.

SCIENTIFIC RIGOR

Just as for quantitative methods, scientific rigor is important to the use of qualitative methods. The terminology is different, although the underlying concepts are comparable. The following four elements of scientific rigor in qualitative methods (Lincoln & Guba, 1985) need to be present for the data to be considered of high quality.

Credibility is roughly equivalent to internal validity and refers to whether one can have confidence in the truth of the findings. Credibility is established through several activities. One is to invest sufficient time in the process so that the findings can be triangulated. Another is to use outsiders, namely individuals other than those who provided or analyzed the data, for insights into the meaning and interpretation of the data. This is sometimes referred to as peer debriefing. Another activity is to refine working hypotheses that are generated during data analysis with negative cases. The process involves actively seeking data that would be evidence that the working hypothesis is not always accurate. Unlike the analysis of qualitative data, working hypotheses are more like hunches that may be influenced by the researcher's bias. Therefore, in qualitative analysis efforts are made to both confirm and disconfirm the working hypothesis.

The act of seeking disconfirming data ensures that the researcher's biases are minimized in the results. Yet another activity is to check findings against raw data, by reviewing the raw data again in light of the findings. Finally, credibility is increased when those who provided the data are asked to review the findings and provide feedback into the accuracy of the interpretations.

Transferability or applicability is similar to external validity in that the findings ought to be applicable to other contexts and respondents. The main technique to increase transferability is to provide in reports thick (detailed, comprehensive) descriptions so that others can independently assess the possibility of transferring the findings to other groups. This stands in contrast to the quantitative technique that focuses on sample selection as a means of increasing the generalizability of findings.

Dependability is roughly equivalent to reliability. The notion is that other researchers and evaluators ought to be able to arrive at the same results if they repeated the study or analyzed the same set of data. Assuring dependability is done primarily by leaving a paper trail of steps in the analysis so that others can see that the findings are supported by the data. Another large aspect of dependability is the use of reliability statistics to demonstrate that, given the same set of data, two researchers would arrive at the same coding of the data. The two most widely used reliability statistics in qualitative research are the percent agreement and the Kappa statistic. Both of these statistics are determined after the codes for the data have been finalized, including having definitions. Percent agreement is the simple percentage of a given data set that two researchers independently code into the same preestablished categories. The numerator is the number of data units that are similarly coded, and the denominator is the total number of data units to be coded. While this is simple to calculate, it does not take into account that both researchers might have assigned a "wrong" code to the same data. To compensate for this shortcoming, the Kappa statistic can be used (Cohen, 1960). The Kappa statistic is based on the ratio of observed (actual) codes used to the expected codes to be used for a given set of data, for any two independently coding researchers.

Confirmability, sometimes referred to as objectivity, connotes that the findings are truly from the respondents, not the researcher's perceptions or biases. As with dependability, the main technique to assure confirmability is to leave an audit trail that others could follow and arrive at the same findings. In addition, there are a variety of techniques for documenting the researcher's impressions, biases, and interpretations, such as making theoretical memos or taking field notes. The use of such techniques adds to the confirmability of the findings because there is greater assurance that the researcher has taken steps to be self-aware of factors that might influence the interpretation of the data, and subsequently the results.

SAMPLING FOR QUALITATIVE METHODS

Qualitative approaches to sampling are guided by a different set of driving forces than those of quantitative approaches. The nonexperimental nature of qualitative designs means that random selection of a sample is not relevant. Power analyses are also not appropriate, because there is no attempt to quantify an effect size or find statistical significance. A different set of criteria exists for establishing the scientific rigor of qualitative design sample selection. Morse (1994) provided some guidelines in terms of numbers. She suggested that at least six participants are needed when trying to understand the experience of individuals, and that 30 to 50 interviews are optimal for ethnographies and ground theory studies.

Generally, the source of the data is intentionally chosen so that the phenomenon of interest is likely to be present. From this premise an explicit set of criteria is established and used, resulting in what is called a purposive sample. When all program staff are interviewed because of their involvement with the health program, a purposive sample is being chosen. The purposive sample allows for data collection from a group that is homogeneous with regard to the criteria used for selection. However, purposive samples might also be chosen to have maximum heterogeneity; to include atypical, extreme, or deviant cases; or to confirm or disconfirm a working hypothesis.

A different approach to sample selection stems from concern with having sufficient heterogeneity that all possible responses, perspectives, or categories of information are likely to be found in the data. This strategy is called sampling for category saturation. At some point, adding more data does not provide more or new information. This point is referred to as saturation and can be desirable as evidence of a minimal possibility that information was missed. Sampling for category saturation requires some degree of flexibility in the number of participants, whether cases or individuals, in the evaluation study. It may be that category saturation is achieved sooner or later than expected, thus allowing a sooner than expected conclusion to enrollment or necessitating the recruitment of additional participants. Similarly, theoretical sampling, which comes from the grounded theory tradition (Charmaz, 2000), is the notion of sampling for ideas and constructs so that theories can be further developed and refined. Like sampling for category saturation, theoretical sampling requires flexibility in determining when enough data have been collected.

QUALITATIVE ANALYSES

Numerous texts provide detailed instructions on analyzing various types of qualitative data (Krippendorf, 1980; Lincoln & Guba, 1985; Miles & Huberman,

1994; Weber, 1990). These and other texts ought to be consulted for detailed instructions on the process of analyzing qualitative data so that scientific rigor is maintained. Remember that program planners and evaluators, whether engaged in qualitative or quantitative data collection, need to make every reasonable effort to achieve scientific rigor as a basis from which claims can be more solidly and confidently made. The following is a brief summary of the steps involved in the immersion into the data and surfacing from the depths of analysis that occur when working with qualitative data.

Overview of the Analysis Process

A note of caution is warranted here. While the steps and procedure outlined are presented in a sequential order, the reality is that in qualitative data analysis most of the steps occur iteratively. It's a bit like taking two giant steps forward and then needing to take three baby steps backward before stepping forward again. This is a normal and expected part of the process of qualitative data analysis.

Before analysis can begin, the data need to be transformed into a format amenable to manipulation and analysis. This may involve transcribing audiotaped interviews, or entering text, audio, or visual data into qualitative analysis software. Once the data are reliably and accurately transformed, analysis can begin.

The first step is to decide upon what the codable units of data are, and then to identify those units within the data. Codable units from in-depth interviews can be words, phrases, or paragraphs, whereas codable units from observation may be facial movements or interactions. In contrast to quantitative data, in which the numeric response to a single question or a lab value is an obvious unit of data, the question of what constitutes a unit of data is not always so obvious in qualitative data. There is a constant struggle to identify the units of data so that they can be categorized based on their properties. The unit of analysis will vary by the method used, the question being asked, and the underlying perspective from which the question is being asked. Also, the unit of analysis can evolve as the analysis proceeds, becoming either larger or smaller in terms of the amount or complexity of what is considered the codable unit of analysis.

The next step is to understand the meaning of what was said, observed, or read. Qualitative methods and their corresponding data analysis approaches have their own terminology. Manifest versus implied meanings are critical in qualitative data. Manifest meanings are the obvious, unambiguous meanings, whereas implied meanings are the unspoken innuendos and the metaphors and references that color the meaning and interpretation. Data analysis relies on making this distinction and being faithful to whether the data are being coded based on manifest or implied meanings.

Based on the meanings, a discovery process begins in which groups of data with similar meanings begin to form categories. This process is rather idiosyncratic, with each researcher having a preferred style. Some begin with broad, overarching categories and gradually generate more specific subcategories. Others prefer to begin with many discrete categories and, based on grouping similar categories, evolve toward broader, overarching categories. Either approach is fine, as they both result in having a nested set of categories, not unlike having an outline of nested ideas that has broad topics and more specific subheadings. The process of generating categories involves constantly comparing the data to be coded with the data that have already been categorized. Constant comparison is a trademark of qualitative data analysis. The process results in the feeling of being immersed in data, lost among the trees in the forest. As the categories evolve, a paper trail is generated that is necessary for dependability.

At the point at which sufficient data have been analyzed for categories to develop, naming the categories is next. This step is likely to occur along with the sorting of data into groups or categories. A category is a classification of concepts in the data. As more and more data are reviewed for the meaning and grouped, properties and dimensions of the categories begin to surface. A dimension implies that the quality of the data exists along a continuum, whereas a property is a discrete attribute or characteristic. As more data are added to the categories, new data are constantly compared with data already in the category, and adjustments are made. Exhibit 12.4 shows an example of some interview text, the coded units, and the categories to which those data units have been assigned.

Once the categories are reasonably well established, definitions of the categories are developed. Based on the properties and dimensions, definitions help establish criteria for whether data belong to that category, and they are used as the guide for whether new data are added to that category or a different category. Definitions are considered good if they enable the categories to meet two standard criteria for category development: mutually exclusive and exhaustive. Mutually exclusive category definitions allow for data to be in one and only one category; there is no other choice for the category that best reflects the data. Exhaustive category definitions prohibit the use of "other" as a category; all data have a place, a category in which they belong. Using the concepts of mutually exclusive and exhaustive categories is very helpful as a gauge for definition clarity and for determining whether more data need to be collected. If a considerable amount of data cannot be categorized, then either the categories need to be changed (broadened or narrowed) or more data

Exhibit 12.4 Example of Interview Text with Final Coding

Interview Text	Final Coding
Interviewer: OK. Thinking specifically about how case management may have affected you or made a difference to you. Uh, how do you think case management has affected your health or your pregnancy or the baby's health? How has it made a difference?	
Respondent: Uh, it really didn't make me no difference.	Outcome coding: case management made no difference to me.
Interviewer: OK. You couldn't identify any ways that it made a difference?	
Respondent: No.	
Interviewer: OK, how has case management affected uh, your thoughts or feelings about yourself?	
Respondent: Uh, I have had when I was pregnant I was depressed and everything and talking to my case manager made me feel better about myself.	Risk coding: expressed psychosocial thoughts about the baby and pregnancy.
	Outcome coding: increased self-concept attributed to case manager involvement.
Interviewer: Uh-huh. How did that happen? How did she make you feel better about yourself?	
Respondent: Uh, she just told me that don't think about nothing else and let it upset you and just think about what you got inside of you because I was under a lot of stress and she said that if I be stressed out too much I could harm the baby.	Risk coding: expressed psychosocial thoughts about the baby and pregnancy.
So, I thought about that and that was serious. If my pregnancy hadn't been stressed out and depressed like that.	Outcome coding: patient demonstrates a change in knowledge.

need to be collected so that the category properties, characteristics, and dimensions can be more fully understood.

Depending on the qualitative method and perspective taken, a step sometimes taken at this point is to present the findings to the participants in the study. They are offered the opportunity to confirm the results and discuss alternative interpretations of the data. This step adds to the confirmability of the final results.

The step that is typically considered the final step is to generate explanations or working theories based on the data. In terms of program planning and evaluation, this may involve revisiting the process theory or the effect theory, or any element of those theories. For example, findings from a qualitative evaluation may lead to a revision of the key contributing or determinant factors of the health problem, as well as a revision of the notion of what intervention is more effective. It is also quite reasonable for a separate model of the health problem to be developed based on the findings. Ultimately, the results need to be considered in reference to the purpose of the study and the questions that were asked at the outset.

Triangulation

Using qualitative data for health program planning and evaluation can involve another step, which is the integration of qualitative data with quantitative data. The term "triangulation" can refer to several ways in which different perspectives are in some way reconciled (Thurmond, 2001). An example of triangulation used for program planning is the needs assessment that was conducted for a program in Chicago (Levy et al., 2003). They used focus groups, key informant interviews, observational data, and quantitative data from the BRFSS to arrive at a set of concerns regarding diabetes and cardiovascular disease in a Latino and an African-American community. They were able to demonstrate areas of overlap and disagreement in the data, which contributed to a better understanding of the communities and what might be optimal programmatic interventions.

Software

Several software programs are commercially available for use in managing qualitative data and facilitating its analysis. The programs commonly used in qualitative research are NUD*IST©, Ethnograph©, and ATLAS-TI©, although several other programs are also available. Articles have been written comparing their capabilities (Barry, 1998; Lewis, 1998), and Exhibit 12.5 provides

Exhibit 12.5   Contact Information for Purchasing Qualitative Research Software

Name of Software	Website
ATLAS/ti	www.atlasti.de/
Ethnograph	www.scolari.com
NUD-IST / N5	www.qsr.com.au/home/home.asp

information about where these programs can be purchased. These programs have features such as the ability to diagram relationships among categories, count units of analysis per category, and code within coded text. Their functions include searching for text, text-based management in terms of linking text to information about that text, coding and retrieving, allowing for higher-order coding to support theory building, and building networks of concepts in graphic representations. While software programs can greatly facilitate the management of potentially overwhelming amounts of data, the conceptual work remains for the evaluator. The interpretation of meanings so that codes are applied to appropriate codable units, and the ongoing development and refinement of categories, domains, and properties are some of the tasks that cannot be done by the computer software. Also, these programs, like any software program, require training for use.

Issues to Consider

Given the traditional and normal reliance on numbers, one issue when reporting qualitative findings is whether to report numbers—in other words, "to count or not to count." Hildebrandt (1999) analyzed focus group data regarding the perceptions of vulnerable adults about community health care. Eight themes were identified in the data. In addition, comments were classified as either positive or negative, and the percentages of positive and negative comments about those eight themes were shown graphically. A bar graph was provided that showed the frequency of positive and negative comments about the themes. Although there were 24 participants in the focus group, the frequency bars seemed to range from 5 to 145. These data must be interpreted very cautiously, as one or two vocal individuals with many negative comments could easily skew the percentages. It is a question of choosing an appropriate denominator when reporting numbers from qualitative data. In the Hildebrandt example, the choice of the denominator was between the number of all coded comments or the number of focus group participants. Equally important is what is an appropriate numerator; it could be either the number of participants who mentioned a category or the number of times a category is mentioned throughout the study. These choices greatly influence how the findings are portrayed and interpreted.

Qualitative methods are notorious for being messy, confusing, and repetitive. While many of these qualities can be managed using available software for qualitative data management, the nature of the data requires iterative category development. This can prove challenging because the quantities of data are often overwhelming, and there can be potentially conflicting interpretations of data by the various stakeholders and evaluation participants. The evaluator, program planner, and relevant stakeholders need to be committed to obtaining and using the qualitative data. Otherwise the delays and frustrations will overcome the ultimate value of the data, and the data will be set aside.

Then there is the cost. Budgets for the collection and analysis of qualitative data must take into account all possible expenses. There is travel time and mileage to and from the sites where the data are collected. Interviews that are recorded need to be transcribed and typed verbatim. This activity is roughly equivalent to data entry from a close-ended survey. However, for every hour of interview there is approximately three hours of transcription. If independent coders are used to establish the reliability of coding data, they may need to be paid for their time and efforts.

A major issue for conducting any qualitative research is the need to have highly trained data collectors and analyzers. Training encompasses learning not only how to collect data that are consistent, reliable, and unbiased, but also how to acknowledge personal preferences and interpretations that may influence the analysis of the data. Training for data collection is important for in-depth interviewing to minimize the use of nonverbal or verbal cues that might lead the interviewee to respond in the way he or she thinks the interviewer wants. Humans are very good at reading other humans, and subtle facial movements and body language can alter the response of an interviewee. Training for data analysis is more complicated and is best accomplished by using a team approach to the data analysis. Team members can challenge each other, seek clarification on interpretations of data, and provide checks and balances during the process.

PRESENTATION OF FINDINGS

As with findings based on quantitative data, the findings of qualitative data analysis need to be communicated to the relevant stakeholders and presented in a manner that both conveys the scientific soundness of the findings and is understandable. One aspect of conveying the scientific soundness of the findings is to include descriptions of the context in which the data were collected in order to show transferability. Tables can be constructed that show the evolution of category development and can help demonstrate dependability and confirmation. Most important is including the words of the study participants alongside the category; this helps show confirmation. Stories, descriptions, explanations, and statements provided in the words of the participants are more powerful than numbers, and they make the numbers more human. The statements can be quite powerful as tools for marketing the program and for fundraising. The final step of generating explanations may result in diagrams of relationships among categories that can provide a visual means of understanding the overall findings. To the extent that the data can be associated with the logic model of the program or the program theory, the findings will be viewed as more immediately relevant.

ACROSS THE PYRAMID

At the direct services level of the public health pyramid, qualitative methods, particularly interviews, are used to answer questions about individual perspectives, interpretations, perceptions, and meanings. Observational methods can also be readily used for process monitoring evaluations (Exhibit 12.6).

At the enabling services level, qualitative methods are likely to focus both on questions about individual perceptions and interpretations and on more aggregatewide perceptions. To obtain individual perceptions for either planning or impact evaluations, in-depth interviews would be appropriate. To ascertain the more common perceptions of members of an aggregate, focus groups would be quite useful.

At the population-based level, qualitative methods are more likely to be used during the assessment phase of the planning and evaluation cycle. Qualitative methods can provide detailed and specific information on cultural understandings related to health, illness, and prevention. These population-level, or aggregatewide, cultural findings can then be used to better design population-based services.

At the infrastructure level, qualitative methods have been used for a variety of purposes. Goodman, Steckler, Hoover, and Schwartz (1993) did a multiple-case study to identify ways in which the PATCH (see Chapter 4) needed to be improved. Bloom and associates (2000) used focus groups of state health department personnel to assess the use of the BRFSS. In other words, the focus group data were helpful in understanding issues related to the information resources of the infrastructure. Westmoreland, Grigsby, Brown, Latessa, and Huber (1998) used a qualitative method to evaluate an infrastructure building

Exhibit 12.6   Suggested Qualitative Methods by Pyramid Level and Planning Cycle

Pyramid Level	Assessment	Planning	Monitoring	Impact Evaluation
Direct services	Interview	Interview	Survey question	Interview, observation
Enabling services	Focus group	Focus group	Survey question	Interview
Population based	Focus group	Focus group	Focus group	Focus group
Infrastructure	Case study, narrative	Case study	Case study	Case study, interview, focus groups

program that was implemented in two different states. The comparative case study approach led to a set of policy recommendations for enhancing the success of implementing the specific workforce development program. As these reports demonstrate, qualitative methods can be used at all stages of the planning and evaluation cycle when the focus is at the infrastructure level.

DISCUSSION QUESTIONS

1. Which qualitative method(s) do you believe would be ideally suited to use at each stage of the planning and evaluation cycle? Justify your answer.

2. If you had a very limited budget but were committed to collecting and using some type of qualitative data to get at the perceptions of program participants, what might your best option be? Explain.

3. List the four criteria for assessing the rigor of qualitative studies. Imagine that you are planning to conduct in-depth interviews of program participants to assess program impact. For each criterion, give one example of how you would address that criterion in your plan for the impact evaluation.

4. Discuss the circumstances under which you would and would not use numbers in the presentation of results from each of the types of qualitative methods reviewed.

References

Bakeman, R., & Gottman, J. M. (1997). *Observing interaction: An introduction to sequential analysis* (2nd ed.). New York: Cambridge University Press.

Barry, C.A. (1998). Choosing qualitative data analysis software: ATLAS/ti and NUD*IST Compared. *Sociological Research Online, 3*(3). *http://www.socreonline.org.uk/3/3/4.html* (accessed 2/2/02).

Bloom, Y., Figgs, L. W., Baker, E. A., Dugbatey, K., Stanwyck, C. A., & Brownson, R. C. (2000). Data uses, benefits, and barriers for the behavioral risk factor surveillance system: A qualitative study of users. *Journal of Public Health Management and Practice, 6,* 78–86.

Charmaz, K. (2000). Grounded theory: Objectivist and constructionist methods. In N. K. Denzin & Y. S. Lincoln (Eds.), *Handbook of qualitative research* (2nd ed.). Thousand Oaks, CA: Sage Publications.

Clapp, J. D., & Early, T. J. (1999). A qualitative exploratory study of substance abuse prevention outcomes in a heterogeneous prevention system. *Journal of Drug Education, 29*(3), 217–233.

Cohen, J. (1960). A coefficient of agreement for nominal scales. *Educational and Psychological Measurement, 20,* 37–46.

D'Emidio-Caston, M., & Brown, J. H. (1998). The other side of the story: Student narratives on the California Drug, Alcohol, and Tobacco Education Programs. *Evaluation Review, 22*(1), 95–117.

Goodman, R. M., Steckler, A., Hoover, S., & Schwartz, R. (1993). A critique of contemporary community health promotion approaches: Based on a qualitative review of six programs in Maine. *American Journal of Health Promotion, 7*(3), 208–220.

Goodman, R. M., Steckler, A., & Alciati, M. H. (1997). A process evaluation of the National Cancer Institute's Data-Based Intervention Research Program: A study of organizational capacity building. *Health Education Research, 12*(2), 181–197.

Goodson, P., Gottlieb, N. H., & Smith, M. N. (1999). Put prevention into practice: Evaluation of program initiation in nine Texas clinical sites. *American Journal of Preventive Medicine, 17*(1), 73–78.

Green, L., & Lewis, F. M. (1986). *Measurement and evaluation in health education and health promotion.* Palo Alto, CA: Mayfield Publishing.

Hildebrandt, E. (1999). Focus groups and vulnerable populations: Insight into client strengths and needs in complex community health care environments. *Nursing and Health Care Perspectives, 20*(5), 256–259.

Issel, L. M. (2000). Women's perceptions of outcomes from prenatal case management. *Birth, 27,* 120–126.

Issel, L. M., Searing, L. M., & Fleming, S. (2002). *Community Landscape Asset Mapping for community-level health assessment.* Working Paper.

Kirk, J., & Miller, M. (1986). *Reliability and validity in qualitative research.* Thousand Oaks, CA: Sage Publications.

Kissman, K. (1999). Respite from stress and other service needs of homeless families. *Community Mental Health Journal, 35*(3), 241–249.

Krippendorf, K. (1980). *Content analysis: An introduction to its methodology.* Beverly Hills, CA: Sage Publications.

Krueger, R. A. (1994). *Focus groups: A practical guide to applied research.* Thousand Oaks, CA: Sage Publications.

Levy, S. R., Anderson, E., Issel, L. M., Willis, M. A., Dancy, B. L., Jacobson, K. M., et al. (2004). Using multi-level, multi-source needs assessment data for planning community interventions. *Health Promotion Practice.*

Lewis, B. R. (1998). ATLAS/ti and NUD-IST: A comparative review of two leading qualitative data analysis packages. *Cultural Anthropology Methods, 10*(3), 41–47. *http://www.acadimage.com/Field_Methods/articles.lewis.htm* (accessed 2/2/02).

Lincoln, Y. S., & Guba, E. G. (1985). *Naturalistic inquiry.* Beverly Hills, CA: Sage Publications.

Miles, M. B., & Huberman, A. M. (1994). *Qualitative data analysis: An expanded sourcebook* (2nd ed.). Thousand Oaks, CA: Sage Publications.

Morgan, D. L. (1998). *The focus group guidebook.* Newbury Park, CA: Sage Publications.

Morse, J. M. (1994). Designing funded qualitative research. In N. K. Denzin & Y. S. Lincoln (Eds.), *Handbook of qualitative research.* Thousand Oaks, CA: Sage Publications.

Schram, S. F., & Soss, J. (2001). Success stories: Welfare reform, policy disclosure, and the politics of research. *Annals of American Academy of Political and Social Science, 577,* 49–65.

Shupe, A. K., Smith, A. E., Stout, C. L., & McLaughlin, H. (2000). The importance of local data in unintended pregnancy prevention programming. *Maternal and Child Health Journal, 4,* 209–214.

Stake, R. E. (1995). *The art of case study research.* Thousand Oaks, CA: Sage Publications.

Stake, R. E. (2000). Case studies. In N. K. Denzin & Y. S. Lincoln (Eds.), *Handbook of qualitative research* (2nd ed.). Thousand Oaks, CA: Sage Publications.

Steward, D. W., & Shamdasani, P. N. (1990). *Focus groups: Theory and practice.* Newbury Park, CA: Sage Publications.

Strauss, A., & Corbin, J. (1990). *Basics of qualitative methods.* Thousand Oaks, CA: Sage Publications.

Thurmond, V. A. (2001). Combined research approaches can enhance interpretations of findings. *Journal of Nursing Scholarship, 33*(3), 253–258.

Veney, J., & Kaluzny, A. (1998). *Evaluation and decision making for health services.* Chicago: Health Administration Press.

Weber, R. (1990). *Basic content analysis* (2nd ed.). Newbury Park, CA: Sage Publications.

Westmoreland, D., Grigsby, K., Brown, L., Latessa, P., & Huber, D. (1998). Replicating Project LINC in two midwestern states: Implications for policy development. *Nursing and Health Care Perspectives, 19*(4), 166–174.

Yin, R. K. (1989). *Case study research: Design and methods* (Rev. ed.). Thousand Oaks, CA: Sage Publications.

Section 5

From Data to Decision

CHAPTER 13

Cost Analyses: The Basics

The choice among alternative programs is not always clear, due to varying degrees of success. Thus, programmatic choices may need to be justified on an economic basis. In this chapter, economic analyses are described so that a health program planner can formulate an economic evaluation question in a manner that will lead to the optimal economic analysis for the situation at hand. Fundamentally, program evaluators concerned with costs formulate the type of economic analysis based on a set of considerations: whether two programs that address the same health problem are being compared, whether only costs are being considered, or whether costs and outcomes of dissimilar health programs are being compared. Economic analyses can be very complex and involved, and can require a high degree of economics knowledge. This makes it a subspecialty of program evaluation. Nonetheless, those who manage programs and conduct basic program evaluations need to be familiar with the different types of economic analyses, as well as being savvy consumers of published health program economic evaluations.

TYPES OF ECONOMIC ANALYSES

Just as there are different types of program evaluations, there are different types of analyses related to program costs. "Costs" is a generic term used to encompass expenses related to the program. The determination of what is included as expenses is part of the cost side of the economic analysis and is discussed later as part of how to conduct an economic analysis. Types of economic analyses can be classified along two dimensions (Drummond, O'Brien, Stoddart, & Torrance, 1997). One dimension is whether one or more programs are under consideration, and the other is whether costs only or costs and effects are included in the analysis (Exhibit 13.1). Classifying economic analyses of programs along these two dimensions helps to discern the types and the subsequent requirements for conducting each type of analysis.

Exhibit 13.1   Types of Cost Analyses

	One Program	Two or More Programs
Costs Only	Cost description, cost analysis	Cost comparison
Costs and Effects	Cost analysis	Cost-effectiveness, cost-benefit, cost-utility

When only one program is considered and effects are not included, the type of analysis is a cost description. Cost description is the simplest form of economic analysis, in that it is a straightforward presentation of expenses related to the delivery of the health program. Most program managers will conduct a cost description as a matter of routine, particularly for any annual reports that require an accounting of expenses by category or line item. A cost description is best thought of as part of process monitoring, particularly with regard to accountability and the budget aspect of the organizational plan.

When the cost description includes a breakdown of total expenses by an analytic factor, such as time periods, participants, or funding source, it becomes a cost analysis. A cost analysis is also useful as a process monitoring tool. It essentially analyzes costs by other elements of either the organizational plan or the service utilization plan. In this way the findings of a cost analysis begin to provide information about the efficiency of a program. For example, a cost analysis reveals the dollars spent per program participant. These findings can be compared to published reports, benchmarks, or the original program plan in order to interpret the extent to which the program is more or less efficient than similar programs.

Other cost descriptions may compare the costs of two or more programs without looking at impacts or outcomes. These cost comparisons may focus on the costs per participant for the programs being considered. Cost comparisons might be done by a single agency with multiple health programs as the basis for deciding which program to continue. For example, Jerrell and Hu (1996) reported on a comprehensive analysis of costs associated with clients in three types of mental health and substance abuse prevention programs administered by one agency; a 12-step program, a behavioral skills program, and case management. Their study was longitudinal and data were collected at baseline, and then 6, 12, and 18 months after participants started the program.

The next three types of economic analyses involve comparing two or more programs and a measure of effect, whether impact or outcome. Each of these is discussed more fully later. Briefly, cost-effectiveness analysis (CEA) always compares the costs of two programs against one type of impact that is measured the same way in both programs. The programs are compared on the basis of a cost per unit of outcome. A cost-benefit analysis (CBA) also compares two programs, but the programs need not address the same health problem. The program effects are compared based on larger societal benefits in addition to the impacts and outcomes of the program. The two dissimilar programs are compared on a cost per dollar value of benefits achieved. The most complex and theoretical economic analysis is a cost-utility analysis (CUA). It is complex because it measures the outcome of health programs in terms of the potential participant's preference for the health impact. The programs are compared on a cost per unit of preference, called utility, as discussed in Chapter 3.

These economic analyses are not mutually exclusive, nor are they the only way to typify economic evaluations. Program personnel are likely to perform cost descriptions and cost analyses and possibly, with the help of a program evaluator, a cost-effectiveness analysis (if it is a mature program and there is good accounting for the program costs). It is unlikely that program personnel and most program evaluators will perform a cost-benefit or cost-utility analysis. These are more likely to be done by researchers, but because they may be used to establish health policy and influence program choices, program planners and managers need to be aware of how these economic analyses are done. This will enable them not only to critique these studies but also to actively participate in the conceptualization and execution of CBAs and CUAs.

The following three sections present basic information that is specific to CEA, CBA, and CUA. Again, this discussion is intended to provide sufficient information about these economic evaluations to allow a program evaluator or program manager to be a savvy consumer of economic evaluations and an informed team member in more-sophisticated efforts to conduct an economic analysis of the program. While these are presented as discrete, distinct types of economic analyses, the lines between them are often blurred, and they are not mutually exclusive; for example, a CEA may be part of a CBA.

Cost-Effectiveness Analysis

A cost-effectiveness analysis, or CEA, as described here, answers the question of whether program A or program B has more effect for the dollars expended. Another way of stating this is to ask which treatment or intervention is the best for the money, or which costs less per unit of impact. A CEA is focused on the cost related to a single, common effect that may differ in magnitude between the alternative programs. It is used to rank alternatives based on their resultant cost-effectiveness ratio (CER). Sometimes the term "cost-effectiveness analysis" is used as a generic category that encompasses CEA, CBA, and CUA. For the sake of clarity, CEA, in this book, refers only to the specific type of economic analysis in which two programs are compared on the basis of one health impact indicator.

Costs include, at a minimum, all direct and indirect expenses related to the delivery of the program or intervention (Exhibit 13.2). They may include start-up costs for a new program. The inclusion of indirect program costs can alter the results of the CEA (Garpenholt, Silfverdal, & Levin, 1998). Other costs that are typically included are medical costs related to the health problem being prevented by the intervention or program, including both hospitalization costs if the health problem is not prevented and outpatient visits. If the accounting perspective taken is societal, then along with program and medical costs, nonmedical costs such as opportunity and secondary costs will be included. The sum of all these costs is estimated.

On the effectiveness side of the equation, impacts of the program are measured in natural or physical units that are common to both programs. Because

Exhibit 13.2   Summary of Cost-Effectiveness Analysis (CEA), Cost-Benefit Analysis (CBA), and Cost-Utility Analysis (CUA)

Type	Basic Formula	Impacts, Outcomes, and Benefits	Costs and Expenses
CEA	$CER = \dfrac{\text{Total cost \$}}{\text{Health effect unit}}$	Program direct health impacts	Program direct and indirect costs
CBA	Net benefit = Total benefit \$ − Total cost \$	Dollar values of program direct impacts + indirect program outcomes + long-term societal consequences, willingness to pay, life expectancy	Program direct and indirect costs + medical costs + nonmedical costs + opportunity costs + other societal costs
CUA	$CUA = \dfrac{\text{Total cost \$}}{\text{Utility units}}$	Preferences for health state	Program costs + medical costs + nonmedical costs

the impacts are common to both programs, they are also quite specific to the health problem being addressed. For example, if two diabetes education programs are being compared with regard to diabetes prevention and management, the impacts common to both programs are likely to be blood glucose levels and a score on diabetes knowledge. In addition to the program-specific impacts, both programs may have broad, more generic impacts on the quality of life, disability levels, and the length of healthy years of life for those program participants. If quality-adjusted life years (QALYs), disability-adjusted life years (DALYs), or healthy life years (HLYs) are considered impacts of the program, they are used along with other program impacts. The program logic model can be very helpful in identifying and justifying what impacts ought to be monetized in the CEA, specifically the variables included in the intervention and determinant theories.

The basic formula to be estimated for each program being compared is as follows (Newbold, 1995):

Cost-effectiveness ratio =

$$\frac{(\text{total costs of program A}) - (\text{total costs of program B})}{(\text{effects of program A}) - (\text{effects of program B})}$$

The results of the CEA lead to a statement regarding the cost per unit of effect for each program. The CER is the incremental price to get one unit of effect compared to the alternative. A low CER is considered a "good buy."

The formula given above is the ideal and the most inclusive. However, specific evaluations may derive more realistic applications of the formula. For example, Windsor and colleagues (1990) conducted an evaluation of a health education program to improve medication adherence. They measured the effect of the program with a reliable and valid scale of adherence. They then used the following simple formula to determine the cost-effectiveness of the intervention: (cost of the intervention) / (percentage improvement on the adherence scale). Although their cost did not include indirect costs, their results were easy to interpret and provided clear evidence in favor of the health education intervention.

Cost-effectiveness studies need not be limited to existing programs. They can be done to assess the value or merit of initiating screening tests. The study by Randolph and Washington (1990) is one such example. They used costs associated with screening and treatment and the cure rates to assess the merit of screening adolescent males for chlamydia. Despite the cost-effectiveness demonstrated by their study, the lack of widespread adoption of this screening attests to the fact that practice decisions are not always dictated by the findings of economic evaluations.

Cost-effectiveness analyses might also focus on the specific impacts. Sevick and colleagues (2000) conducted a cost-effectiveness analysis of two exercise interventions for adults. They calculated the cost for each increment of improvement in a set of impact measures and indicators, such as amount of weight loss, number of additional flights of stairs walked, and blood pressure. The approach they use is based on another modification of the CEA formula:

Incremental improvement in cost-effectiveness =

$$\frac{\text{program cost per participant}}{\text{amount of change in a specific impact indicator}}$$

Exhibit 13.3 shows the usefulness of conducting an incremental improvement cost analysis. The three hypothetical programs vary in the program cost per participant and the degree to which the three impact indicators are changed by participation in the program. The cost per impact objective varies, suggesting that the choice of impact to be costed and considered is crucial in selecting the "best" health program.

Cost-Benefit Analysis

The intent of a cost-benefit analysis, or CBA, is to determine which of two different programs will have the greater social benefit, given their separate costs. A CBA answers questions regarding whether the benefits gained are worthwhile to society, given the costs. It is used to assess the inherent worth of a program, and because of its societal focus, the findings of a CBA are used for policy decision making (Szucs, 2000). Often the program under consideration is compared to a do-nothing option. A CBA is useful when comparing programs at different levels of the public health pyramid because it can be used to compare dissimilar programs. For example, a CBA could compare a mass immunization program (population level) with cognitive therapy sessions at a nursing home (direct services level). In addition, because a CBA compares programs in dollars, programs from different sectors of society can be compared, such as a health program and a military program.

A CBA results in a ratio, expressed in dollars. Outcomes included in a CBA are the benefits (impacts) as measured in market value, willingness to pay, or life expectancy (Exhibit 13.2). A key feature of a protypical CBA is that it takes into account all outcomes, thereby considering the broadest possible social consequences of the program. Therefore, all outcomes and benefits must be monetized, including intangibles and benefits of the program. This allows for a direct comparison of two dissimilar programs, using dollars as the basis of

Exhibit 13.3   Example of Simple and Incremental Cost-Effectiveness of Three Hypothetical Programs

	Program A (usual care, control)	Program B (experimental program)	Program C (alternative experimental)
Total program costs	$400	$1000	$700
Number of participants per program	100	100	100
Total program cost per participant	**$4**	**$10**	**$7**
Total amount of overall improvement	5 units	25 units	20 units
Program cost-effectiveness ratio	$80 per unit	$40 per unit	$35 per unit
Program cost-effectiveness per participant	$8 per unit per participant	$4 per unit per participant	$3.50 per unit per participant
Cost-effectiveness ratio comparing programs	—	A with B	A with C
(cost control program − cost experimental program)/ (effect control program − effect experimental program)	n.a.	($400 − $1000 / 5 − 25) = $30 saving per unit	($400 − $700 / 5 − 20) = $20 saving per unit
Incremental cost effectiveness analyses			
Amount of improvement in impact objective #1: increase in perceived health status score	2 units	5 units	10 units
Cost per unit of higher perceived health status per participant	$2.00 per unit per participant	$2.00 per unit per participant	$0.70 per unit per participant

Exhibit 13.3   Example of Simple and Incremental Cost-Effectiveness of Three Hypothetical Programs *(continued)*

	Program A (usual care, control)	Program B (experimental program)	Program C (alternative experimental)
Amount of improvement in impact objective #2: additional minutes of exercise	3 minutes	20 minutes	15 minutes
Cost per additional minute of exercise per participant	$1.33 per minute per participant	$0.50 per minute per participant	$0.47 per minute per participant
Amount of improvement in impact objective #3: diastolic blood pressure decrease	2mm Hg	4mm Hg	4mm Hg
Cost per mm Hg decrease in blood pressure per participant	$2.00 per mm Hg per participant	$2.50 per mm Hg per participant	$1.75 per mm Hg per participant

comparison. Tangible benefits are those that are directly observable and measurable, whereas intangible benefits are those that are indirect, less measurable, and more likely to be secondary benefits. The costs associated with the programs include both the direct programmatic costs and the indirect costs in terms of the program and society. Opportunity costs can also be included in a CBA.

As with the CEA, the program logic model, particularly the impact theory, becomes critical as the conceptual and theoretical basis for identifying the direct and tangible program benefits. Because the CBA encompasses distal and societal effects of the program, the effect theory becomes critical as a starting point for conceptualizing additional programmatic impacts, effects, and influences on alternative contributing factors. Shaw (1995) aptly pointed out that impacts are beneficial if they are favorable to the program recipients but are costs if they are unfavorable. The effect theory provides a basis for assigning an impact as a benefit or as a cost.

The results of a CBA are expressed as a ratio of benefit dollars to cost dollars. The ratio yields a value that ranges from a negative value to zero or a positive value. If the ratio has a positive value, then the program will provide or is providing a net benefit to society, whereas if the ratio has a negative value, the program will be more costly than the benefits to society. In short, the program with the higher positive ratio is preferred, as it has the greater societal benefit. The formula for the ratio can be expressed as follows:

Benefit-cost ratio =

$$\frac{\text{(dollar value of tangible benefits + dollar value of intangible benefits)}}{\text{total costs associated with program}}$$

Some impacts, such as averted illness, can be valued as either benefits or costs, depending on one's perspective. Averted illness can be a benefit in terms of wages earned but a cost in terms of lost revenue for a clinic. Therefore, the recommendation is to use the net benefit, as it avoids the difficulties of determining which costs belong in the numerator and which belong in the denominator. The net benefit is calculated as follows:

Net benefit = (dollar value of tangible benefits + dollar value of intangible benefits) − (direct costs + indirect costs)

The values of the net benefit of the programs are then compared to determine which program has a greater societal benefit given the costs. Whether the ratio or net benefit is calculated, the decision makers are ultimately comparing programs that are dissimilar on an equal basis. This enables decision makers to make difficult choices regarding allocation of resources to one program over another.

Cost-Utility Analysis

Cost-utility analyses, or CUAs, are less common than either CEAs or CBAs. A CUA is used to answer the question of how much it is worth in dollars to have a particular state of health. Like the CBA, the CUA compares programs with different outcomes. There are three conditions under which it would not be wise to undertake a CUA: if intermediate program impacts are of interest, if quality of life is not measurable with a single variable, or if it is costly to obtain utility data. Also, CUAs are difficult to use for planning or policy because of the idiosyncratic nature of preferences that are the basis of CUAs.

The preferences for health states tend to be related to specific illnesses and thus are idiosyncratic. However, a CUA is a good choice when quality of life is an important programmatic outcome, as would be the case with a program for patients with arthritis or for a neonatal intensive care unit. Cost-utility studies are more commonly done as a means of comparing medical treatments for different illnesses, because of the idiosyncratic nature of preferences.

The outcome considered in a CUA is utility, specifically a preference for a state of health, which is achieved as an impact from the program. The population preferences discussed in Chapter 4 in terms of program planning are applicable to a CUA. Preference or utility assessment provides a way to integrate the preferences or values attributed to the worth of life at a given point in time with the quality of life spent in various health states (Patrick & Erickson, 1993). The data gathered from the methods used to ascertain the utility, such as standard gamble and timed trade-off, are used in the CUA. Examples of paired comparisons used to determine utility preference are, Would you rather have severe, chronic hypertension or Type II diabetes? Would you rather lose your right leg or your left hand? Would you rather lose your left hand or have Type II diabetes? A CUA is concerned with the utility of health states, whether in terms of preferences or labor market value. Utility values are obtained through judgment, through values from literature, and from participants. In addition to preferences, QALYs, DALYs, lives saved, and disability days averted can be used in a CUA. However, the multidimensionality of quality of life and the relative importance of those dimensions of quality of life (Bowling, 1995) add considerable complexity to conducting a CUA. In addition, there continue to be methodological debates and advances in making CUA, and the use of QALYs more health policy friendly (Ubel et al., 2000). Nonetheless, the results of the CUAs reflect the relative importance of the health program outcome.

As with CEAs and CBAs, CUA findings are expressed as a ratio of the program costs to the level of preference for the health state offered by the program. The formula is as follows:

$$\text{Cost-utility ratio} = \frac{\text{total costs associated with the program}}{\text{utility units}}$$

The results of the analysis, in the form of the ratio, show how much each unit of additional health value costs with the specific program. As with the economic analyses of programs, the ratio allows decision makers to compare programs on the basis of dollars.

Gabriel et al. (1999) found that the preference for a health state varied based on the health experiences of those being surveyed. This variation had an effect on the estimated cost utility of interventions to prevent osteoporosis in women. Such findings hint at the relative and sensitive nature of preferences and the subsequent difficulty in arriving at one definitive cost-utility ratio.

BASIC STEPS INVOLVED IN CONDUCTING ECONOMIC EVALUATIONS

As with any study and analysis, there is a prescribed set of steps that can be used to guide the process (Barry & DeFriese, 1990; Gold, Seigel, Russell, & Weinsten, 1996; Shepard & Thompson, 1979). The following steps are generic but provide the basis for developing and conducting an economic analysis. The initial steps are similar to the steps involved in any research study and program evaluation, but they diverge when attention to costs is required. The first step is to define the problem.

Define the Problem

Defining the problem involves being explicit about the purpose of the economic analysis, as the purpose determines which type of economic evaluation should be done. This is similar to defining the evaluation question or research study question. The target population and the health problem that the program is addressing need to be clearly specified. Another familiar aspect of defining the problem is delineating limitations that affect the resources available for the economic analysis. For example, the experience and expertise available to conduct the economic evaluation may require that a less complex economic evaluation be conducted.

Stipulate Comparison Parameters

If only one program is the subject of the economic analysis, this step is irrelevant. Nonetheless, it is important to explicitly state that the economic evaluation question does not involve comparison, as that justifies conducting a cost description or a cost analysis. If two programs are being compared, then one must clearly explain and justify which programs are being compared. If the economic evaluation question is posed in terms of comparisons, then each of the two alternatives must be fully detailed. In particular, the interventions to be evaluated must be understood. It is also very helpful to state the program goals and objectives of each alternative. Comparisons need not be between new or innovative programs; one of the programs included in the comparative economic evaluation can be the do-nothing option or the standard treatment. The cost study by Jerrell and Hu (1996) is an example in that one of the programs being compared with the other two is an AA/12-step program, which is often considered a standard or widely used intervention for alcohol abstinence.

Develop Decision Rules

As with any evaluation or study, an economic analysis makes assumptions about the health problem, about the interventions, and about the methods used. If those assumptions are made explicit, their potential consequences can then be anticipated and corrections made. One aspect of decision rules is definitions of key parameters of the economic evaluation. For example, when comparing programs with varying degrees of intensity (a single weak intervention versus multiple intensive interventions) and duration (e.g., annual versus monthly), Torrance, Siegal, and Luce (1996) recommended using in the analysis all levels that are realistically feasible. This is one type of decision rule that needs to be explicit. Another type of decision may involve the time frame during which the costs and the effects/benefits/utility will be measured. The breadth of program costs to be included also ought to be a decision rule, based in part on the accounting perspective chosen.

Another decision rule may focus on the age groups to be included in the analysis. As the results from Prosser and associates (2000) found, the cost-effectiveness ratio of primary prevention of high LDL cholesterol decreases as the number of those receiving the primary prevention intervention increase. Their results also highlight the differences in the cost-effectiveness ratio for men and for women. Therefore, characteristics of program participants ought to be a point of discussion and decision, particularly if the program effects may vary by those characteristics in ways that can affect the economic analysis.

Choose an Accounting Perspective

An accounting perspective is the theoretical point of view taken, which then guides the decisions as to what factors will be included as costs and as outcomes (Exhibit 13.4). One perspective consists of the views of individual participants and members of the target audience regarding the costs of and gains from the program. Factors important from this accounting perspective include out-of-pocket costs, opportunity costs of program participation, and externalities experienced and valued by participants. Opportunity costs refer to purchases that cannot be made because of having spent the money on something else. In terms of participants, because they are paying, in some form, for being in the program, they no longer have that money to spend on

Exhibit 13.4   Examples of Costs and Benefits Related to Accounting Perspectives

Perspective	Costs	Benefits and Outcomes
Participants	Medical costs, treatment and medication costs, costs of participation, opportunity costs	Program-specific impacts, secondary effects on family, quality of life
Program	Program costs, opportunity costs for the organization	Visibility and good will (marketing value), increase program or agency funding
Societal	Lost taxes, disability support, criminal justice	Gain in taxes, reductions in public services (i.e., police, fire), reductions in costs to family members related to health problem (lost wages, lost taxes, out of pocket), reductions in costs to support family due to health problem

something else. In other words, they do not have the opportunity to spend the money that is going to program participation. Opportunity costs become critical in decision making, particularly if resources are scarce or severely limited. For example, if a mother takes her child for immunizations, the cost of getting to the clinic and the co-payment may cost her the opportunity (the money) to purchase new clothes for that child. The inclusion of opportunity costs in the analysis can alter the final results (Zivolich, Shueman, & Weiner, 1997). Costs, from the point of view of program participants, would include losses or gains in work productivity, the family burden related to the health problem or program, out-of-pocket expenses related to participation, and such. For example, to attend an immunization program, a mother may need to pay for transportation, babysitting, and baby Tylenol, as well as missing half a day of work. Fiedler and associates (2000), in a cost study of a nutrition fortification program, found that the opportunity costs of volunteers were 41% of personnel costs and 30% of total program costs. These findings reinforce the importance of factoring in opportunity costs, including those to volunteers participating in the health program.

Another accounting perspective is that of program sponsors. They are more concerned with wise expenditures, accountability of program managers, and return on their investments. This translates into an emphasis on factors such as administration expenses and other indirect costs, and direct program expenses. A third perspective is that of the communal aggregates and society. This accounting perspective is very complex and comprehensive but a bit more neutral. From the societal perspective, factors to include in the economic analysis would include taxes, costs of morbidity, and opportunity costs to provide other social or human services programs.

Each accounting perspective has its advantages and disadvantages, as well as being more appropriate for some economic evaluations than for others. For example, a simple cost description would not include the societal perspective, but a cost-benefit analysis would be deficient if a societal perspective was not taken. For some economic analyses, it may be appropriate to combine accounting perspectives, within reasonable limits. To avoid a systematic bias in underinclusion or overinclusion of program costs, refer to the service utilization and program theory as guides to determining what ought to be included as program costs.

Monetize and Compute Program Costs

The majority of costs are related to the program and would include the resources utilized by the program and by participants. Detailed program expenditures are used as the basis for computing the indirect and direct costs associated with providing the program. The program theory provides a guide for identifying program costs, especially the process theory (Exhibit 13.5). Depending on the type of analysis, the cost associated with antecedent, determinant, and contributing factors in the effect theory may need to be considered (Exhibit 13.6). Some cost analyses, particularly of population-based services, may use cost data that are not directly from each program. For example, Schramm (1992), in a cost study of prenatal care, used Medicaid claims data to generate the cost of prenatal care. For large population studies, claims data may be the only cost data available, but it inherently represents the amount paid by an insurer, not the full costs to provide the service. Most providers would argue that Medicaid or Medicare claims data grossly underestimate the actual costs of providing the service. Whether the claims data used to monetize program costs are from federal or private insurers, the claims payments represent only the amount that the insurer is willing to pay relative to the charge for the service, not the actual cost of providing the program.

If costs or expenses to the participant are included in the economic analysis, it may be necessary to monetize items for which a dollar value is knowable, as well

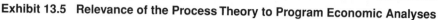

Exhibit 13.5   Relevance of the Process Theory to Program Economic Analyses

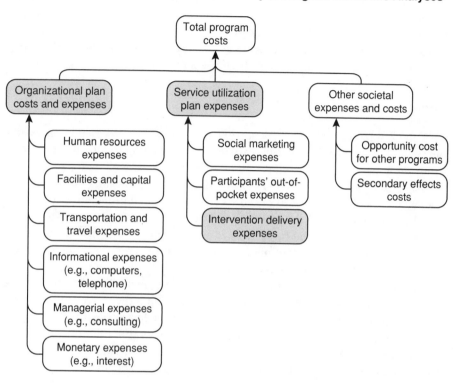

Exhibit 13.6   Relevance of the Effect Theory to Program Economic Analyses: Conceptualizing Costs and Savings Based on Effect Theory

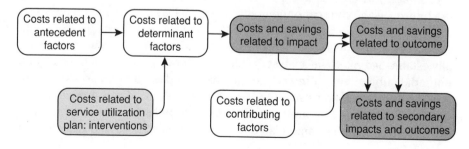

as those for which the dollar value is less obvious. Knowable costs for program participants would include new or special equipment (i.e., handrails or cooking utensils), educational materials (i.e., books or magazine subscriptions), transportation, or child care while attending the program. Other costs and expenses may not be easy to monetize. For example, participation in a substance abuse program may cost the participant older friendships based on substance use activities.

Adjust for Time

Time is a factor that affects costs, just as it can affect program impacts and outcomes. Therefore, it is necessary to decide upon a time period during which program impacts and outcomes will be considered, as well as for projecting program expenses and costs. In addition, time changes the value of money and the value of health benefits. Economists have developed procedures for taking time into account. All of the procedures attempt to convert a monetary value either in the past or in the future into a current value. The procedures most commonly used in economic analyses of health programs are discounting, adjusting for inflation, and depreciation.

Discounting is the process of converting future health benefits and future dollars to the present value. It is done by decreasing the current value by a rate, usually between 1% and 3%, on an annual basis. In a sense it is the reverse of interest. In this way, expenses and health benefits that might be expected in 2 or 20 years are all valued on a par with one another. This facilitates interpretation of the values and makes it simpler to see the costs so that decision makers can make choices based on data that are, so to speak, standardized.

Two adjustments for time are typically applied only to expenses or costs: inflation and depreciation. The most familiar is inflation. Inflation is the rate at which current dollars will have a lower value in the future, and thus a set number of additional dollars will be needed in the future to have the same value as now. Inflation is applied to program expenses. Adjustment for inflation is readily noted when reports state the year for dollar amounts, such as "$500 (in 1986 dollars)." Depreciation is the decreasing value of capital equipment into the future, just as your car or computer is worth less the longer you own it.

Each of these adjustments uses a rate. The rate chosen can be an estimated rate, the rate used by the organization providing the program, or the federally established rate. The analyst decides which rate to use, which hints at the potential subjectivity of the economic analyses. Despite this area of discretion, each of these adjustments for time has a standardized procedure and economic formulas that are applied. Most textbooks on economic analyses provide these formulas, and related tables. Nonetheless, the rate selected and the items to which the rates are applied involves both theoretical and practical knowledge of the program, its costs, and its potential effects.

Identify and Measure Program Effects

The choice of what to use in the economic analysis, as an indicator of program effect would have been made when the effect evaluation was designed. For this reason, generally, economic analyses of a program rely on data already collected as part of the impact evaluation. Those data or results can be used as the basis for the next step. If an impact evaluation has not been conducted, then the action and conceptual theories of the program effect are essential for justifying what outcomes would be likely to occur, and hence what should be measured.

Not all program effects are part of the program theory. There can be secondary effects, whether anticipated or not, and the effects can spill over to individuals not participating in the program. These are called externalities. Externalities may be indirect or even unanticipated consequences of the program, whether beneficial or harmful. Including them can be important in economic analyses that attempt to monetize a broad range of program-related effects, specifically CBAs. Externalities are identified by conducting a "thought experiment" in which one imagines possible programmatic effects on the target audience as a whole, irrespective of participation. Identifying externalities is important because they then become effects (if beneficial) or costs (if harmful or in some way costly). Including externalities provides a more comprehensive, and thus more accurate, economic analysis.

Monetize the Effects

There are many ways to assign dollar values to intangible health program impacts and outcomes. A decision must be made as to which of the various methods of monetizing program impacts and outcomes to use. Exhibit 13.7 lists the possible approaches. The choice depends upon the information available and is influenced by the overall accounting perspective of the economic analysis and the level and type of expertise of those doing the economic evaluation.

That a variety of methods are possible for monetizing outcomes highlights the possible difficulties in conducting economic evaluations of health programs. One of many possible complications in monetizing outcomes is that not all impacts or benefits are equally important, yet monetizing the impacts and benefits treats them as equal in terms of dollars.

Exhibit 13.7   Approaches to Monetizing Impacts and Outcomes

Approach	Method
Market value of any state of health or ongoing medical treatment for illnesses	Obtain price for treatments, wages
Client willingness to pay for the service	Observe choices that are made by program participants or members of the target audience
Policy maker's view of the value	Ask policy maker to estimate the dollar value of the impact
Practitioner's view of the value	Ask health professional to estimate the dollar value of the impact

Conduct an Analysis

This step essentially involves doing the math. It is possible to perform the calculations for many economic analyses, particularly cost analyses and CEAs, using readily available software, such as Excel. This requires that the spreadsheet be set up in a manner that includes all the key parameters of the economic analysis.

Conduct a Sensitivity Analysis

A sensitivity analysis is the systematic alteration of any parameter of the economic analysis for the purpose of determining the point at which the conclusions would become substantively different (Drummond et al., 1997). The purpose of conducting a sensitivity analysis is to identify the parameter that is most influential in altering the conclusion, as well as to establish the range wherein changes in the costs related to either the program or the outcomes have minimal effect. In conducting any economic analysis, there are uncertainties regarding factors such as the mortality and morbidity prevented, or regarding the actual costs. Another way to think of sensitivity analysis is that it helps deal with the uncertainties of CBA, CEA, and CUA because it allows one to do "what if" scenarios and thus gain additional information for decision making. Because it varies and tests the values of key parameters, a sensitivity analysis helps to identify dependence upon assumptions. It thus provides additional information for determining a break point around which decision making is more important. For example, in a study of the cost-effectiveness of care for very low birth weight (VLBW) infants, Rogowski (1998) found that the cost-effectiveness ratio varied by category of VLBW. This type of analysis reflects the overlap between sensitivity analyses and the use of decision rules mentioned earlier regarding characteristics of program participants. A sensitivity analysis is done as a final step because all of the variables that are to be monetized have then been identified and monetized in the primary analysis.

Conducting a sensitivity analysis requires deliberately varying one or more key parameters, one at a time, along a range of values. The economic analysis is then repeated using the new range of values for the key parameter. For example, in a cost-effectiveness study of pneumococcal vaccination of infants and children, Lieu and associates (2000) conducted a sensitivity analysis. They varied the following parameters used in their CEA: the incidence rate of pneumococcal infection, the rate of serious subsequent infection, the rate of a secondary infection (otitis media), the vaccine efficacy, the cost of vaccine administration, the cost of clinic visits and hospitalizations, the discount rate, the rate at which infants and children were covered by the vaccination, and the cost of medical care and work loss of the parents due to adverse reactions to the immunization. By varying each of these key parameters, the authors were able to identify which parameter was most critical in altering the results of the CEA. They found that using assumptions that favored the efficacy and coverage rates altered the "bottom line" recommendation, compared to less favorable assumptions. This highlights the critical importance of conducting a sensitivity analysis.

Disseminate the Findings

As with the process evaluation and the impact evaluation, the findings of the economic analysis need to be distributed to relevant program stakeholders and to policy makers. The method of dissemination ought to be suited to the level of rigor used to conduct the economic analysis. In some cases, dissemination can be through academic venues, such as professional journals, especially if the findings are new or provocative. It may also be important to disseminate the findings more rapidly through electronic venues that are accessible by those interested in the health problem or program, such as Listservs and websites. The assumption is that dissemination, particularly to the stakeholders and decision makers, leads to programmatic decisions based on the findings. Prosser, Koplan, Neumann, and Weinstein (2000) suggested that a lack of understanding about economic evaluations may be one barrier to the use of the findings. This suggests that to have a programmatic effect, the dissemination of the findings ought to be accompanied by some education of the decision maker.

ASSESSING ECONOMIC EVALUATIONS

Not all publications and reports of program economic evaluations are what they seem or do what their titles say they do. In addition, Deverill, Brazier, Green, and Booth (1998) found that reports of economic evaluations fell short of meeting established criteria for being ideal reports. Therefore, it is important to become a savvy consumer of economic evaluations. The following are widely accepted criteria for assessing published economic evaluations (Drummond et al., 1997; Carande-Kulis et al., 2000; Gold et al., 1996). These criteria can be used to determine whether the published report warrants merit and therefore can be used for programmatic decision making.

The first factor to consider is the framework for the study, with regard to whether the economic question is well defined. A study that is not founded on either economic theory or program theory is likely to contain scientific flaws, especially with regard to monetizing impacts and externalities.

Descriptions of alternative programs that are being compared must be included. These descriptions ought to address the extent to which the effectiveness of the interventions has been established. Preferably, strongly recommended or recommended interventions, practices, or programs are being evaluated. However, it may be that the study is of a new or alternative intervention that is not yet recommended or strongly recommended as practice. In such a study, the efficacy of the new intervention, practice, or program must then be well established.

The data and methods used in the economic analysis ought to be critiqued. Both the costs and consequences, or programmatic impacts, need to have been identified for the programs being considered. In addition, the appropriateness of units of measure ought to be critiqued, particularly in terms of the type of economic analysis being done. The dollar values need to be credible for both the program costs and the program benefits, impacts, and peripheral effects. A carefully done economic analysis will also have taken into account adjustments for time, specifically discounting, inflation, and depreciation. Moreover, a thorough report will state the base year and type of currency used in the analysis. The type of software used to conduct the analysis should also be mentioned.

The results section must be carefully reviewed. In particular, a sensitivity analysis ought to have been conducted and the results of that separate analysis included in the report. A well-done report will include a graphical presentation of the results. If any secondary analyses were conducted, there also ought to be a description of how those were done and the findings.

Finally, scrutinize the discussion section of the study. This section should acknowledge and explain the limitations of the study. Policy implications of the findings need to be explicit, and programmatic intervention implications need to be addressed. Overall, the discussion section ought not to include new results but should provide new insights based on the findings.

ACROSS THE PYRAMID

At the direct services level of the public health pyramid, a CEA is more likely than a CBA or a CUA to be used to choose between two comparable programs or treatments for the same health condition. Most medical economic evaluations are of interventions intended to be delivered at this level.

At the enabling services level, economic evaluations are more likely to be of a CBA or CUA nature, because of the intangible aspect of enabling services. Economic evaluations of enabling services programs are probably the most challenging for several reasons. One reason is that the enabling service is likely to entail considerable intangible benefits, many of which may be difficult to quantify and to monetize. Also, enabling services programs have considerable indirect costs that may not be obvious until the program is scrutinized. For example, volunteer time may be a key indirect cost of a less visible component in a larger program. Another reason that economic evaluations of enabling services are challenging is that there are likely to be considerable and varied family benefits and costs to take into account. This translates into needing to address more secondary costs and benefits, as well as more externalities and opportunity costs for program participants. Yet another reason that economic evaluations of enabling services are challenging is that these services are often "hidden" within programs, making it difficult to conduct the economic evaluation. For example, providing a referral for GED classes can be part of the WIC program, yet the GED referral and attendance at GED classes may never be measured in the WIC program.

At the population-based level, all types of economic evaluations can be used to evaluate population-level programs. A CEA would be appropriate for comparing two screening programs that will be used with a population, such as mammogram versus breast self-examination, vaccine A versus vaccine B for a given infectious disease, or nutritional supplements in flour versus nutritional supplements in bread. A CBA would be appropriate for comparing two dissimilar full-coverage programs. For example, WIC might be compared with a bicycle helmet law, or a newborn hearing screening might be compared to a new workplace safety regulation, or Medicare might be compared with universal health insurance. A CUA would be appropriate if the overall health of a community is of concern, because it takes into consideration general preferences and because the preferences are usually measured in terms that are used to describe the quality of life and the overall health of a community. Examples would be comparing a motorcycle helmet law to no law, a proposed workplace safety regulation versus no new regulation.

At the infrastructure level, all economic evaluations can help guide health services or health policy decisions, and as such they are most aptly thought of as applying primarily at the infrastructure level. There might be economic evaluations of programs to strengthen the workforce, in which case a simple cost analysis of health personnel would be appropriate, such as the cost of using nurse practitioners or lay case managers to provide a service. Cost analyses indicate how to make the program more efficient and how to make the public health sector more efficient.

DISCUSSION QUESTIONS

1. Compare and contrast CEA, CBA, and CUA with regard to the costs that are included in the analysis. What effects would an underestimation of costs have? What effects would an overestimation of costs have?

2. Conduct a brief literature search for cost analyses or economic evaluations related to school health programs and for breast cancer prevention programs. Which types of economic evaluations tend to be used for each? At what level of the pyramid do these economic evaluations tend to occur?

3. Select one of the articles you found in your search of the literature for Question 2. Read the article and critique the report using the criteria provided. What is your overall assessment of the report?

4. Discuss possible methodological, ethical, or moral issues involved in monetizing outcomes.

References

Barry, P. Z., & DeFriese, G. H. (1990). Cost-benefit and cost-effectiveness analysis for health promotion programs. *American Journal of Health Promotion, 4,* 448–452.

Bowling, A. (1995). What things are important in people's lives? A survey of the publics' judgments to inform scales of health related quality of life. *Social Science and Medicine, 41,* 1147–1162.

Carande-Kulis, V. G., Maciosek, M. V., Briss, P. A., Teutsch, S. M., Zaza, S., et al. (2000). Methods for systematic reviews of economic evaluations for the Guide to Community Preventive Services. *American Journal of Preventive Medicine, 18*(IS), 75–91.

Deverill, M., Brazier, J., Green, C., & Booth, A. (1998). The use of QALY and non-QALY measures of health-related quality of life: Assessing the state of the art. *Pharmacoeconomics, 13,* 411–420.

Drummond, M. F., O'Brien, B., Stoddart, G. L., & Torrance, G. W. (1997). *Methods for the economic evaluation of health care programmes* (2nd ed.). Oxford: Oxford University Press.

Fielder, J. L., Dado, D. R., Maglalang, H., Juban, N., Capistrano, M., & Magpantay, M. V. (2000). Cost analysis as a vitamin A program design and evaluation tool: A case study of the Philippines. *Social Science & Medicine, 51,* 223–242.

Gabriel, S. E., Kneeland, T. S., Melton, L. J., Moncur, M. M., Ettinger, B., & Tosteson, A. N. (1999). Health-related quality of life in economic evaluations for osteoporosis: Whose values should we use? *Medical Decision Making, 19,* 141–148.

Garpenholt, O., Silfverdal, S. A., & Levin, L. A. (1998). Economic evaluation of general childhood vaccination against Haemophilus influence type B in Sweden. *Scandinavian Journal of Infectious Diseases, 30,* 5–10.

Gold, M. R., Seigel, J. E., Russell, L. B., & Weinstein, M. C. (Eds.). (1996). *Cost-effectiveness in health and medicine.* Oxford: Oxford University Press.

Jerrell, J. M., & Hu, T. (1996). Estimating the cost impact of three dual diagnosis treatment programs. *Evaluation Review, 20,* 160–180.

Lieu, T. A., Ray, G. T., Black, S. B., Butler, J. C., Kleinm, J. O, Brieman, R. F., et al. (2000). Projected cost-effectiveness of pneumococcal conjugate vaccination of healthy infants and young children. *Journal of the American Medical Association, 283,* 1460–1468.

Newbold, D. (1995). A brief description of the methods of economic appraisal and the valuation of health states. *Journal of Advanced Nursing, 21,* 325–333.

Patrick, D. L., & Erickson, P. (1993). *Health status and health policy: Allocating resources to health care.* New York: Oxford University Press.

Prosser, L. A., Koplan, J. P., Neumann, P. J., & Weinstein, M. C. (2000). Barriers to using cost-effectiveness analysis in managed care decision making. *American Journal of Managed Care, 6,* 173–179.

Prosser, L. A., Stinnett, A., Goldman, P., Williams, L., Hunink, M., Goldman, L., and Weinstein, M. (2000). Cost-effectiveness of cholesterol-lowering therapies according to selected patient characteristics. *Annals of Internal Medicine, 132,* 769–779.

Randolph, A. G., & Washington, E. (1990). Screening for chlamydia trachomatis in adolescent males: A cost-based decision analysis. *American Journal of Public Health, 80,* 545–550.

Rogowski, J. (1998). Cost-effectiveness of care for very low birth weight infants. *Pediatrics,* *102*(1 pt. 1), 35–43.

Schramm, W. F. (1992). Weighing costs and benefits of adequate prenatal care for 12,023 births in Missouri's Medicaid Program, 1988. *Public Health Reports, 107,* 647–652.

Sevick, M., Dunn, A., Morrow, M., Marcus, B., Chen, G. J., & Blair, S. (2000). Cost-effectiveness of lifestyle and structured exercise interventions in sedentary adults: Results of Project ACTIVE. *American Journal of Preventive Medicine, 19,* 1–8.

Shaw, J. (1995). Cost benefit analysis in the human services. *Australian Psychologist, 30,* 144–148.

Shepard, D. S., & Thompson, M. S. (1979). First principles of cost-effectiveness analysis in health. *Public Health Reports, 94,* 535–543.

Szucs, T. (2000). Cost-benefits of vaccination programmes. *Vaccine, 18*(Suppl. 1), S49–51.

Torrance, G. W., Siegel, J. E., & Luce, B. R. (1996). Framing and designing the cost-effectiveness analysis. In M. R. Gold, J. E. Seigel, L. B. Russell, & M. C. Weinstein (Eds.), *Cost-effectiveness in health and medicine.* Oxford: Oxford University Press.

Ubel, P. A., Nord, E., Gold, M., Menzel, P., Prades, J. L., & Richardson, J. (2000). Improving value measurement in cost-effectiveness analysis. *Medical Care, 38,* 892–901.

Windsor, R., Bailey, W., Richards, J., Manzella, B., Soong, S., & Brooks, M. (1990). Evaluation of the efficacy and cost effectiveness of health education methods to increase medication adherence among adults with asthma. *American Journal of Public Health, 80,* 1519–1521.

Zivolich, S., Shueman, S., & Weiner, J. (1997). An exploratory cost-benefit analysis of natural support strategies in the employment of people with severe disabilities. *Journal of Vocational Rehabilitation, 8,* 211–221.

CHAPTER 14

Continuing the Cycle

Chapter 1 described the program planning and evaluation process as a cycle, as reflected in Exhibit 1.3, which depicts feedback loops from impact evaluation to the assessment and planning stages. Information from an evaluation does not magically or automatically become a feedback loop; rather, intention and effort are needed to create and maintain the connection between evaluation findings and subsequent planning. Factors that influence the existence and strength of the feedback loops include making persuasive arguments, disseminating information, contextual elements, and ethics. This chapter finishes the cycle by focusing on the facts that constitute and strengthen the feedback loop.

DATA AND INFORMATION

It is incumbent upon the evaluator to disseminate information about the evaluation in order to complete the feedback cycle. Several considerations influence the dissemination of program evaluation findings. The first concern is with making a persuasive argument based on the data. Once a set of persuasive statements about the program is developed, the next consideration is the logistics of the report format. Finally, there is the possibility that the evaluation will be misused. Each of these considerations is discussed in this chapter.

Persuasion and Information

A major factor determining the effectiveness of feedback loops is the persuasiveness of the data and the resulting information. Although the word "persuasion" has negative connotations, the reality is that for change to occur and for decisions to be based on evaluation findings, individuals with decision-making authority need to be persuaded by the "facts." Unless the statements made based on the process monitoring and impact evaluation data are persuasive, there will not be any feedback loops; rather, there will be discrete, disconnected, and unused information.

When using statistical results, Abelson (1995) suggested that there are five properties of statements that govern the degree to which they are persuasive. One property is the magnitude of the intervention effect—in other words, the amount of change attributable to the program. The amount of change that can be attributed to the program influences the extent to which the statistical data are perceived as persuasive. One way to think about this is that people are more inclined to believe good news, and therefore larger intervention effects increase the persuasiveness of evaluation findings. A corollary of this is that people are less likely to be persuaded by small program effects, regardless of the potential clinical significance of a small effect. While it would be unethical to conduct an impact evaluation that is highly biased in favor of the program, the design and methods need to be such that the largest effect theorized can be identified.

Another property of a statement is the degree to which it is articulate in explaining the findings. Articulate statements have both clarity and detail. This speaks directly to the quality of the written or verbal report, sometimes referred to as style. Recipients of the findings must perceive that the report is clear, regardless of whether the producer of the report feels it is clear. Clarity can be achieved through style, language, use of graphs, and careful delineation of ideas and issues. Similarly, consumers of the evaluation report may have a different need for details compared to the producers of the evaluation report. One strategy for arriving at the optimal level of detail to be persuasive is to have someone not involved in the evaluation review the report and make suggestions as to what needs to be included. In other words, involve a few stakeholders in the development of any written reports that will be disseminated to their peers.

The third property of a statement that contributes to its persuasiveness is the generality of the conclusions. This means that the wider the applicability of the findings, the more likely the findings are to be persuasive. The notion that having highly generalizable findings makes the findings more persuasive runs counter to a more popular line of reasoning in the health field: that results must be tailored to the unique characteristics of the program participants, especially race, ethnicity, sexual orientation, and such. While it is imperative to consider the effect of the unique needs and perspectives of the program recipients in order to have an effective program, when it comes to influencing decisions, decision makers want information that will make the decision widely applicable. Thus, the decision makers often seek results that are generic, rather than specific. In addition, there is an intuitive sense that if something applies to many, there must be some underlying truth. Whether this line of reasoning is accurate is less important than acknowledging that as human beings we may instinctively think this way.

The fourth characteristic of persuasive statements is the degree to which the findings are interesting with regard to challenging current beliefs. When the findings are a surprise, more attention is paid to them. Similarly, if the findings are about important claims or behaviors, the statements will receive more attention and be more persuasive. Another way of thinking about this characteristic is that if the evaluation does not answer the "so what?" question, or only confirms the obvious, the findings are less persuasive. Findings that are surprising, unexpected, or not immediately explainable, and those that are important, become sound bites that are used to get attention and influence perceptions.

Lastly, if the findings have credibility in terms of being based on rigorous and sound methods and a coherent theory, the findings are more persuasive. The bottom line is if the evaluation methods, design, data collection, or analyses are flawed, the findings lose credibility and persuasiveness. It is worth reinforcing that a coherent theory is also needed for the findings to have credibility and persuasiveness. A coherent theory explains the findings in terms of relationships among the program intervention and impacts and outcomes. Such a theory decreases the possibility of claims that the findings happened by chance.

Patton (1997) suggested that both the strength of the evaluation claim, like the first of Abelson's statement properties, and its importance to the decision makers is crucial to the evaluation being of value. If we extend Patton's two dimensions to encompass intervention effect and interest values, the result is a matrix demonstrating that the influence of these characteristics on decision making varies (Exhibit 14.1). Unimportant claims that are not interesting and that reveal a low level of intervention effect based on weak rigor are quickly forgotten. Claims that are important and interesting, are based on good science, and show large program effects are readily used as the basis for decision making. The matrix hints at the challenges that must be overcome to generate claims that will be used in decision making, including subsequent program or evaluation decisions.

Information and Sense Making

Steps taken to turn data into persuasive information are important, but so is the process by which sense is made of information. Sense making (Weick, 1979, 1995) involves attributing meaning to information. Understanding the

---

Exhibit 14.1   Effect of Rigor and Importance of Claims on Decision Making*

	Quality of Claim	
Strength of Claim	Major importance, high interest	Minor importance, low interest
High rigor and effect	Ideal for making decisions	Becomes "factoid"
Low rigor and effect	Cause for concern, need to study further, tentativeness to decisions	Ignored, forgotten, unspoken

*Adapted from Patton, 1997.

psychological processes used by individuals to interpret information in order to make decisions is the other side of the persuasion coin. Data become information when they are given meaning. The process of giving meaning involves various human perceptual and judgment-making processes. These processes ultimately influence the decision-making process and are therefore important for health program planners and evaluators.

Several well-recognized phenomena are now widely accepted as affecting decision making, such as the unconscious use of a set of heuristics in making judgments (Tversky & Kahneman, 1974), and the use of hindsight bias and consequences to make judgments (Chapman & Elstein, 2000; Fischhoff, 1975), is also called retrospective sense making (Weick, 1979, 1995) or the one-of-us effect (Hastorf & Cantril, 1954). Each of these cognitive processing phenomena has potential consequences for program planners and evaluators. For example, Lipshitz, Gilad, and Suleiman (2000) studied the effect of having information about the outcomes on the perception of events. They found that the perception that the subject was "one of us" dramatically altered whether the subject's success or failure was met with reward or punishment. The findings from their study underscore the importance of the sociocultural context of decision making, especially with regard to situations in which there are clear failures and successes and when both rewards and sanctions are possible. These findings have relevance to the presentation of evaluation information.

They suggest that if the evaluator is *not* viewed as "one of us," then failures of either the program or the evaluation are more likely to be met with sanctions. In other words, evaluators who become aligned with the stakeholders are less likely to experience repercussions. This same psychological phenomenon applies to program staff; if the policy and organizational decision makers view program staff as "one of us," then the program staff are less likely to experience sanctions if the program is not successful.

Culture is another factor that can affect interpretation of data. Culturally based values, ways of thinking, and experiences influence the meaning attributed to results. One key area in which this may become evident is in discussions about what program changes need to occur. Just as there is a need for cultural competence in the design of the health program, there is a need for cultural competency in terms of organizational competence to make or guide the implementation of program changes based on data about the program theory or the effect theory.

A recognition of the cognitive elements in interpreting data, whether related to decision making or culture, highlights the intricate nature of facts and interpretations. It is easy to believe that having factual data will result in a detached, logically derived decision. However, evidence from decision science and psychology (not to mention one's own experience) does not fully support this proposition. Evaluators and program planners need not only to attend to the science of their work, but also to apply the science of decision making and attribution.

REPORTS

Evaluators are required to generate written reports and perhaps to make an oral presentation of the findings. The notions of persuasiveness and the malleable nature of interpretations are part of the context for these. Typically, the format of a report is tailored to the evaluation and overall situation. However, there are instances in which the format is very specific and the evaluator has minimal flexibility in the report format, as with state or federal grants. Increasingly, these reports are submitted over the Internet, using predetermined forms that have severe limits on the number of words or characters. If the evaluator is not the one submitting the forms, it will be critical to work with program personnel in advance so that they have the information required for reporting to the funding agency. In addition to the reporting required by the funding agency, the evaluator may be asked to prepare a longer narrative report.

To the extent possible, a report ought to relate findings to the program process and impact objectives. This might be done in a table format, in which each objective is listed and the corresponding evaluation results are presented. Such a table will provide a visual context in which the audience can clearly see the areas in which the program was more and less successful in meeting its objectives.

Evaluation reports generally contain an executive summary, background on the program and evaluation, a description of the program, a description of the evaluation, and a summary and recommendations. The content and style used for writing the report ought to be tailored to its audience. Gabriel (2000) argued that because of the ever evolving nature of the evaluations of health programs, evaluation reports and reporting strategies ought to forgo the usual research format that emphasizes data analysis and instead should focus on providing evaluation information to the decision makers and program stakeholders as expediently as possible.

An executive summary is the portion of the report that is most likely to be copied and distributed and hence most widely read. It ought to contain enough information to convince any reader that the program and evaluation designs were appropriate. It is also the section in which recommendations are summarized, and it therefore can be used as a tool for decision making about the program. Executive summaries vary in length from one page to several pages. The length of the executive summary depends on its anticipated use, reporting requirements, and agency preferences.

Evaluators will often be asked or required to give oral presentations of the evaluation plan or results. The first consideration when preparing such a presentation is the audience. Will it be staff, program participants, policy makers, or other researchers? The answer will influence the content to be covered, as well as the choice of which details will be of greatest interest to the audience. Use of software such as Microsoft's PowerPoint can greatly facilitate generating an outline of the presentation and can simplify making appropriately designed overheads. Overheads ought to be in large print, with no more than one idea per slide and no more than seven or eight lines of text. Audiences have also become accustomed to receiving handouts of the presentation, but carefully consider what is on the overheads and whether it is wise and timely to make that information widely available. If the evaluation has been done in a manner that has involved the stakeholders throughout the process, there should not be any surprises, and release of the information will not be an issue. In less ideal situations, caution may be in order.

The use of charts and graphics is important when writing reports. The old adage that a picture is worth a thousand words is true, and exhibits are more likely to be remembered than text. While not every number needs to be graphed, having no graphic representations makes reports dense, potentially boring, and less persuasive. Exhibits, whether graphs, charts, figures, or tables, ought to be designed to facilitate remembering critical points. Findings that are surprising, confirming, alarming, or interesting are appropriate choices for being illustrated with exhibits. Readily available software makes generating exhibits and integrating them into written reports quite easy. Exhibits should follow convention regarding which variable is on which axis. For example, time is best plotted on the horizontal (or y) axis. It is essential that some explanatory text accompany all exhibits, as not all readers will be able to interpret graphic presentations. The rationale for including the exhibit needs to be explicit. The choice of what is presented graphically is in part a way to influence perceptions, attention, and hence decision making.

Performance Measures

The format for reporting on the progress and evaluation of health programs may be predetermined by the funding agency. In particular, state health programs that receive federal funding are required to report on a standard set of performance measures. The development and use of performance measures across the Department of Health and Human Services (DHHS) has become ubiquitous, and performance measures are now required of federally supported state health programs. A performance measure is "a quantitative indicator that can be used to track progress toward an objective" (Perrin & Koshel, 1997, p. 5). Exhibit 14.2 gives definitions of the terms used in federal performance measures. These terms are required of state programs funded by the Bureau of Maternal and Child Health. However, each funding body will have a similar set of performance measures and definitions.

The language of performance measures is different from that used by evaluators, potentially causing tension and confusion. Because state health programs that receive federal funding are required to develop and report on these types of performance measures, evaluators and program planners need to consciously translate the more pure evaluation science language of objectives and program theory into the federal language of performance measures (Exhibit 14.3). The translation is not always a direct one; this is an additional reason to involve the stakeholders throughout the process of program development and evaluation. Also, while the funding agency may need standard reports from all programs, the data reported may not be in a format that the program managers find helpful in their program management. In such cases, evaluations may have a dual focus of providing the performance measure data and generating information that is more immediately useful for program management, development, and improvement.

Exhibit 14.2   Definitions of Terms Used in Federal Performance Measures

Performance Measure Element	Definition
Measure Type	Broad health status that the performance measure is intended to describe
Measure	Statement in measurable terms of the desired health status or behavior, as it relates to the measurement type
Numerator	Definition by which to assign individuals into the numerator in order to quantify the measure
Denominator	Definition by which to assign individuals into the denominator in order to quantify the measure
Rationale for Measure	Brief explanation of relationship of the measure to the measurement type. Includes reference to the appropriate *Healthy People 2010* objective
Limitations of Measure	Statement of possible key factors that can contribute to the potential failure of the program, and that would be captured in the measure
Use of Measure	Suggestions for how the measure might be used in program development or policy making
Data Resources	Relevant sources of data for estimating the measure
Limitations of Data	Brief statement as to possible factors that may contribute to inaccurate, not valid, or not reliable data from the data resource listed

Making Recommendations

Making recommendations, whether in a report or verbally, can tax the interpersonal and political skill of an evaluator. Recommendations can focus on the positive aspects that were identified through the evaluation as well as on areas needing change or improvement. They must be based on and be a

Exhibit 14.3   Comparison of Performance Measurement and Evaluation Language and Terms

Performance Measurement Language	Evaluation Terms
Measure type	Goal
Measure	Process or impact objective
Numerator	Sample
Denominator	Sampling frame, sample population
Rationale for measure	Hypotheses from the outcome theory
Limitations of measure	Confounding factors related to program implementation
Use of measure	Specific utilization-focused application of the evaluation
Data resources	Data collection methods
Limitations of data	Validity and reliability issues

direct and clear outgrowth of the evaluation data. Recommendations ought to be linked to the program theory and should address the organizational and service utilization plan (Exhibit 14.4), identifying specific elements in need of improvement. As well, the recommendations can address elements of the effect theory (Exhibit 14.5) by specifying which of the hypotheses seem not to be supported by the evaluation data and indicating alternative hypotheses that could be used to explain the findings. Framing the recommendations in accordance with the way the program was conceptualized will help program managers and other stakeholders make decisions regarding what needs to be or can be done and in what order of priority. Also, recommendations that are linked to elements of the program theory are more likely to be readily understood and hold higher credibility. The following information regarding recommendations frames the dos and don'ts suggested by Hendricks and Papagiannis (1990) within the context of program theory.

Exhibit 14.4   Making Recommendations Related to the Organizational and Service Utilization Plans

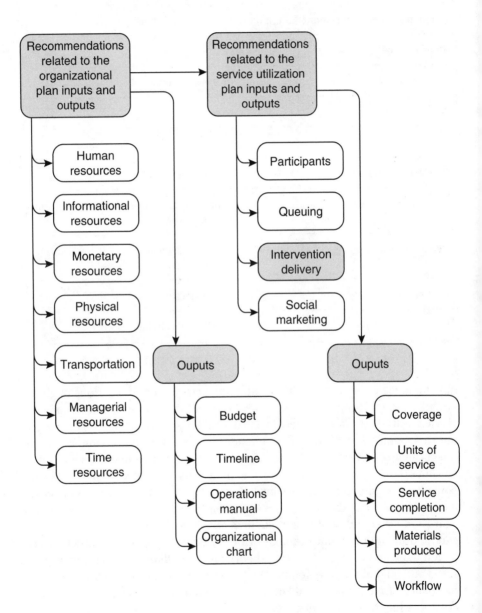

Exhibit 14.5 Making Recommendations Related to the Effect Theory

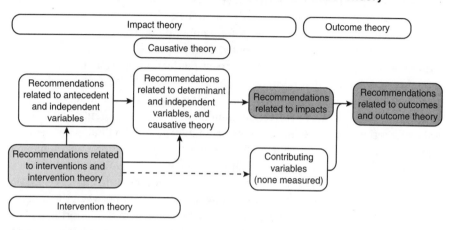

Throughout the development and evaluation of the health program, recommendations can be collected so that good ideas and insights are not lost or forgotten. Also, a wide variety of resources can be the basis of making recommendations, including existing scientific literature, program staff, and program stakeholders. Drawing on such sources for explanation or justification of the recommendations adds to their credibility. It almost goes without saying that it is important to work closely with the program decision makers, including during the process of developing the recommendations. This will minimize the possibility of surprises being included in the report, thus decreasing the risk of being perceived as undermining the program. Working with the decision makers also begins to build support for the recommendations.

Recommendations ought to make sense in the larger context in which the program and the evaluation occurred, including the social, political, and organizational context, as well as within the context of the technical knowledge available when the program was conceived. Recommendations that show knowledge of the contextual influences can more easily be accepted as applicable and may lead to changes in various elements of the program theory. Recommendations that are realistic in the view of the stakeholders are more likely to be accepted and implemented. This does not negate the need to make appropriate recommendations that may take time to implement or that could be implemented under different circumstances. In this sense, not all recommendations need to be equal in the effort that acting upon them might require, nor are all recommendations equal in terms of specificity and generality. Decision makers generally prefer choosing from a set of recommendations, thus enabling them to maintain their positions as decision makers.

Recommendations that require a fundamental change, such as to the program theory, are less likely to be accepted or implemented than ones that are less extensive. Such recommendations are best made in an incremental format so that they are simplified and, therefore, more acceptable and useful to the decision makers. It also helps to have some accompanying statements or insights into future implications of the recommendations, whether potential benefits or implementation strategies. Again, this type of information facilitates the decision making regarding which recommendations to act upon. Of course, recommendations that are easy to understand will receive more attention and acceptance. Techniques for improving the ease of comprehension include categorizing the recommendations in meaningful ways, drawing a boundary between the findings and the recommendations, placing the recommendations in the report in a place that is meaningful and appropriate, and presenting the recommendations in ways that the decision makers are accustomed to receiving information.

Misuse of Evaluations

Given the pressures to sustain programs and to meet funding mandates, evaluation results may be misused. Misuse can occur in many ways, but it is generally understood as the manipulation of the evaluation in ways that distort the findings or that compromise the integrity of the evaluation. Misuse can occur at any point during the evaluation process, beginning with an inappropriately chosen design that will bias findings, and extending to interference with data collection and the outright alteration of the evaluation findings (Stevens & Dial, 1994). Evaluators, program management, program staff, stakeholders, and program participants involved in an evaluation can be susceptible to a variety of pressures that may result in a less than unbiased evaluation. These pressures include biases based on resource constraints and self-interest, as well as external political and funding agency pressures. Pressures can also come from within the organization providing the health program. Such pressures affect not only the evaluation design and execution, but also the manner in which the results are interpreted, used, and disseminated or suppressed.

Patton (1997) argued that increases in the use of evaluation information are accompanied by an increase in the misuse of the information. This is a function of the increased opportunity for the pressures leading to misuse to be present. It is important to acknowledge that misuse can be both intentional, such as falsifying client satisfaction responses, and unintentional, such as not having time to distribute client satisfaction surveys on busy days. Sometimes the pressures for misuse are subtle and responses are almost subconscious, and the intention might even be to help the program. Such complexities add to the difficulty of detecting and avoiding misuse. One way to minimize misuse is to involve program stakeholders and educate them about the evaluation and its appropriate use. For example, it may be important not only to publicize favorable findings, but also to acknowledge unfavorable findings and the plans to address those findings. In addition, sharing with the stakeholders and program staff the standards to which evaluators are held by their professional organization may help them realize that the use of evaluation is not only a funding or sustainability issue but also an ethical issue.

ETHICS

With recent attention at the federal level and in the press on research involving human subjects, ethics has become a foremost concern in health care. Ethics is the discipline or study of rights, morals, and principles that guide human behavior. Issues become ethical when basic human rights are involved or when dilemmas arise as to what might be the moral and principled course of action. In terms of health program development and program evaluation, the potential for ethical concerns is omnipresent.

Choices regarding who will or will not receive the health program can raise ethical questions. For example, if random assignment is planned, then the ethical question is what to do for those who are not to receive the program. Also, the choice of the target population can be subject to ethical questioning. What makes one high-risk or vulnerable group of individuals more or less worthy of receiving a health program can be an ethical issue. It is possible that conflicts regarding the development of a health program are implicitly conflicts of ethical perspectives.

Institutional Review Board Approval and Consents

For evaluation, ethical issues are most likely to surface with regard to the need to have participants in the evaluation provide informed consent. Informed consent is the agreement to voluntarily and willingly participate in a study based on a full disclosure of what constitutes participation in the study and the risks and benefits involved in participating. Whether or not informed consents are used in the evaluation is based on a set of factors: the requirements of the funding agency, the requirements of the agency providing the program, and the intent of the evaluation. If the evaluation will be used only for internal managerial purposes and will not be used to generate knowledge, then the evaluation is not research and informed consent is not required.

However, if the evaluation is done with the intent of generating generalizable knowledge, then the evaluation is considered research. For example, if the findings of the evaluation are to be shared beyond the program agency, as in an academic journal, the evaluation is considered research. In that case, evaluators, as researchers, are obligated to comply with federal regulations regarding obtaining informed consent. Universities and health care organizations that receive federal research grants have Institutional Review Boards (IRBs) that review the proposed research for compliance with the federal regulations governing research involving human subjects. IRBs are composed of researchers, nonresearchers, and representatives from the community at large.

The process of gaining IRB approval for conducting an evaluation is not a trivial issue and warrants serious attention. Even students who are conducting evaluation research need to obtain IRB approval of their research. There are three levels of IRB review (Exhibit 14.6), with full review being the most comprehensive and involving all members of the IRB. Research may either qualify for expedited review by two members of the IRB or be exempt from IRB review but still required to be registered as human subject research. Although the exact procedures and forms will vary slightly among IRBs, the responsibilities and reviews are essentially the same because the IRB is following federal regulations, specifically the 45 CFR 46. According to these regulations, informed consent has eight elements (Exhibit 14.7), each of which must be addressed in the consent form, preferably at an eighth-grade reading level. These eight elements can be addressed in brief letters for anonymous surveys or may entail extensive, multiple-page details for medical studies.

The highly formalized and bureaucratic procedures involved in obtaining IRB approval often cloud the underlying need to assure that researchers, and evaluators, act ethically and that all persons involved in evaluation research be protected from needless harm. Therefore, if the evaluation is expected to generate knowledge, the evaluator either is obligated or is just plain smart to gain IRB approval. However, IRB approval is needed before the evaluation begins, and hence it can be a major issue in the timeline of conducting program evaluation.

Ethics and Evaluation

Marvin (1985) stressed that evaluators have a responsibility to program participants and to evaluation participants to explain how the evaluation has

Exhibit 14.6 Comparison of Types of IRB Reviews

Type of Review	Definition and Criteria	Process
Full (review by all IRB members)	Involves more than minimal risk, involves knowing the identity of the participants, data are sensitive or may put the participant at risk	Requires completing a full IRB application, must provide copies of all materials (i.e., surveys, consents, recruitment flyers, data abstraction forms, interview questions) that will be used in the research
Expedited (review by two IRB members)	Involves no more than minimal risk and may involve knowing the identity of participants	Requires completing a full IRB application, must provide copies of all materials (i.e., surveys, consents, recruitment flyers, data abstraction forms, interview questions) that will be used in the research
Exempt (no IRB review required)	Involves no more than minimal risk, the identity of participants is not known or knowable, routine educational research, food tasting research	A brief form is submitted that describes the research, one member of the IRB determines its exempt status

the potential to harm them and future program participants. One point he made is particularly relevant to IRBs and consent forms. If the evaluation has potential implications for future programs and their availability, participants have the right to be aware of this.

Many health programs are designed for and delivered to children. Hence, the evaluation necessitates the collection of data from children. This can pose special ethical and IRB problems. Children who are old enough to understand that they are being asked to participate in a study must provide assent to be in the study; this would include being in evaluation research. The refusal of either the child or the parent to be in the evaluation study must be honored. This becomes complicated as the child becomes older and is increasingly capable of making decisions independently of his or her parents. For example, adolescents in safe-sex education programs may be willing to be in an evaluation

Exhibit 14.7   Eight Elements of Informed Consent, as Required in the Federal Regulations 45 CFR 46

1. Statement that makes it clear that the participant is being asked to volunteer to be in a research study (and that they can withdraw if they choose).

2. Explanation of the purpose of the research.

3. Description of the research procedures that details what is expected of the participant (tasks, length of participation in the intervention and the research, type of data to be collected, etc.).

4. Specification of the risks or discomforts that are possible or likely from being in the study.

5. Explanation of the direct benefits to the participant, if any are possible or likely, from being in the study.

6. Statement of confidentiality and how it will be maintained.

7. Description of any compensation or payment for being in the study.

8. Phone numbers where the participant can get more information about the research, about their rights as research participants, and assistance if there is an injury or other problem resulting from being in the research.

study but may not want their parents to know they are in the program. The evaluator must carefully consider the consequences and creatively develop means of including children without denying parental or child rights. One major consequence of including children in evaluation research is that participation rates may decline when parental consent is required for participation either in the program or in the evaluation. Esbensen and associates (1996) studied the effect of requiring parental consent on participation in an evaluation of a gang prevention program. They achieved a participation rate of 65%, which varied by program site. They were unable to determine the reason that parents failed to provide consent for their children. Similarly, Johnson and associates (1999) were able to achieve 70% written parental consent in only 7 of 10 schools involved in a health promotion program. They found that in order to get parental consent for children to participate in a school program evaluation, a school-based strategy was most cost-effective in reaching the goal of 80% written parental consent. Dynarski (1997) further complicated the situation by reminding that consent is needed in experimental evaluations, as occurs when schools are randomized to experimental and control conditions.

Just as children are considered a special vulnerable population, there are many other vulnerable groups for whom health programs are designed and offered. The special circumstances of these groups need to be considered with regard to obtaining consents. For example, Gondolf (2000) found that in evaluating domestic violence programs focused on the batterers, several issues needed to be addressed: maintaining the safety of the victim, tracking in longitudinal studies, and obtaining consent from both the present and past batterers and their corresponding victims. Taking precautions to address these issues resulted in a low refusal rate and few safety problems for participants. Evaluators can use this and similar studies to better estimate the highest possible participation rates and ethical techniques to use for increasing the participation of children and other highly vulnerable groups in health program evaluations.

Evaluators and program managers also may need to deal with ethical issues related to program staff. Such issues emerge when the health program involves community outreach and the safety of program staff is a major concern. Also, if program staff are participants in the program evaluation, as is likely to occur in process monitoring evaluations, their rights as study participants need to be taken into account. These rights include confidentiality with regard to the information they provide. Program staff may themselves face ethical issues with regard to legally mandated reporting of occurrences, such as child abuse and specific infectious diseases (i.e., syphilis, tuberculosis) that they may feel need to be balanced against their safety or the safety of others involved.

Other factors contributing to ethical issues are financial arrangements, conflicts of interest, multiple relationships, level of competence, and deadlines. Each of these factors has the potential to create an ethical dilemma. Another consideration is highlighted by the findings of one study in which evaluators who were employed in private or consulting businesses had different views of what constituted unethical behavior compared to evaluators employed in academic settings (Morris & Jacobs, 2000). These results are a stark reminder that ethics is both contextual and highly individualized. While principles may be agreed upon, their application may not. It is reasonable to also expect that evaluators working closely with stakeholders may find a wide range of opinions about ethical behavior. As always, open dialogue and discussion of the ethical issues inherent in the health program or evaluation are the optimal approach to reaching either consensus on actions or comfortable disagreements.

HIPAA and Evaluations

In April 2003, the Health Insurance Portability and Accountability Act (HIPAA) went into effect (Center for Medicaid and Medicare Services, 2003;

Department of Health and Human Services, 2003). The purpose of HIPAA is to protect personal information related to having received health care. Personal information includes birth date, any element of an address, dates on which services were received, and diagnoses. Health providers must take specified steps to protect personal identifier information, including having secure fax lines and getting written permission to share personal information with others, whether insurance companies or consulting providers.

The effects of HIPAA on the evaluation of health programs depend on whether the evaluator is an employee of the organization and the evaluation is part of routine care, or whether the evaluator is an outsider and the findings of the evaluation will be public in any way. In the first situation, the evaluation is likely to be small scale and involve an existing program being conducted by program staff. Because personal information about clients or patients is not being shared, there is no need to take additional steps with regard to the HIPAA regulations. This situation is similar to the one in which an informed consent would not be needed because the evaluation is not research. However, if client data are being provided to an external evaluator or the evaluation is federally funded (National Institutes of Health, 2003), then the HIPAA regulations would require that each client be informed that his or her information is provided to others and provide a signed authorization of information release. As implementation of the HIPAA regulations becomes part of the routine functioning of health care organizations, there will be key individuals who can provide guidance on how to meet the HIPAA regulations.

HIPAA regulations apply only to a specific group of health care organizations, typically hospitals, clinics, and physician offices. The regulations do not apply to organizations that do not provide medical care. Thus, their health programs do not fall under the regulations, and evaluations of programs in exempt organizations do not require steps beyond the basic ethical considerations discussed earlier.

CONTEXTUAL CONSIDERATIONS

The evaluation process occurs within the context of organizations and other processes that exist to improve programs. Understanding the relationship of these to the evaluation has considerable benefits.

Organization-Evaluator Relationship

The relationship between the evaluator and the organization is one that requires attention, whether the evaluator is an employee or an external consultant. Several factors can influence or shape the relationship. One such factor is that the evaluator may be a third party between the program or organization and the funding agency. In this situation, third-party dynamics come into play. That is, two parties may form a coalition against the third. The most likely scenario would be for the program manager to align with the funding agency in any dispute with the evaluator. Another factor influencing the evaluator-organization relationship is the different levels of priority given by the evaluator and the organization to the health program, and possible changes in these priorities. The differences in priorities lead to different timelines, different expectations, and different levels of commitment in terms of attention and resources. Yet another factor affecting the relationship between the evaluator and the organization is differences in professional and organizational cultures and in the language used to describe the health program and the evaluation. Divergences in any of these areas can become a source of tension and conflict, especially if the divergence is not explicitly acknowledged. This is not an exhaustive list of possible factors affecting the relationship of the evaluator and the organization of the health program, but it reveals the complexities of the relationship, which deserve attention and merit the development of strategies and dialogues to optimize the relationship.

Another area of possible divergence is the broader purpose of the evaluation. Owen and Lambert (1998) suggested that evaluation for management is different from evaluation for leadership. They proposed that evaluation for management focuses on individual units or programs for the purpose of making ongoing adjustments with an emphasis on performance and accountability. This is essentially a process monitoring evaluation. In contrast, evaluation for leadership focuses on the whole organization, with a long-term perspective and collection of information across programs. They also noted that the roles of evaluator and organizational development consultant become blurred, particularly if the evaluator is asked to provide recommendations. In fact, Patton (1999) argued that there are numerous opportunities for evaluators to act as organizational development consultants. He explained that because programs are embedded in organizational contexts, improving programs may require attention to that organizational context. He found, through a case study, that the attainment of project goals was not necessarily related to the extent to which the program contributed to the fulfillment of the organizational mission. In other words, some programs are very good at doing the wrong thing when viewed from the perspective of the organization's business strategy. Being aware of this potential paradox and addressing it is one way in which evaluators contribute to organizational development.

Evaluators may see themselves, or be seen by others, as organizational change agents. Evaluators, as change agents, need to be conscious about how change occurs; a prerequisite for change is organizational readiness. The type of organization being changed is a further consideration, namely whether it is a small, community-based not-for-profit agency or a large federal bureaucracy. Evaluators can influence organizational decision making by first having affected or changed the perceptions held by those who are decision makers for the program. This can occur through the recommendations made at the end of an evaluation, or through continual rather than sporadic involvement with the program. Education of stakeholders throughout the planning and evaluation cycle, and through personal perseverance with regard to dissemination of information and accessing decision makers can all contribute to some degree of organizational change. In the end, the evaluator's skills in generating an understanding of what is needed from the organization must be matched to the organizational type, culture, and readiness for change.

An early point of discussion between the planner/evaluator and the hiring organization needs to focus on who owns the data gathered and analyzed throughout the planning and evaluation cycle. Generally, planners and evaluators who are hired as consultants have very limited proprietary rights over the data. The contract with the hiring organization will specify who owns the data and what can and cannot be done with it. An external evaluator needs some leeway and latitude so that potentially unfavorable findings can be seen by those who need to know about them. Getting the information to the decision makers is essential if the evaluation, whether a process monitoring or impact evaluation, is to serve as a feedback loop that fosters the development of the health program and the organizational functioning. Evaluators who cannot express concerns to key decision makers will be frustrated and are essentially divested of their proper responsibility. Ownership of data and dissemination of findings can become not only an internal political issue but also an ethical issue in terms of getting the results to decision makers and to making public the research findings, which can influence choices. The underlying issue is that evaluators may have a different perspective and interpretation of the evaluation results from those of the hiring organization, leading to conflict and tensions.

The organization is also a context for ethical dilemmas. Mathison (1999) suggested that there are minimal differences in the ethical dilemmas faced by internal and external evaluators. However, they live in different environments, which influence their actions or responses to ethical situations. Ultimately, evaluators need to be clear on their relationship with the organization and their role vis-a-vis ethical factors.

Evaluation and CQI/TQM

Within the health care industry, there has been an evolving focus on ways to improve the quality of care and services, beginning with Donabedian in 1966. Donabedian (1980) was the first in health care to suggest taking a systems approach by investigating structure, processes, and outcomes. Physiological health outcomes are comparatively easy to document and are familiar to practitioners. In contrast, organizational processes involved in providing care had no standardized reporting and were less familiar. Thus, well-developed approaches to studying processes became accepted as a means of improving organizational efficiency and effectiveness.

Two such approaches are continuous quality improvement (CQI) (Juran, 1989) and total quality management (TQM) (Deming, 1982). During the 1990s both approaches became popular as a means of enhancing organizational effectiveness. CQI and TQM are based on the premise that problems are best addressed through attention to the system as a whole and that employees are the best source of possible solutions. For the most part, these approaches focus on examining organizational processes using statistical and other tools. Since the 1990s, CQI and TQM have become commonplace in health care organizations (Shortell et al., 2000), and they are already being replaced by subsequent popular methodologies, such as Six Sigma, which is a process to reduce variation in clinical and business processes (Lazarus & Neely, 2003). Evaluators working in health care will, no doubt, experience a continual adoption of more-current approaches to improving the processes and outcomes of health care organizations. Because such methodologies direct attention toward solving problems, program evaluators need to be sensitive to how current process improvement approaches might influence program development and implementation and, hence, the evaluation. Organizational process improvement approaches differ from evaluation with regard to the underlying philosophy, the purposes, who does the activity, and the methods used (Exhibit 14.8).

Evaluations can be affected by the presence of CQI and TQM in several ways. Mark and Pines (1995) suggested that the evaluation will be influenced by whether an organization is engaged in CQI or TQM because employees will already be sensitized to the use of data, will have had an introduction to data analysis methods, and will be accustomed to participating in analytic and change activities. Staff, because of their participation in CQI or TQM teams, may expect to be involved in the development of a program and its evaluation. Thus, involving program staff may be slightly easier in organizations using CQI or TQM. It also may be easier to develop program theory in organizations using CQI or TQM because staff will already have training and knowledge of

Exhibit 14.8   Comparison of Improvement Methodologies and Program Evaluation

	Organizational Process Improvement Methodologies	Program Evaluation
Philosophy	Organizations can be more effective if they use staff expertise to improve services and products	Programs need to be justified in terms of their effect on participants
Purpose	Systems analysis and improvement are focused on identified problem areas from the point of view of customer needs	Need to determine whether a program was provided as planned and if it made a difference to the participants (customers)
Approach	Team-based approach to identifying and analyzing the problem	Evaluator-driven approach to data collection and analysis
Who does it	Staff: employees from any or all departments, midlevel managers, top-level executives	Evaluators, with or without the participation of stakeholders
Methods	Engineering approaches to systems analysis	Scientific research methods

techniques that can be very useful in program planning, especially PERT charting, Fishbone diagramming, and the use of control charts. PERT charting involves diagramming the sequence of events against a specific timeline and thus shows when tasks need to be accomplished. Fishbone diagrams, or cause diagrams, are representations of sequential events and major factors at play at each stage. Control charts show an average, with upper and lower confidence intervals and standard deviations. They show whether a variable is within the acceptable parameters, and they result in a heavy focus on setting and staying within control limits and parameters for a select set of impact indicators. These skills help articulate and then construct a diagram of underlying processes, especially in the process theory. They also make the CQI/TQM way of thinking and methods helpful and useful in designing and conducting process monitoring evaluations. This is especially the case because CQI/TQM methods facilitate identifying problems related to the implementation of the service utilization plan and deficiencies in the organizational plan.

Organizations with strong process improvement processes, nonetheless, need program evaluations, especially outcome or summative evaluations. Quality improvement methodologies that are focused primarily on service delivery or program implementation have as a major weakness not being able to causally link the program with impacts and outcomes. Thus, evaluators working in organizations with CQI/TQM processes contribute scientific rigor and knowledge to studying program impacts and outcomes.

META-EVALUATION

The term "meta-evaluation" has been used since at least 1982 (Feather, 1982). Meta-analysis is the analysis and synthesis of findings from previous studies in order to draw conclusions across a variety of data sets and samples about the strength of relationships among variables or the effectiveness of an intervention. This type of meta-evaluation is very similar to evidence-based approaches to medicine, in which the optimal, most effective intervention is sought based on a synthesis of existing research. In fact, the methodology for conducting meta-evaluations is similar to that for generating evidence-based practice guidelines.

The steps in a meta-evaluation essentially begin with a comprehensive search for existing evaluations on the topic or intervention of interest. The advent of electronic databases of published evaluation research makes it easy to search for existing evaluations from which to draw conclusions about effective interventions and programs. Once all relevant research has been located, using a variety of techniques (Cooper, 1998), a systematic review of each publication is conducted. From the information abstracted about the studies reviewed, a synthesis is done that results in a conclusion based on all the relevant research or evaluations. The conclusions drawn from meta-evaluations and evidence-based reviews are valuable because the techniques overcome the pitfalls inherent in relying on only one study or evaluation to make decisions. In addition, when meta-analytic statistics are used in conjunction with the review, the meta-evaluation results are adjusted for variations in the sample sizes of the original studies or evaluations.

Meta-evaluations have a place in health program planning and evaluation. Boyd and Windsor (1993) did a meta-analysis of prenatal nutrition programs and later of smoking cessation programs among pregnant women (Windsor, Boyd, & Orleans, 1998). Both of these would be considered systematic literature reviews according to Cooper (1998), rather than meta-analyses, because they did not present any summative statistics across the evaluations. Nonetheless, the use of these meta-evaluation and evidence-based approaches has led to some proactive thinking about health programs. For example, Robinson, Patrick, Eng, and Gustafson (1998) proposed a framework for reporting evaluations of the use of interactive health communications, such as websites. The purpose of their framework is to systematically develop a body of information that can be used to determine the effectiveness of the interactive health communications. Because such coordinated efforts are not likely to be widely adopted, reliance on the diverse evaluation studies is likely to remain the primary source of meta-evaluations and evidence-based reviews.

Another type of meta-evaluation focuses on programs either funded by or provided by a particular agency; this type of meta-evaluation seeks to understand the overall effectiveness of programs associated with that agency. The agency-based meta-evaluations are done using existing evaluations conducted by programs related to that agency. Major philanthropic foundations and large public health agencies are the types of agencies likely to engage in this type of meta-evaluation.

Whether meta-evaluations are conducted using extensive published evaluations or in-house reports, they are a means of synthesizing information across programs, across agencies, or across recipient populations. A major step in conducting meta-evaluations and evidence-based reviews is determining the quality of the evaluation research included in the systematic review. Tools and criteria have been developed for use in systematically evaluating the quality of the intervention and evaluation research (Farrington, 2003).

QUALITY OF EVALUATION

Various criteria can be used to assess and define the overall quality of program evaluations. Similar criteria have been established for use with systematic meta-evaluations and evidence-based reviews. Criteria have been established by groups concerned with evaluations (i.e., Advisory Committee on Head Start Research and Evaluation, 1999). Researchers have similarly established criteria and rating scales for the quality of research (Brown, 1991). Across the criteria, the following elements are areas commonly identified as needing to be thoroughly addressed for an evaluation to be considered of high quality. Of course, each of these elements can be addressed to varying degrees, and rarely will any one evaluation address all elements to perfection. The criteria also provide an outline for being more successful in avoiding evaluation failure (Exhibit 10.7) and ought to serve as a reminder of the challenges inherent in program evaluation. Along with this abbreviated list of elements of high-quality evaluations are the chapters in which that element is discussed.

One element is that the conceptual foundation of the evaluation ought to be explicitly stated, including the use of biological, social, psychological, or other theories relevant to the program effect theory (Chapter 5) and references made to previous evaluations of the same health problem. Another is that the evaluation question should be clearly stated and should focus on identifying the effect of the program (Chapter 9). The emphasis on effect and outcomes is consistent with the purpose of meta-evaluations and evidence-based reviews—to identify the most effective intervention for the stated health problem. Next, the evaluation design must be valid, credible, and feasible (Chapter 10). In other words, the scientific rigor of the design is evident in the published findings or the report. A high-quality evaluation of outcomes also includes attention to multiple domains of the outcome, using existing reliable measures (Chapter 9) and multiple modes of data collection when necessary or scientifically justified (Chapters 9 and 12). The attention to multiple domains is a recognition of the multiple components and multiple domains of health that might be affected by the health program. An optimal design includes random assignment to the program but does not compromise the provision of the health service to those not receiving the program. It also includes careful selection of program sites and careful attention to incentives for participating in the evaluation. Lastly, the data analysis methods must be appropriate for the data collected and the evaluation question (Chapter 11).

The Joint Commission on Standards for Educational Evaluation created standards for evaluation practice, and they were presented in Exhibit 1.2. These standards of utility, feasibility, propriety, and accuracy remain cornerstones for assessing the quality of health program evaluations. Evaluations need to be useful in meeting the needs of the program stakeholders, program audiences, and funding agencies. This requires communication, dialogue, and negotiation. Evaluations must be doable in terms of cost, political and diplomatic factors, and timelines. To achieve the feasibility standard, the evaluation must be developed and implemented with the same careful planning as that required to develop and implement the health program. Evaluations must be conducted in ethical and legal ways that are unbiased and sensitive to the vulnerability and rights of all program and evaluation participants. This requires attention to ethical and legal parameters, as well as to moral ones. Lastly, evaluations must collect appropriate and accurate data that are consistent with the purpose of the evaluation and the health program being evaluated. The scientific rigor of the evaluation is thus only one of four criteria by which a health program evaluation can be assessed.

ACROSS THE PYRAMID

At the direct services level of the public health pyramid, the concern is with how the processes discussed in this chapter ultimately can affect the quality, type, and existence of the direct services health program. Most of the processes discussed occur at the infrastructure level but can subsequently affect decisions regarding what is done at this level of the pyramid. Nonetheless, informed consent from program and evaluation participants is most likely to be obtained at this level of the pyramid because health programs at the direct services level involve individuals who are accessible for obtaining consent. Meta-evaluations, along with evidenced-based reviews, are likely to focus on direct services and programs, as they are widely studied and evaluated.

At the enabling services level, obtaining informed consent for participation in the health program and evaluation may be feasible and thus necessary. As with the direct services level, the processes that occur at the infrastructure level, such as processing information for decision making, ultimately affect the types of enabling services offered by health programs and the form they take.

At the population-based level, the issue of informed consent becomes blurred with the implementation of health policy because consent is almost implied by the passage of the health policies. Nonetheless, as Davis and Lantos (2000) pointed out, ethical considerations pervade population-level services. They cautioned that if sanctions are attached to a failure to comply with required services, such as immunization, harm may be done. Unfortunately, the nature of the harm is likely to be overlooked by policy makers when health policy is formulated and evaluated because they are focused on the benefits. Because population-based services are more closely linked to health policy, the processes that occur at the infrastructure level are critical in determining the nature and scope of health programs at this level of the pyramid. However, the growing body of evaluations of population-based health services, often couched as health policy studies, can lead to meta-evaluations and evidence-based practice for population-based services.

At the infrastructure level, although sense making occurs within individuals, the collective processes by which organizations and policy makers come to a shared understanding and interpretation of evaluation findings leads to policy decisions regarding health programs. Policy adoption and program implementation are two possible uses for evaluations (McClintock & Colosi, 1998). Recommendations are given to the decision makers, and decisions regarding health program implementation are made, and in this process the organizational, contextual issues become evident. Beck, Meadowcroft, Mason, and Kiely (1998) described the process of implementing a statewide system for monitoring outcomes. Their report is a reminder that statewide information systems are a key component of the infrastructure level, but that unless the data are used, collecting and warehousing them may be counterproductive in terms of improving programs and developing new ones. Also, approaches to improving organizational processes are essentially infrastructure processes that have consequences for programs at the other levels of the pyramid. Decision makers, who are part of the infrastructure, may need to reconcile differences between organizational process improvement and evaluation with regard to perspectives and recommendations. Lastly, procedures for dealing with ethical issues and IRB and HIPAA procedures must emanate from the infrastructure level and be consistently applied throughout the pyramid levels.

DISCUSSION QUESTIONS

1. At each level of the pyramid, identify at least two factors that can affect the acquisition of informed consent from those involved in providing evaluation data about a health program.

2. At what points in the planning and evaluation cycle would CQI/TQM techniques and processes be helpful to health program planners and evaluators? Explain your response.

3. In what ways might evidence-based practice (of any of the health disciplines) benefit from a meta-evaluation of programs to address a given health problem?

4. Using evaluation findings as part of feedback loops to improve or sustain health programs is predicated on a set of assumptions about humans and decision makers. What might be some of the assumptions that underlie this perspective? What, if anything, can be done to overcome, address, or deal with those assumptions in order to create the feedback loops?

References

Abelson, R. P. (1995). *Statistics as principled argument.* Hillsdale, NJ: Lawrence Erlbaum Associates.

Advisory Committee on Head Start Research and Evaluation. (1999). *Evaluating Head Start: A recommended framework for studying the impact of the Head Start Program.* Department of Health and Human Services, Administration for Children and Families. *http://aspe.hhs.gov/* (accessed 7/27/00).

Beck, S. A., Meadowcroft, P., Mason, M., & Kiely, E. S. (1998). Multiagency outcome evaluation of children's services: A case study. *Journal of Behavioral Health Services and Research, 25*, 163–176.

Boyd, N. R., & Windsor, R. A. (1993). A meta-evaluation of nutrition education intervention research among pregnant women. *Health Education Quarterly, 20*, 327–345.

Brown, S. (1991). Easy to use tool to assess the quality of a study. *Nursing Research, 40*, 352–355.

Center for Medicaid and Medicare Services. (2003). The Health Insurance Portability and Accountability Act of 1996 (HIPAA). *http://cms.hhs.gov/hipaa* (accessed 6/27/03).

Chapman, G. B., & Elstein, A. S. (2000). Cognitive processes and biases in medical decision making. In G. B. Chapman & F. A. Sonnenberg (Eds.), *Decision making in health care: Theory, psychology, and applications.* Cambridge: Cambridge University Press.

Cooper, H. (1998). *Synthesizing research.* (3rd ed.). Thousand Oaks, CA: Sage Publications.

Davis, M. M., & Lantos, J. D. (2000). Ethical considerations in the public policy laboratory. *Journal of the American Medical Association, 284*, 85–87.

Deming, W. E. (1982). *Quality, productivity, and competitive position.* Cambridge, MA: MIT Press.

Department of Health and Human Services. (2003). Office for Civil Rights-HIPAA. *http://www.hhs.gov/ocr/hipaa* (accessed 6/27/03).

Donabedian, A. (1980). *Explorations in quality assessment and monitoring, Volume 1: The definition of quality and approaches to its assessment.* Ann Arbor, MI: Health Administration Press.

Dynarski, M. (1997). Trade-offs in designing a social program experiment. *Children and Youth Services Review, 19*, 525–540.

Esbensen, F-A., Deschenes, E. P., Vogel, D. E., West, J., Arboit, K., Harris, L., et al. (1996). Active parental consent in school-based research: An examination of ethical and methodological issues. *Evaluation Review, 20*, 737–753.

Farrington, D. (2003). Methodological quality standards for evaluation. *Annals of the American Academy of Political and Social Science, 587*, 49–68.

Feather, J. (1982). Using macro variables in program evaluation. *Evaluation and Program Planning, 5*, 209–215.

Fischhoff, B. (1975). Hindsight =/= foresight: The effect of outcome knowledge on judgments under certainty. *Journal of Experimental Psychology: Human Perception and Performance, 1*, 288–299.

Gabriel, R. M. (2000). Methodological challenges in evaluating community partnerships and coalitions: Still crazy after all these years. *Journal of Community Psychology, 28*, 339–352.

Gondolf, E. W. (2000). Human subject issues in batterer program evaluation. *Journal of Aggression, Maltreatment and Trauma, 4*, 273–297.

Hastorf, A., & Cantril, H. (1954). They saw a game: A case study. *Journal of Abnormal and Social Psychology, 49*, 129–134.

Hendricks, M., & Papagiannis, M. (1990). Dos and don'ts for offering effective recommendations. *Evaluation Practice, 11*, 121–125.

Johnson, K., Bryant, D., Rockwell, E., Moore, M., Straub, B. W., Cummings, P., et al. (1999). Obtaining active parental consent for evaluation research: A case study. *American Journal of Evaluation, 20*, 239–250.

Juran, J. M. (1989). *Juran on leadership for quality: An executive handbook.* New York: The Free Press.

Lazarus, I. R., & Neely, C. (2003). Six Sigma: Raising the bar. *Managed Healthcare Executive, 13,* 31–33.

Lipshitz, R., Gilad, Z., & Suleiman, R. (2000). The one-of-us effect in decision evaluation. *Acta Psychologica, 108,* 53–71.

Mark, M. M., & Pines, E. (1995). Implications of continuous quality improvement for program evaluation and evaluators. *Evaluation Practice, 16,* 131–139.

Marvin, G. (1985). Evaluation research: Why a formal ethics review is needed. *Journal of Applied Social Sciences, 9,* 119–135.

Mathison, S. (1999). Rights, responsibilities, and duties: A comparison of ethics for internal and external evaluators. *New Directions for Evaluation, 82,* 25–34.

McClintock, C., & Colosi, L. A. (1998). Evaluation of welfare reform: A framework for addressing the urgent and the important. *Evaluation Review, 22,* 668–694.

Morris, M., & Jacobs, L. R. (2000). You got a problem with that? Exploring evaluators' disagreements about ethics. *Evaluation Review, 24,* 384–406.

National Institutes of Health. (2003). Impact of the HIPAA privacy rule on NIH processes involving the review, funding, and progress monitoring of grants, cooperative agreements and research contracts. Notice NOT-OD-03-025. *http://grants.nih.gov/guide/2003/03.02.07/index.htm* (accessed 6/27/03).

Owen, J. M., & Lambert, F. C. (1998). Evaluation and the information needs of organizational leaders. *American Journal of Evaluation, 19,* 355–365.

Patton, M. Q. (1997). *Utilization focused evaluation* (3rd ed.). Thousand Oaks, CA: Sage Publications.

Patton, M. Q. (1999). Organizational development and evaluation. *Canadian Journal of Program Evaluation* (special issue), 93–113.

Perrin, E. B., & Koshel, J. J. (1997). *Assessment of performance measures for public health, substance abuse, and mental health.* Washington, DC: National Academy Press.

Robinson, T., Patrick, K., Eng, T. R., & Gustafson, D. (1998). An evidence-based approach to interactive health communication: A challenge to medicine in the information age. *Journal of the American Medical Association, 280,* 1264-1269.

Shortell, S. M., Jones, R. H., Rademaker, A. W., Gilles, R. R., Dranove, D. S., Hughes, E. F. X., et al. (2000). Assessing the impact of total quality management and organizational culture on multiple outcomes of patient care for coronary artery bypass graft surgery patients. *Medical Care, 38,* 207—217.

Stevens, C. J., & Dial, M. (1994). What constitutes misuse? *New Directions for Program Evaluation, 64*(Winter), 3–14.

Tversky, A., & Kahneman, D. (1974). Judgement under uncertainty: Heuristics and biases. *Science, 185,* 1124–1131.

Weick, K. E. (1979). *The social psychology of organizing.* Reading, MA: Addison-Wesley.

Weick, K. E. (1995). *Sensemaking in organizations.* Thousand Oaks, CA: Sage Publications.

Windsor, R. A., Boyd, N. R., & Orleans, C. T. (1998). A meta-evaluation of smoking cessation intervention research among pregnant women: Improving the science and art. *Health Education Research, 13,* 419–438.

Index

L

Lafayetteville example
  determinants, antecedents, and
    contributing factors for, 128
  developing determinant theory
    for, 165
  needs assessment, 116
  statement of need or problem,
    143, 144
LaLonde, M., 74–75
Lambert, F. C., 455
Language
  data collection from health pro-
    grams and, 44, 46–47
  ethnicity, culture, and measure-
    ment of, 43–44
  questionnaires reflecting diversi-
    ty in, 299
Lantos, J. D., 462
Latent needs, 133–134
Latessa, P., 407–408
Lay sector of health providers, 54
Leadership
  as managerial skill, 221
  selection of planning group, 93
Legal accountability
  organizational plan and, 213–214
  process evaluation and, 269, 270,
    271
Legal standards, target values and,
    191
Legge, C., 48
Lew, R., 48
Lewis, F. M., 239, 363, 380, 387
Lickert scales, 99, 292
Liddle, H. A., 176
Lientz, B. P., 62
Lieu, T. A., 431
Lifestyle behavior domain, data
    sources for intervention
    effect evaluations, 300
Liller, K. D., 331
Lincoln, Y. S., 6, 387, 398, 400

Linked data, 360–361
Lippmann, M., 305
Lipsey, M. W., 152, 237
Literature, 133, 169–171, 298
Logic model
  goals, objectives and, 185
Lorig, K. R., 131
Luce, B. R., 424
Lumsdaine, A., 363
Lundle, J., 301

M

MacKay, G., 301
MacLehose, R. F., 98
Macro health problems, 159–160
Magnitude
  in descriptive statistics, 136
  significance and, 371
Maibach, E. W., 230
Maisto, S. A., 290
Managerial resources
  monitoring, 245, 246
  as organizational plan input,
    219–221
Manalo, V., 345
Manifest meanings, implied mean-
    ings *versus*, 401–402
Manipulability, of interventions,
    161–162
MAPP (Mobilizing for Action
    through Planning and Part-
    nership), 76–77
Mark, M. M., 457
Marketing
  assessment of, 120, 121
  inclusion parameters in plan for, 181
  social, 171, 229–230
Marvin, G., 450–451
Mason, M., 462–463
Matching variables, 361
Materials produced
  as service utilization plan output,
    233

Program theory, 151–152
  communication base and, 175
  effect theory and, 19, 154–155
  espoused theory in development
    of, 172
  explanations from, 174–175
  functions of, 172–175
  goals, objectives and, 185
  guidance from, 173–174
  impacts, outcomes and, 163–172
  interventions and, 155–163
  logical model of, 153
  personnel training and, 255
  process theory and, 152–154
  qualitative formation of, 387
  as scientific contribution, 175
  validity assumptions for, 172
Project directors, usefulness of
    evaluations for, 15
Promotion, social marketing and, 230
Proportions, in descriptive statis-
    tics, 136–137
Proprietary data, collection of, 132
Propriety standard, 10
Prospective evaluations, 323
  two groups, 337–339
Prosser, L. A., 424, 431–432
Providers, data collection from,
    131–132
Public data, collection of, 131
Public health (needs assessment)
    model, 116, 117, 118
Public health pyramid
  components of, 21–22
  cost analyses, 433–434
  data analysis and interpretation,
    382–383
  development of, 20
  diversity in, 65–67
  as ecological model, 23–25
  feedback cycle, 462–463
  health program planning and
    evaluation in, 31–33

impact evaluation design,
    353–354
intervention effect evaluations
    and, 313
intervention typology and, 157,
    158
needs assessment, 145–147
planning and, 106–108
program implementation logis-
    tics, 233–234
program objectives and target
    setting, 208
program process evaluation and
    monitoring, 271–273
program theory for interventions
    and, 175–176
qualitative methods, 407–408
use of, 22–23
Published literature, 133, 169–171,
    298
Purposive samples, 346, 347, 348
Put Prevention into Practice pro-
    gram, 391–392

Q
Qualitative analysis, 400–401
  issues with, 405–406
  overview of, 401–404
  software for, 404–405
  triangulation, 404
Qualitative methods, 387
  across the pyramid, 407–408
  benefits and challenges to using,
    391
  case studies, 388–392
  focus groups, 395–397
  functions of, 387–388
  in-depth individual interviews,
    394–395
  narrative, 397–398
  observation, 392–394
  presentation of findings, 406–407
  sampling for, 400